ECTOPIC PREGNANCY – MODERN DIAGNOSIS AND MANAGEMENT

Edited by **Michael Kamrava**

Ectopic Pregnancy – Modern Diagnosis and Management
Edited by Michael Kamrava

Published by InTech
Janeza Trdine 9, 51000 Rijeka, Croatia

Publishing Process Manager Dragana Manestar

Technical Editor Teodora Smiljanic

Cover Designer InTech Design Team

Additional hard copies can be obtained from orders@intechopen.com

Ectopic Pregnancy – Modern Diagnosis and Management, Edited by Michael Kamrava
p. cm.
ISBN 978-953-307-648-5

For EU product safety concerns:
IN TECH d.o.o., Prolaz Marije Krucifikse Kozulić 3, 51000 Rijeka, Croatia,
info@intechopen.com or visit our website at intechopen.com.

Meet the editor

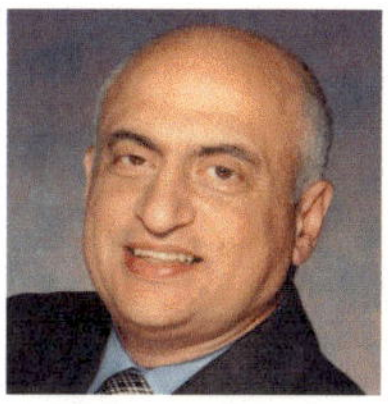

Michael Kamrava, M.D., earned a Bachelor of Science in physiology with high honors from University of Illinois, USA, and graduated from Case Western Reserve Medical School in 1976 with honors in Endocrinology. Following a residency in OB/GYN, he finished a fellowship in Reproductive Endocrinology and Infertility at Beth Israel Hospital, Harvard medical school, Boston, MA. He has served at the faculty position and been involved with teaching resident and medical school students at UCLA. He was the principal investigator on the use of pulsatile subcutaneous GnRH in ovulation induction. He has been on the editorial staff of different national and international scientific journals, and has authored and co-authored many scientific journal articles. In addition, he has been an invited speaker at numerous national and international talks and conferences and has conducted international workshops. He was awarded the "Golden Telescope" for introducing the SEED technique for embryo implantation..

Contents

Preface XI

Part 1 Epidemiology, Morbidity and Mortality 1

Chapter 1 **Differential Diagnosis of Ectopic Pregnancy - Morbidity and Mortality 3**
Panagiotis Tsikouras, Marina Dimitraki, Alexandros Ammari, Sofia Bouchlariotou, Stefanos Zervoudis, Panagiotis Oikonomidis, Constantinos Zakas, Theodoros Mylonas, Anastasios Liberis, Vasileios Liberis and Georgios Maroulis

Part 2 Causes of Ectopic Pregnancy 11

Chapter 2 **Tubal Damage, Infertility and Tubal Ectopic Pregnancy: *Chlamydia trachomatis* and Other Microbial Aetiologies 13**
Louise M. Hafner and Elise S. Pelzer

Chapter 3 **Ectopic Pregnancy and Assisted Reproductive Technologies: A Systematic Review 45**
Anastasia Velalopoulou, Dimitrios Peschos, Mynbaev Ospan, Eliseeva Marina, Ioannis Verginadis, Yannis Simos, Tsirkas Panagiotis, Spyridon Karkabounas, Vicky Kalfakakou, Angelos Evangelou and Ioannis P. Kosmas

Chapter 4 **Hysteroscopic Endometrial Embryo Delivery (HEED) 79**
M.M. Kamrava, L. Tran and J.L. Hall

Chapter 5 **Ectopic Pregnancy Following Reconstructive, Organ-Preserving Microsurgery in Tubal Infertility 87**
Cordula Schippert, Philipp Soergel and Guillermo-José Garcia-Rocha

Chapter 6 **Persistent Ectopic Pregnancy After Laparoscopic Linear Salpingostomy for Tubal Pregnancy: Prevention and Early Detection 97**
Shigeo Akira, Takashi Abe and Toshiyuki Takeshita

Part 3 Diagnosis of Ectopic Pregnancy 107

Chapter 7 **Management and Outcome of Ectopic Pregnancy in Developing Countries 109**
Buowari Yvonne Dabota

Chapter 8 **Clinical Application of One-Step Diagnosis for Ectopic Pregnancy by HCG Ratio: Hemoperitoneum Versus Venous Serum 137**
Yu-dong Wang, Wei-wei Cheng and Xiao-ping Wan

Chapter 9 **Inhibins and Activins as Possible Marker of Ectopic Pregnancy 151**
Blazej Meczekalski and Agnieszka Podfigurna-Stopa

Chapter 10 **Term Extra-Uterine Pregnancy 163**
Ismail A. Al-Badawi, Osama Al Omar and Togas Tulandi

Part 4 Management of Ectopic Pregnancy 175

Chapter 11 **Clinical Treatment of Unruptured Ectopic Pregnancy 177**
Julio Elito Junior

Chapter 12 **MTX Could Be First-Line Therapy Even in Cases Where hCG Level is Greater than 5,000 IU/ml 209**
Yoshiki Yamashita, Sousuke Katoh, Yoko Yoshida, Satoe Fujiwara, Sachiko Kawabe, Mika Hayashi, Atsushi Hayashi, Yoshito Terai and Masahide Ohmichi

Chapter 13 **The Treatment of Ectopic Pregnancy with Laparoscopy-Assisted Local Injection of Chemotherapeutic Agents 217**
Ching-Hui Chen, Peng-Hui Wang, Li-Hsuan Chiu and Wei-Min Liu

Chapter 14 **Fertility-Preserving Surgery for Cervical Ectopic Pregnancy, from Past to Present 225**
Seiryu Kamoi, Nao Iwasaki and Toshiyuki Takeshita

Chapter 15 **Modern Management of Cornual Ectopic Pregnancy 237**
Maged Shendy and Rami Atalla

Preface

The objective in compiling this book has been to bring more worldwide awareness of this important cause of maternal morbidity and mortality. In addition to the sexually transmitted diseases, as advanced reproductive technologies have become available everywhere, occurrence of ectopic pregnancies has also increased more than before. With better understanding of the causes of this condition, earlier diagnosis and earlier treatment of sexually transmitted diseases, along with employing improved reproductive technologies, has led to more non-invasive treatment options and improved outcome in the management of these, potentially life-threatening, situations.

This book is dedicated to all our patients from all over the world who have given us the impetus for giving them hope for having a family. Also, I would like to thank my wife, Soheila, and our children Mitchell and Michelle for their patience, understanding and encouragement in taking on this task.

Michael Kamrava
West Coast IVF Clinic, Inc.
CA, USA

Part 1

Epidemiology, Morbidity and Mortality

1

Differential Diagnosis of Ectopic Pregnancy - Morbidity and Mortality

Panagiotis Tsikouras et al.,*
Department of Obstetrics and Gynecology , Democritus University of Thrace Greece

1. Introduction

The term ectopic pregnancy refers to a gestation in which the fertilized ovum implants on any tissue other than the endometrial membrane lining the uterine cavity. Fig 1 presents the various types of ectopic pregnancy and their relative frequencies The classic clinical symptoms of ectopic pregnancy are pelvic pain, amenorrhea, and vaginal bleeding , spotting (40-50%). However, only 50% of patients present typical symptomatology. Patients may present with other symptoms common to early pregnancy, including nausea (frequently after rupture), breast fullness, fatigue, abdominal pain, heavy cramping, shoulder pain, and recent dyspareunia . Physical findings during examination should be pelvic unilateral tenderness, especially on movement of cervix (75%), enlarged uterus or palpable adnexal mass; crepitant mass on one side or in culde-sac (50%). Approximately 20% of patients with ectopic pregnancies are hemodynamically compromised at initial presentation, which is highly suggestive of rupture. Body temperature ranges from 37.2 to 37.8 ^{0}C while the pulse is variable: normal before but rapid after rupture. Today, using modern diagnostic techniques, most ectopic pregnancies may be diagnosed prior to rupturing [1].

Diagnosis of ectopic pregnancy has been greatly improved by the advent of rapid serum beta-human chorionic gonadotropin (beta-HCG) tests and then the widespread adoption of transvaginal pelvic ultrasonography (TVUS) [2].

Serum beta-HCG levels can definitively rule out pregnancy if negative, although there have been case reports of pathology-proven ruptured ectopic pregnancy and hemorrhagic shock despite an undetectable serum beta-HCG [3]. In the early stages of a normal intrauterine pregnancy (IUP), the serum beta-HCG rises along a well-defined curve. Therefore, serial beta-HCG tests can be useful for determining the ultimate location of a pregnancy of unknown location. The lower limit of normal rise in beta-HCG (using a 99% confidence interval) is 53% in 2 days [4]. Patients with a beta-HCG level that falls more than 50% in 2

*Marina Dimitraki[1], Alexandros Ammari[1], Sofia Bouchlariotou[1], Stefanos Zervoudis[2], Panagiotis Oikonomidis[2], Constantinos Zakas[2], Theodoros Mylonas[1], Anastasios Liberis[1], Vasileios Liberis[1] and Georgios Maroulis[1]
[1]*Department of Obstetrics and Gynecology , Democritus University of Thrace, Greece*
[2]*Department of Obstetrics and Gynecology, Rhea Hospital, Athens, Greece*

days are at low risk of having an ectopic pregnancy [5].As ruptured ectopic pregnancies have been reported at a wide range of beta-HCG levels, the beta-HCG level should not be a factor in determining whether or not transvaginal ultrasonography should be performed. (The prevalence of false-positive serum hCG results is low, with estimates ranging from 0.01-2%. False-positive serum hCG results are usually due to interference by non-hCG substances or the detection of pituitary hCG. Some examples of non-hCG substances that can cause false-positive results include human LH, antianimal immunoglobulin antibodies, rheumatoid factor, heterophile antibodies, and binding proteins. Most false-positive results are characterized by serum levels that are generally less than 1000 mIU/mL and usually less than 150 mIU/mL[6].)

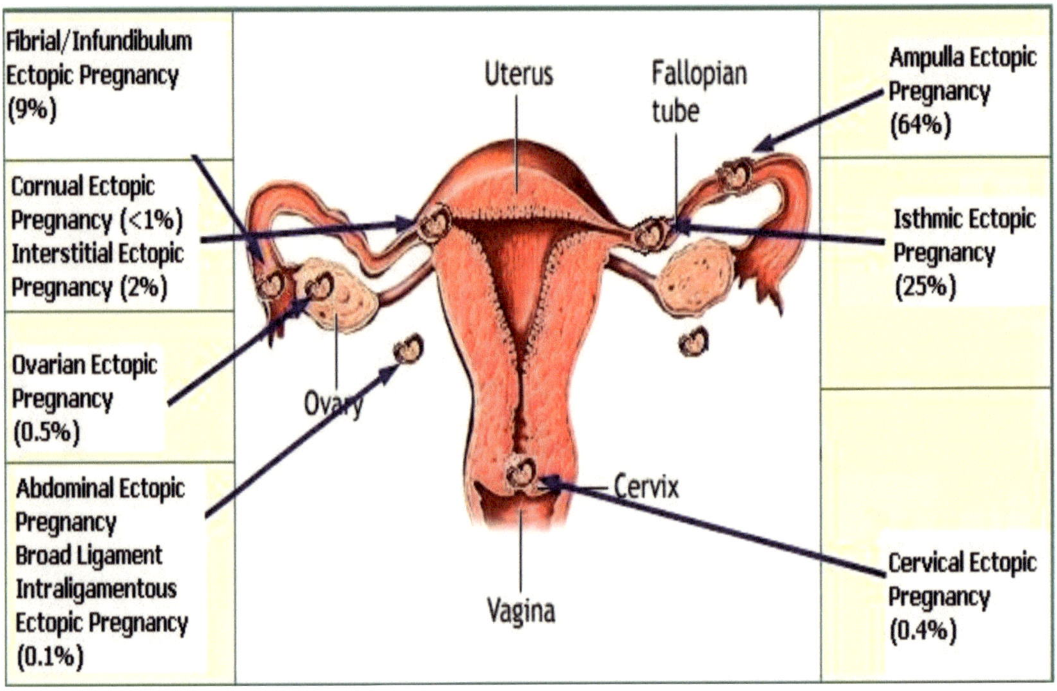

Fig 1. Various types of ectopic pregnancy and their relative frequencies

Serum progesterone levels tend to be stable over time during the first trimester and concentrations are higher in normal intrauterine pregnancy. A single serum progesterone level has been used alone to discriminate between normal and failing intrauterine pregnancies, but it cannot accurately discriminate between intrauterine and ectopic pregnancies [7]. Levels of <5ng/ml are associated with a viable pregnancy in 0.16% of cases . Low progesterone levels in combination hCG levels is "essentially 100% predictive of a□with an abnormal rise in nonviable pregnancy" (intra or extrauterine) . A progesterone level of less than 15 ng/ml is seen in: 81% of ectopics, 93% of abnormal intrauterine pregnancies, 11% of normal intrauterine pregnancies [8].

The human chorionic gonadotropin (hCG) ratio of hemoperitoneum to venous serum ($R_{P/V}$) has been demonstrated to improve early diagnosis of ectopic pregnancy, according to a recent study. Investigators observed that the $R_{P/V}$ was higher in ectopic pregnant subjects (median 4.07) than in patients with hemoperitoneum and intrauterine pregnancy (hIUP; median 0.6), with 1.0 as their suggested threshold value for differential diagnosis [9].

Research is ongoing concerning CA 125, pregnancy-associated plasma protein-A, vascular endothelial growth factor and creatine kinase. None of them have yet shown superiority to serial beta-HCG measurements in distinguishing between intrauterine pregnancy and ectopic pregnancy [10].

Furthermore , pelvic sonography is the imaging test of choice to investigate early pregnancy complaints. As sonogram findings of early normal IUP development (<7 weeks) are well correlated with beta-HCG level, the absence of a normal IUP on sonogram together with a beta-HCG level above the discriminatory zone virtually rules out a normal IUP.

Pelvic sonography is usually conducted first using the transabdominal approach (which can reliably identify intrauterine pregnancies at a beta-HCG level above 6500 mIU/mL), and then the transvaginal approach (which can extend the discriminatory zone down to 1500 mIU/mL). M-mode imaging is useful for measuring the fetal heart rate. Color Doppler ultrasonography can help identify some ectopic pregnancies by identifying a placental blood flow pattern in the adnexa. The following sonographic findings are of special interest : An intrauterine gestational sac containing a yolk sac, or fetal pole: A definitive IUP virtually rules out ectopic pregnancy (aside from heterotopic pregnancies). An intrauterine gestational sac larger than 16 mm without a fetal pole, or larger than 8 mm without a yolk sac; or an intrauterine fetal pole larger than 5 mm without heart motion: These findings are indicative of failed intrauterine pregnancy. A gestational sac with a mean sac diameter less than 5 mm greater than the crown-rump length has an 80% risk of pregnancy loss [11]. An extrauterine sac containing a yolk sac or a fetal pole, with or without heart motion Fig 2: Although definitive for ectopic pregnancy, only 16-32% of ectopics have this finding on transvaginal sonogram [12].

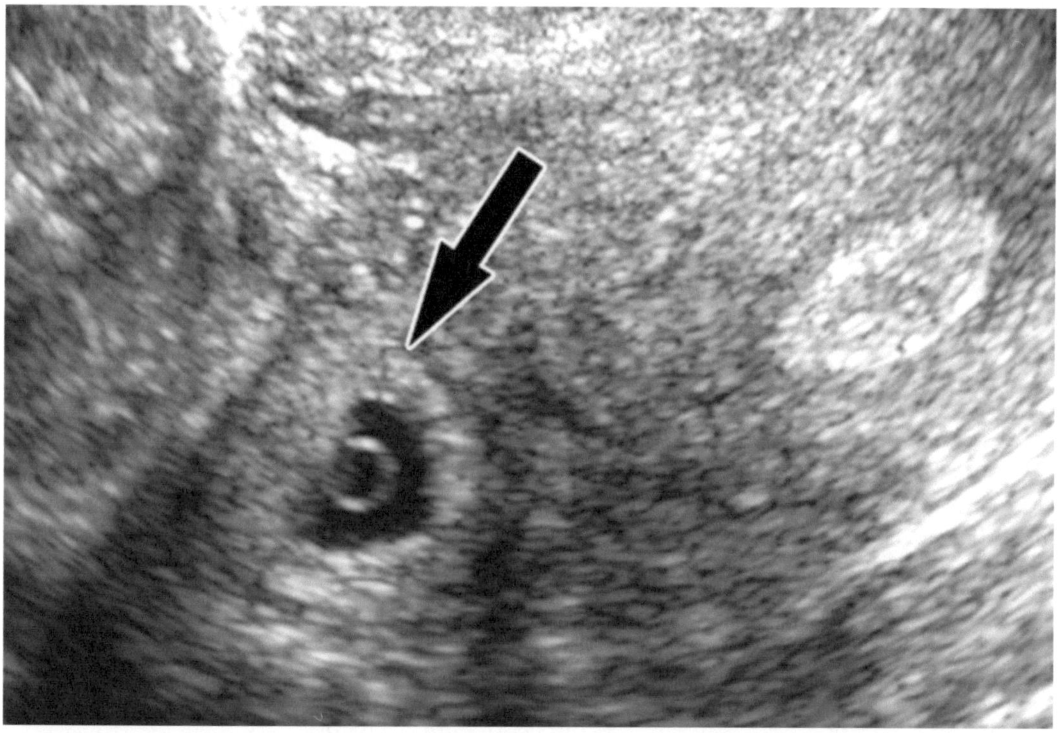

Fig. 2. Vaginal Ultrasound showing gestational sac with yolk sac in extra uterine location.

Tubal ring is a thick-walled cystic structure in the adnexa, independent of the ovary and uterus, and is highly predictive of ectopic pregnancy [13]. It can sometimes be confused with a corpus luteum cyst when the ovary is not well visualized. The corpus luteum cyst wall tends to be thinner and less echogenic than the endometrium and the cyst tends to contain clear fluid [14]. When surrounded by free fluid, it can sometimes be confused with a hemorrhagic ovarian cyst [15]. A complex adnexal mass is the sign most frequently found in ectopic pregnancies [16]. It can be somewhat cystic-appearing or entirely solid in nature, surrounded by free fluid, and ill-defined. If it cannot be moved independently of the ovary, it is unlikely to be an ectopic pregnancy [17]. A moderate amount of anechoic free fluid (tracking more than one third of the way up the posterior wall of the uterus), or any echogenic free fluid, has a higher chance of being ultimately diagnosed as an ectopic pregnancy [18].

Culdocentesis is the transvaginal needle aspiration of fluid from the posterior cul-de-sac of Douglas. A positive result means aspiration of 0.5 ml of nonclotting blood, while negative result is accociated with aspiration of 0.5 ml of serous fluid.. If no fluid is aspirated ,the test is inadequate. In positive cases ,if the hematocrit of aspirated fluid is over 15%, ruptured ectopic pregnancy is possible ,while a hematocrit of aspirated fluid below 15% is usually in favor of other causes of intraabdominal hemorrhage, such as hemorrhagic corpus luteum cyst, tubal reflux of intrauterine blood , previous attempt at culdocentesis or(19-21). A positive culdocentesis is found in 70-90% of cases in ectopic pregnancy. A positive culdocentesis indicates the presence of a hemoperitoneum ,(21) but does not give the source of the blood and does not necessarily indicate tubal rupture .The volume of blood recovered does not correlate with the volume of the hemoperitoneum. A positive culdocentesis test in combination with a positive pregnancy test predicts the presence of an ectopic pregnancy, in approximately 95% of cases. (22-3) However double decidual sac sign, or gestational sac <8 mm without yolk sac or fetal pole is in favor of the diagnosis of ectopic pregnancy. While considered diagnostic of IUP by experienced sonographers, this can be easily confused with the pseudogestational sac found in ectopic pregnancy (caused by breakdown of stimulated endometrial lining) and lead to falsely ruling out of ectopic pregnancy [12]. The pseudogestational sac (seen in 10-20% of ectopic pregnancies [24] can be differentiated by its central location in the uterus, oval shape, thin echogenic rim, and lack of double decidual sac sign [11]. A thin endometrial stripe (<8 mm) appears to be somewhat predictive of eventual diagnosis of ectopic pregnancy in patients with a beta-HCG below 1,000 mIU/Ml [25] but there is sufficient overlap with eventual failed IUPs and normal IUPs that this is a poor diagnostic test [26].

Numerous conditions may have a presentation similar to an extrauterine pregnancy (EP). The most common differential diagnosis hemmoragic are: a ruptured corpus luteum cyst or ovarian follicle (RC), and a spontaneous abortion or threatened abortion (SA). Other differential diagnosis are appendicitis (A), salpingitis(S), ovarian torsion(OT), and urinary tract disease(UD): cystitis, ureteric colic. Intrauterine pregnancies with other abdominal or pelvic problems such as degenerating fibroids must also be included in the differential diagnosis.

Specifically, differential diagnosis of ectopic pregnancy includes : Miscarriage (Includes anembryonic gestation, threatened abortion, incomplete abortion, complete abortion, missed abortion.) Often presents with vaginal bleeding in the first trimester, accompanied by abdominal discomfort secondary to uterine contractions. History may yield disappearance of pregnancy symptoms such as breast tenderness and nausea. Ultrasound shows intrauterine pregnancy or products of conception. Pelvic examination may note dilation of the cervix, as well as presence of tissue at the cervical os. Consecutive serum chorionic gonadotrophin levels often do not rise appropriately (66% in 48 hours), and progesterone levels often <15.9 nmol/L (<5 ng/mL). Acute appendicitis: Anorexia and periumbilical pain followed by nausea, RLQ (Right Lower Quadrant) abdominal pain, tenderness localizing at Mc Burney' s point; rebound tenderness and vomiting usual , precedes shift of pain to right lower quadrant. Vaginal bleeding in appendicitis occur unrelated to menses , temperature is 37.2-37.8 C and pulse are variable. No masses founded by pelvic examination. Ultrasound sensitivity of 85% to 90% and specificity of 92% to 96%; may show appendix with outer diameter >6 mm, no compressibility, lack of peristalsis, or periappendiceal fluid. WBC >10,000 cells/ µl (rarely normal) ;red cell count normal; sedimentation rate slightly elevated. Ovarian torsion: Sudden onset, severe, unilateral lower abdominal pain that worsens intermittently over many hours. Peritoneal signs are often absent. Ovarian enlargement secondary to impaired venous and lymphatic drainage is the most common sonographical finding in ovarian torsion. Absence of arterial blood flow may also be used for diagnostic purposes, but this is often absent in the early stages of torsion. PID (pelvic inflammatory disease) or tubo-ovarian abscess: Lower abdominal tenderness on palpation, pain usally in both lower quadrants, with or without rebound, adnexal tenderness, adnexal masses only when pyosalpinx or hydrosalpinx is present and cervical motion tenderness. May also have body temperature >38.4°C?[MORE THAN 38] and abnormal cervical or vaginal discharge. Occurrence of hypermenorrhea or metrorrhagia or both. Nausea and vomiting are infrequent . Although rare in pregnancy, can occur in the first 12 weeks of gestation before the decidua seals off the uterus from ascending bacteria. WBC often >10,000 cells/mm^3 ; red cell count normal; sedimentation rate normal. Ultrasound not used in uncomplicated PID, but is a valuable adjunct in diagnosis of tubo-ovarian abscess. Ruptured corpus luteal cyst or follicle : Non-specific nausea, vomiting, low fever, and pelvic pain, which is often sharp, intermittent, sudden in onset, and severe unilateral ,becoming general with progressive bleeding. At times the ruptured cyst may lead to profuse bleeding and result in haemorrhagic shock. Period delayed, then bleeding , often with pain. Temperature not over 37.2 ; pulse normal unless blood loss marked, then rapid. Laboratory findings : white cell count normal to 10.000 /µl ; red cell count normal ; sedimentation normal. Doppler ultrasonography usually diagnostic, especially when transvaginal and transabdominal modalities are used together. Nephrolithiasis: Classically writhing in pain, pacing about, and unable to lie still, in contrast to a patient with peritoneal irritation, who remains motionless to minimise discomfort. Often presents with unilateral or bilateral flank pain. Haematuria (presence of >1 RBC/hpf) and pyuria (>5 WBC/hpf on a centrifuged specimen) common. Due to potential risks to the fetus, the only imaging modalities used in pregnant women are ultrasonography (direct visualisation of the stone, hydroureter > 6 mm in diameter, and perirenal urinoma suggesting calyceal rupture) and MRI (if ultrasound is non-diagnostic). UTI (urinary tract disease): Dysuria with accompanying urinary urgency, frequency, and abdominal discomfort along the surface of the bladder. May have pyuria (>5 WBC/hpf on a centrifuged specimen). Presence of nitrites is highly specific for a UTI, but its absence should not exclude the diagnosis.

Finally , bowel colitis ,inguinal or crural hernia and muscular pain should be included in the differential diagnosis of abdominal pain in lower quadrants.

Ectopic pregnancy is responsible for a significant proportion of maternal mortality and morbidity. According to the WHO, ectopic pregnancy accounts for 0.1 to 4.9% of the total maternal deaths worldwide. [27] The range varies in different regions of the world, exhibiting the highest prevalence in developed countries. Table 1 . [27] It should be mentioned at this point that in developing countries, hemorrhage is the leading cause of maternal deaths.

It is responsible for an enormous amount of hospital admissions, surgical interventions and blood transfusions worldwide.

The mortality rate has declined from 35.5 maternal deaths per 10,000 ectopic pregnancies in 1970 to only 3.8 maternal deaths per 10,000 ectopic pregnancies in 1989. [28]Mortality from ectopic pregnancy is the commonest cause of maternal death, replacing mortality resulting from illegal abortion. [29]

World Region	Percentage (%)
Asia	0.1
Africa	0.5
Latin America	0.5
Developed countries	4.9

Table 1. Variability of maternal deaths due to ectopic pregnancy in different regions of the world.

Studies have shown that African-American women have a mortality ratio 3 to 18 times higher than white women [29-30]

Delay of treatment and misdiagnosis are the main factors that lead to mortality. Approximately 50 percent of ectopic pregnancies are misdiagnosed at the initial visit to an emergency department. [31-2]

The significant fall of maternal mortality is due to modern diagnostic advances and minimally invasive treatments.

2. References

[1] Vicken PS., Wood E, Ectopic Pregnancy, emedicine.medscape.com Updated: Mar 8, 2011

[2] Cohen HL, Moore WH. History of emergency ultrasound. J Ultrasound Med. Apr 2004;23(4):451-8.

[3] Grynberg M, Teyssedre J, Andre C, Graesslin O. Rupture of ectopic pregnancy with negative serum beta-hCG leading to hemorrhagic shock. Obstet Gynecol. Feb 2009;113(2 Pt 2):537-9.

[4] Barnhart KT, Sammel MD, Rinaudo PF, Zhou L, Hummel AC, Guo W. Symptomatic patients with an early viable intrauterine pregnancy: HCG curves redefined. Obstet Gynecol. Jul 2004;104(1):50-5.

[5] Dart RG, Mitterando J, Dart LM. Rate of change of serial beta-human chorionic gonadotropin values as a predictor of ectopic pregnancy in patients with indeterminate transvaginal ultrasound findings. Ann Emerg Med. Dec 1999;34(6):703-10.

[6] Ackerman R, Deutsch S, Krumholz B. Levels of human chorionic gonadotropin in unruptured and ruptured ectopic pregnancy. Obstet Gynecol 1982;60:13-14.

[7] Mol BW, Lijmer JG, Ankum WM, van der Veen F, Bossuyt PM. The accuracy of single serum progesterone measurement in the diagnosis of ectopic pregnancy: a meta-analysis. Hum Reprod. Nov 1998;13(11):3220-7.

[8] Lipscomb GH, Stovall TG, Ling FW. Non surgical treatment of ectopic pregnancy. NEJM 200;343(18):1325-1329

[9] Wang Y, Zhao H, Teng Y, Lu L, Tong J. Human chorionic gonadotropin ratio of hemoperitoneum versus venous serum improves early diagnosis of ectopic pregnancy. Fertil Steril. 2008 .

[10] Cabar FR, Fettback PB, Pereira PP, Zugaib M. Serum markers in the diagnosis of tubal pregnancy. Clinics (Sao Paulo). Oct 2008;63(5):701-8.

[11] Dighe M, Cuevas C, Moshiri M, Dubinsky T, Dogra VS. Sonography in first trimester bleeding. J Clin Ultrasound. Jul-Aug 2008;36(6):352-66.

[12] Patel MD. "Rule out ectopic": Asking the right questions, getting the right answers. Ultrasound Q. Jun 2006;22(2):87-100.

[13] Brown DL, Doubilet PM. Transvaginal sonography for diagnosing ectopic pregnancy: positivity criteria and performance characteristics. J Ultrasound Med. Apr 1994;13(4):259-66.

[14] Stein MW, Ricci ZJ, Novak L, Roberts JH, Koenigsberg M. Sonographic comparison of the tubal ring of ectopic pregnancy with the corpus luteum. J Ultrasound Med. Jan 2004;23(1):57-62.

[15] Hertzberg BS, Kliewer MA, Bowie JD. Adnexal ring sign and hemoperitoneum caused by hemorrhagic ovarian cyst: pitfall in the sonographic diagnosis of ectopic pregnancy. AJR Am J Roentgenol. Nov 1999;173(5):1301-2.

[16] Frates MC, Brown DL, Doubilet PM, Hornstein MD. Tubal rupture in patients with ectopic pregnancy: diagnosis with transvaginal US. Radiology. Jun 1994;191(3):769-72.

[17] Blaivas M. Color doppler in the diagnosis of ectopic pregnancy in the emergency department: is there anything beyond a mass and fluid?. J Emerg Med. May 2002;22(4):379-84.

[18] Dart R, McLean SA, Dart L. Isolated fluid in the cul-de-sac: how well does it predict ectopic pregnancy?. Am J Emerg Med. Jan 2002;20(1):1-4.

[19] Glezerman M, Press F, Carpman M. Culdocentesis is an obsolete diagnostic tool in suspected ectopic pregnancy.Arch Gynecol Obstet. 1992;252(1):5-9

[20] Wyte CD.Diagnostic modalities in the pregnant patient. Emerg Med Clin North Am. 1994 Feb;12(1):9-43. Review
Cartwright PS, Vaughn B, Tuttle D. Culdocentesis and ectopic pregnancy. J Reprod Med. 1984 Feb;29(2):88-91.

[21] Falfoul A, Makni MY, Bellasfar M, Tnani M, Kaabar N, Kharouf M. [The role of culdocentesis in the diagnosis of ectopic pregnancy. Prospective study of 478 cases].J Gynecol Obstet Biol Reprod (Paris). 1991;20(7):917-22. French.

[22] Romero R, Copel JA, Kadar N, Jeanty P, Decherney A Hobbins JC. Value of culdocentesis in the diagnosis of ectopic pregnancy.Obstet Gynecol. 1985 Apr;65(4):519-22

[23] Nyberg DA, Laing FC, Filly RA, Uri-Simmons M, Jeffrey RB Jr. Ultrasonographic differentiation of the gestational sac of early intrauterine pregnancy from the pseudogestational sac of ectopic pregnancy. Radiology. Mar 1983;146(3):755-9.

[24] Dart RG, Dart L, Mitchell P, Berty C. The predictive value of endometrial stripe thickness in patients with suspected ectopic pregnancy who have an empty uterus at ultrasonography. Acad Emerg Med. Jun 1999;6(6):602-8.

[25] Seeber B, Sammel M, Zhou L, Hummel A, Barnhart KT. Endometrial stripe thickness and pregnancy outcome in first-trimester pregnancies with bleeding, pain or both. J Reprod Med. Sep 2007;52(9):757-61.
Khan KS, Wojdyla D, Say L, Gülmezoglu AM, Van Look PF. WHO analysis of causes of maternal death: a systematic review. Lancet. 2006 Apr 1;367(9516):1066-74. Review.

[26] Goldner TE, Lawson HW, Xia Z, Atrash HK. Surveillance for ectopic pregnancy--United States, 1970-1989. MMWR CDC Surveill Summ 1993.

[27] Dorfman SF. Epidemiology of ectopic pregnancy. Clin Obstet Gynecol. 1987 Mar;30(1): 173-80.

[28] Anderson FW, Hogan JG, Ansbacher R. Sudden death: ectopic pregnancy mortality. Obstet Gynecol. 2004 Jun;103(6):1218-23.

[29] Abbott J, Emmans LS, Lowenstein SR. Ectopic pregnancy: ten common pitfalls in diagnosis. Am J Emerg Med 1990;8:515-22.

[30] Kaplan BC, Dart RG, Moskos M, Kuligowska E, Chun B, Adel Hamid M, et al. Ectopic pregnancy: prospective study with improved diagnostic accuracy. Ann Emerg Med 1996;28:10-7.

Part 2

Causes of Ectopic Pregnancy

2

Tubal Damage, Infertility and Tubal Ectopic Pregnancy: *Chlamydia trachomatis* and Other Microbial Aetiologies

Louise M. Hafner and Elise S. Pelzer
Institute of Health and Biomedical Innovation, (IHBI),
Queensland University of Technology (QUT)
Australia

1. Introduction

Infertility is a worldwide health problem with one in six couples suffering from this condition and with a major economic burden on the global healthcare industry. Estimates of the current global infertility rate suggest that 15% of couples are infertile (Zegers-Hochschild *et al.,* 2009) defined as: (1) failure to conceive after one year of unprotected sexual intercourse (i.e. infertility); (2) continual failure of implantation at subsequent cycles of assisted reproductive technology; or (3) persistent miscarriage events without difficulty conceiving (natural conceptions). Tubal factor infertility is among the leading causes of female factor infertility accounting for 7-9.8% of all female factor infertilities. Tubal disease directly causes from 36% to 85% of all cases of female factor infertility in developed and developing nations respectively and is associated with polymicrobial aetiologies. One of the leading global causes of tubal factor infertility is thought to be symptomatic (and asymptomatic in up to 70% cases) infection of the female reproductive tract with the sexually transmitted pathogen, *Chlamydia trachomatis*. Infection-related damage to the Fallopian tubes caused by *Chlamydia* accounts for more than 70% of cases of infertility in women from developing nations such as sub-Saharan Africa (Sharma *et al.,* 2009). Bacterial vaginosis, a condition associated with increased transmission of sexually transmitted infections including those caused by *Neisseria gonorrhoeae* and *Mycoplasma genitalium* is present in two thirds of women with pelvic inflammatory disease (PID). This review will focus on (1) the polymicrobial aetiologies of tubal factor infertility and (2) studies involved in screening for, and treatment and control of, Chlamydial infection to prevent PID and the associated sequelae of Fallopian tube inflammation that may lead to infertility and ectopic pregnancy.

2. Tubal factor infertility

In the absence of functional Fallopian tubes, couples may only conceive through *in vitro* fertilisation procedures. Women with tubal factor infertility may be defined as women who have either (1) damaged/occluded Fallopian tubes or (2) have history of salpingectomy. Ectopic pregnancy is only relevant if the Fallopian tubes remain *in situ*. Previous studies have concluded that salpingitis can accompany early intrauterine pregnancy, often with significant foetal loss (Lara-Torre & Pinkerton 2002; Yip *et al.*, 1993) but that upper genital tract infections do not always result in poor reproductive health outcomes (den Hartog *et al.*, 2006). PID, which is diagnosed in greater than 800,000 women each year in the United States is associated with Fallopian tube inflammation, which can lead to tubal factor infertility in women ranging from 5.8% and 60%, depending upon the microbial aetiology of disease and the number of recurrent infections (Soper, 2010; Westrom, 1980). A recent estimate, not including women with 'silent salpingitis' or asymptomatic infections was that the annual cost of caring for women with PID is US $2 billion (Soper, 2010). PID is known to be caused by the sexually transmitted microorganisms *C. trachomatis, N. gonorrhoeae,* and *M. genitalium* as well as bacterial vaginosis-associated microorganisms consisting predominantly of anaerobic Gram-negative bacilli. Investigations into the levels of antimicrobial compounds in Fallopian tubes or antibodies in sera collected from women with ectopic pregnancy, suggest that immune responses to infectious agents may also predispose for this condition (Refaat *et al.*, 2009; Srivastava *et al.*, 2008).

3. Fallopian tube function

The Fallopian tube plays an essential role in gamete and zygote transport. In parallel with the endometrium, the Fallopian tube also undergoes cyclical changes in response to the steroid hormones oestradiol and progesterone, which alter morphology and the frequency of beating of the ciliary (Critoph and Dennis, 1977a).

The transport of gametes and embryos through the Fallopian tubes relies on contractions of the tubal musculature, ciliary activity and the flow of tubal secretions (Jansen, 1984). Distortions of the luminal architecture of the Fallopian tubes have been associated with tubal ectopic pregnancy, predominantly because of failure of the transport mechanisms to move the gametes/embryos through the tube and into the uterus prior to implantation (Mast, 1999). Microbial infection of the Fallopian tubes is one reason for alterations in the tubal epithelial lining. Tubal disease resulting in infertility is the result of an inflammatory process in or around the Fallopian tube (Mastroianni, 1999). The extent of tubal damage is dependent on the severity and duration of the infection. The disease spectrum ranges from complete tubal occlusion with hydrosalpinx to mild intraluminal adhesions (Mastroianni, 1999).

3.1 Ovulation and oocyte capture

After ovulation, follicular fluid is the major constituent of the Fallopian tube secretions. The overall composition and viscosity of the tubal secretions (including elevated levels of steroid hormones and prostaglandins) enhances the ciliary beat frequency (Blandau *et al.*, 1975). Ciliary beat frequency is different for each part of the Fallopian tube. Elevations in the progesterone concentration in tubal secretions result in a slowing of the ciliary beat to allow fertilisation to occur, however, if the progesterone levels are too high then deciliation occurs and the prolonged delay in ciliary beat may result in implantation of the embryo within the Fallopian tube mucosa (Diaz *et al.*, 1980).

Prostaglandins within the follicular fluid mix with the tubal secretions and also increase the contractility of the fimbriae and the tubo-ovarian ligaments (Morikawa *et al.*, 1980). A controlled, deliberate movement of the tubal fimbriae ensues, initiating contact between the point of ovulation and the cumulus-oocyte-complex gently propelling the ovulated oocyte into the Fallopian tube toward the uterus (Lindblom & Andersson 1985). Transportation of the oocyte and then following fertilisation, the embryo, through the Fallopian tubes takes approximately 80 hours (Croxatto *et al.,* 1972; Croxatto *et al.,* 1978). Inhibition of oocyte capture by the Fallopian tube may result from microbial infections of the tube. The subsequent immune response can form adhesions on the fimbrial end of the Fallopian tubes or cause altered pelvic anatomy, which prevents the physical movement of the tube.

3.2 Steroid hormones (oestradiol and progesterone)

The Fallopian tubes undergo cyclical changes under the influence of the steroid hormones, oestradiol and progesterone (Critoph & Dennis, 1977) and Fallopian tube steroid hormone receptors are expressed in response to the ovulatory cycle (Pollow *et al.,* 1981). Changes in the steroid hormone expression within the Fallopian tube contribute to successful transport and ultimately implantation (Horne *et al.,* 2009).

Progesterone has an inhibitory effect in ciliary movement and tubal smooth muscle contractility, resulting in a reduction in contraction frequency (Paltieli *et al.,* 2000) and ciliary beat (Wanggren *et al.,* 2008), capable of causing delayed transport of the embryo and ectopic implantation. Horne *et al.,* (2009) reported a reduced expression of progesterone receptors in the Fallopian tubes of women with previous tubal ectopic pregnancies. They were also unable to detect expression of an oestrogen receptor on the Fallopian tubes from these same women when compared to Fallopian tubes from non-pregnant women. The alterations in steroid hormone expression in response to the ovulatory cycle were discordant in non-pregnant women, compared with those reported in women with tubal ectopic pregnancies (Horne *et al.,* 2009).

The oestrogen receptor is reportedly a dominant regulator of normal Fallopian tube development (Mowa & Iwanaga 2000) however; expression of the oestrogen receptor remains constant throughout the ovulatory cycle (Horne *et al.,* 2009).

Previous investigations have assessed the effect of oral contraceptives on the risk of ectopic pregnancy. The inhibition of fertilisation or ovulation resulted in a decreased incidence of ectopic pregnancy in women with vasectomised male partners, and in women prescribed combined oral contraceptives. In contrast, the incidence of ectopic pregnancy was elevated in women using progesterone only contraceptives, and highest in those women using progesterone only contraceptive and an intra-uterine device (Franks *et al.,* 1990). This may be due to the effect of progesterone on ciliary beat frequency or in the case of an intra-uterine device; there is an increased risk of ascending infection by commensal microflora.

Finally, the steroid hormones oestradiol and progesterone are growth factors or inhibitors for various microbial species. It has been suggested that the more frequent diagnosis of specific genital tract infections at various stages of the menstrual cycle is due to the concentrations of each of these hormones (Sonnex, 1998).

3.3 Salpingitis and alterations to the Fallopian tube luminal epithelium

The most frequent cause of ectopic pregnancy is previous salpingitis (Lehner *et al.,* 2000). The predominant facultative pathogens identified in tubal fluid from women with salpingitis are coliform bacteria (Holmes *et al.,* 1980; Ledger *et al.,* 1994; Swenson *et al.,* 1974) and the predominant anaerobic species originate from the *Bacteroides* genera. Microorganisms and the immune response may result in scar tissue formation, alter the activity of tubal cilia, result in the partial or complete destruction of cilia, and alter the composition and viscosity of the tubal secretions. Within the Fallopian tube mucosa, the response to microorganisms is not uniform. Each species evokes an individual and specific response (Laufer *et al.*, 1984). For example, *E. coli* cells or lipopolysaccharide cause swelling of the ciliary tips followed by adhesions between shortened and swollen cilia in addition to shortened microvilli on non-ciliated cells (Laufer *et al.*, 1980; Laufer *et al.*, 1984). *C. trachomatis* infection of Fallopian tubes reveals patches of flattened cells mixed with cells with only a single elongated cilium (Patten *et al.*, 1990). The sexually transmitted pathogen, *N. gonorrhoeae* causes invagination in ciliated cells and loss of microvilli in non-ciliated cells (Draper *et al.*, 1980).

4. Effects of microorganisms on the Fallopian tubes

The Fallopian tubes play an integral role in reproduction and undergo cyclical changes in morphology and ciliary activity that are dependent upon ovarian hormones (Lyons *et al.*, 2006). Recent reviews have reported that infection reduces ciliary motion and even destroys cilia within the Fallopian tubes (Lyons *et al.*, 2006; Shaw *et al.*, 2010). Reduced ciliary function can be a cause of infertility and can result in ectopic pregnancy since the embryo relies on cilia to facilitate its propulsion through the Fallopian tubes into the uterus. In addition, inflammation of the lumen of the Fallopian tubes results in tubal occlusion and tubal factor infertility. Whilst much research regarding the microflora associated with Fallopian tube damage continues to focus on sexually transmitted pathogens many other microorganisms have been associated with Fallopian tube pathology and tubal factor infertility.

4.1 Bacterial vaginosis

Bacterial vaginosis is a frequently encountered condition among women affecting from between 10 - 20% of fertile women (Holmes, 2008). Bacterial vaginosis is induced by the change from *Lactobacillus* spp. dominant vaginal flora to vaginal flora dominated by other microorganisms (Holmes, 2008). Several factors contribute to a reduction in the vaginal *Lactobacillus* spp. levels including antimicrobial treatment, hormonal imbalance, douching, use of non-barrier contraception, demographic factors – age and socioeconomic status, and the sexual history of the female – age of commencement of sexual intercourse, and number of previous sexual partners (Tibaldi *et al.*, 2009; Witkin *et al.*, 2007a). Bacterial vaginosis is a polymicrobial condition and an altered immunity hypothesis proposes that bacterial vaginosis develops as a result of the inhibition of Toll-like receptor (TLR) activation. The negative consequences of bacterial vaginosis are facilitated in part by a release and/or inadequate function of the antimicrobial plasma protein, mannose binding lectin (MBL) (Witkin *et al.*, 2007b). Microorganisms that frequently replace the normal *Lactobacillus* dominant lower genital tract flora include *Gardnerella vaginalis, Ureaplasma* spp., *M. hominis, Streptococcus viridans* and anaerobic Gram-negative bacilli from the genera *Prevotella, Porphyromonas, Bacteroides, Fusobacterium* and the coccus, *Peptostreptococcus* (Biagi *et al.*, 2009; Hillier 1993). The quantification of several microorganisms, particularly *G. vaginalis* and *Atopobium vaginae*, allows for a molecular diagnosis of bacterial vaginosis (Menard *et al.*, 2008). Microorganisms infecting the lower genital tract can be transported to the uterus and the Fallopian tubes either by (1) ascending to cause endometritis and subsequent salpingitis or (2) transport by the lymphatic system (Brook, 2002). Bacterial vaginosis has been associated with genital and obstetric infections, including PID (Catlin, 1992; Hay *et al.*, 1992; Soper, 1994), particularly in the presence of other sexually transmitted infections (Hillier *et al.*, 1996; Wiesenfeld *et al.*, 2002) including human papilloma virus infections (Verteramo *et al.*, 2009).

Gaudoin *et al.*, (Gaudoin *et al.*, 1999) reported a strong association between bacterial vaginosis and tubal factor infertility and in a study by Wilson and colleagues (2002) it was concluded that women with tubal infertility were three times more likely to have bacterial vaginosis than women with male factor or unexplained infertility. In a retrospective analysis of a population of 952 women investigated over two years, it was recently reported that the genital discharges of asymptomatic women with infertility consisted of an overgrowth of several aerobic bacteria especially *G. vaginalis* (19.7%), Enterobacteriaceae or Enterococci (12.1%) and *Streptococcus agalactiae* (8.6%) noting a prevalence of *C. trachomatis* of only 0.5% in this cohort of women (Casari *et al.*, 2010).

4.2 Upper genital tract infections

The most frequent method of female upper genital tract infection is by ascension of members of the lower genital tract endogenous microflora, which may first cause disruption to the normal balance such as that seen in cases of bacterial vaginosis or vaginal candidiasis (Population Council, 2003). Following medical intervention, iatrogenic infections may result from the direct inoculation of microorganisms from the lower genital tract into the upper genital tract. Iatrogenic procedures associated with tubal ectopic pregnancy are tubal surgery and trans-vaginal oocyte retrieval for *in vitro* fertilisation (IVF).

Seminal fluid is also reportedly a mechanism of microbial transfer to the female upper genital tract. Furthermore, some microorganisms have the propensity to attach to the surface of spermatozoa, whilst others are obligate intracellular parasites within the spermatozoa *C. trachomatis, N. gonorrhoeae, Mycoplasma* spp., *Ureaplasma* spp., and *E. coli* have all been shown to adhere to the surface of spermatozoa or form intracellular inclusions within the spermatozoa (Friberg *et al.*, 1987; Hickey *et al.*, 2009; James-Holmquest *et al.*, 1974; Murthy *et al.*, 2009; Sanchez *et al.*, 1989; Wolner-Hanssen & Mardh 1984). Further, female partners of infected men with spermatozoa in their ejaculate had a significantly higher incidence of upper genital tract infection compared to infected men who have been vasectomised (Toth *et al.*, 1984). Interestingly it was recently reported that a significantly higher incidence of sperm-immobilizing antibodies (6.4%) was found in sera collected from 273 infertile women with a past *C. trachomatis* infection compared to that found in women without a past chlamydial infection (1.5%) (Hirano & Hoshino 2010). Thus, it may be that the production of sperm-immobilizing antibodies in infertile women is the result of a past *C. trachomatis* infection in these women and this may contribute to their infertility.

4.3 Infections of the female upper genital tract (the endometrium, Fallopian tubes and ovaries)

It is becoming increasingly accepted that the female upper genital tract is not a sterile site, but likely in fact to be asymptomatically colonised or infected with microorganisms (Horne et al 2008; Wira et al 2005). Endometritis, a persistent inflammation of the endometrial lining, has been reported in up to 19% of women (Farooki 1967). Endometritis is frequently asymptomatic, but similarly to other gynaecological infections, endometritis has been shown to reduce conception rates (Feghali et al 2003; Taylor & Frydman 1996). Excessive inflammation in the endometrium at the time of implantation may be a cause of infertility. Endometritis represents an early stage in the continuum from lower genital tract infection through to salpingitis, the most serious form of female genital tract infection with respect to fertility.

Endometritis is a polymicrobial infection caused by the ascension of endogenous microorganisms or sexually transmitted infections. Endometritis is frequently reported in association with an altered lower genital tract microflora, such as that seen in women with bacteria vaginosis (Hillier et al., 1992; (Jacobsson et al 2002) or PID (Centres for Disease Control and Prevention, 2002). Alterations of the lower genital tract microbial milieu are not the only cause of endometiritis as this infection has been reported in women with 'normal' levels of lower genital tract microorganisms (Lucisano et al 1992). Microorganisms can also be introduced into the endometrium iatrogenically, during gynaecological investigations and treatment (Kiviat et al 1990).

PID results from ascension of microorganisms from the vagina to the upper genital tract (Holmes, 1984) causing post-infectious inflammation with potentially long-term sequelae including tubal infertility, ectopic pregnancy and pelvic pain (Cherpes *et al.,* 2006). Reportedly, up to 20% of women will be rendered infertile following a single diagnosis of PID (Westrom *et al.,* 1992) increasing to 50% following multiple episodes (Westrom *et al.,* 1980). In addition, women with a history of PID were twice as likely to have experienced an ectopic pregnancy when compared to women without any history of upper genital tract infection (Miller *et al.,* 1999). Similar to bacterial vaginosis, PID is also frequently polymicrobial. Opportunistic pathogens comprising anaerobic and facultative aerobic bacteria from the normal microflora of the lower genital tract, or species implicated in genital tract infections cause up to 50 % of PID, not the sexually transmitted bacteria *C. trachomatis* or *N. gonorrhoeae* (Soper, 2010).

Salpingitis is an infection in the Fallopian tube(s). A polymicrobial microflora has been reported for Fallopian tube tissue from women with salpingitis (Eschenbach *et al.,* 1975; Soper, 1994). Tubo-ovarian abscesses represent an extension of salpingitis and reportedly occur in up to 16% of women diagnosed with salpingitis.

Tubo-ovarian abscesses are usually complications of PID and represent inflammation of both the Fallopian tubes and the ovaries (Landers & Sweet 1983). The microbial aetiology of tubo-ovarian abscesses is predominantly polymicrobial (Landers & Sweet 1983; Wiesenfeld & Sweet 1993). Microbial invasion of the Fallopian tube(s) initiates an inflammatory response which results in oedema, increased pressure and restricted blood supply to the affected Fallopian tube(s) causing abscess formation and survival of the pathogens in a 'protected' environment (Osborne, 1986).

Numerous sexually transmitted and non-sexually transmitted pathogens have been isolated from infected upper genital tract tissues. Bacterial vaginosis associated bacteria have been detected independently of *C. trachomatis* and/or *N. gonorrhoeae* suggesting that investigations regarding causes of upper genital tract infection, but more specifically in the context of tubal ectopic pregnancy, and tubal damage, should focus on a diverse range of microorganisms.

4.4 *Chlamydia trachomatis*

C. trachomatis is an important pathogen in the aetiology of acute PID and has been isolated from the upper genital tracts of approximately one quarter of patients with this disease. In addition to causing symptomatic PID, *C. trachomatis* is also associated with subclinical upper genital tract disease in women (Horne *et al.*, 2008). The potentially serious sequelae of cervical infection with *C. trachomatis* can include infertility, ectopic pregnancy, pelvic pain and recurrent PID and these have recently been reviewed (Batteiger *et al.*, 2010; Darville and Hiltke, 2010; Haggerty *et al.*, 2010;). The extent to which disease sequelae eventuate following cervical infection with *C. trachomatis* is probably also significantly linked to natural processes that occur in the reproductive tract and include coitus-related phenomena and cyclical hormonal conditions. A novel paradigm that includes consideration of these and other aspects of reproductive biology particularly when using animal models to investigate potential vaccines for chlamydial genital tract infections in women has recently been proposed (Lyons *et al.*, 2009a). Continued investigations into the mechanisms of *Chlamydia*-induced tissue damage are required to further develop our understanding of the pathogenesis of genital tract disease caused by this organism, and to direct research into effective ways to control *C. trachomatis* infection, including vaccine development.

4.4.1 Chlamydia, tubal pathology and tubal factor infertility

In women it has previously been reported that a single chlamydial infection of the genital tract does not result in tubal scarring (Paavonen and Eggert-Kruse, 1999); however, prolonged exposure to *Chlamydia* due to a chronic persistent infection or frequent re-infection has been associated with (1) an autoimmune response to Chlamydial heat shock protein (which shares homology with human heat shock protein) and (2) the chronic inflammation associated with tubal factor infertility (Brunham and Peeling, 1994; Mardh, 2004; Ness *et al.*, 2008). The severity of the inflammatory response to chlamydial infection is enhanced during re-infection, causing inflammation, tissue damage and scarring. Recent studies by Hvid *et al.*, (2007) have concluded that damage to the Fallopian tubes is disproportional to the number of *C. trachomatis* infected cells, suggesting that Fallopian tube cell lysis does not occur as a direct result of infection. In their study, they instead demonstrated that IL-1 had a toxic effect on ciliated Fallopian tube cells.

Based on the results of epidemiological studies, prospective data from studies of infertile women and on results from animal models, *C. trachomatis* infection of the female reproductive tract is known to be causally associated with tubal infertility. In the murine model, a primary chlamydial infection is sufficient to induce tubal damage and infertility (Swenson *et al.*, 1983) with Toll-like receptor 2 being identified as essential for oviduct pathology in this model (Darville *et al.*, 2003; Phillips *et al.*, 1984;). Derbigney and colleagues (2007) reported that *C. muridarum* infection of murine oviduct epithelial cell lines induced a beta-interferon response and implicated Toll-like receptor 3 as the source of this interferon. In female guinea pigs, long-term tissue damage was also caused following the host response to a primary chlamydial infection (Rank and Sanders, 1992), with chlamydial salpingitis also reported in female guinea pigs receiving oral contraceptives (Barron *et al.*, 1988). By contrast, in macaque monkeys a single upper genital tract infection with *Chlamydia* is usually self-limiting with tubal scarring only resulting from repeated episodes of salpingitis (Patton *et al.*, 1987; VanVoorhis *et al.*, 1997). It has been shown that *C. trachomatis* infection in monkeys induced delayed hypersensitivity, which is proposed to be the pathogenic mechanism of tubal damage in this species (Patton *et al.*, 1994).

There have been reports of serologic evidence of past chlamydial infections (Ness and Brooks-Nelson, 1999; Patton *et al.*, 1994b; Robertson *et al.*, 1987) in women with tubal infertility, and it has been reported that interleukin-1 (IL-1) initiates Fallopian tube destruction following a *C. trachomatis* infection (Hvid *et al.,* 2007). In a retrospective study of 84 infertile women with tubal occlusion, the sera collected from 28% of these women were positive for chlamydial anti-IgG antibody, compared to only 11% positivity to the chlamydial anti-IgG antibody in sera collected from 253 infertile controls (Merki-Feld *et al.,* 2007). A study of 114 women with laparoscopically-verified tubal factor infertility (of which 96 cases showed evidence of past infection with *Chlamydia*) was undertaken to further elucidate the mechanisms of tubal damage in women with *Chlamydia*-associated infertility (Ohman *et al.,* 2009). The functional polymorphisms in selected cytokine genes [including IL-10, interferon gamma (IFN-γ), tumour necrosis factor alpha (TNF-α] revealed an increase in severe tubal damage in women with infertility caused by *Chlamydia* when certain IL-10 and TNF-α alleles were present (Ohman *et al.,* 2009). In terms of cytokine secretions in *Chlamydia*-positive infertile women, it has been reported that *Chlamydia*-stimulated cervical cells secreted significantly higher levels of IL-1ß, IL-6, IL-8 and IL-10. This indicated that the cytokine secretion profile of cervical cells may produce vital information to indicate the outcome (i.e. fertile or infertile) of a chlamydial infection of the female genital tract (Agrawal *et al.,* 2009). Others have reported that IL-1β, IL-4, IL-5 and IL-6 as well as IL-10 levels were found to be higher in *Chlamydia* membrane protein (Inc protein)-stimulated cervical cells of *C. trachomatis*-positive infertile women compared to fertile women infected with *Chlamydia* (Gupta *et al.,* 2009). More recently a unique link between elevated levels of anti-Chlamydial caseinolytic protease P (ClpP) and tubal factor infertility was identified in 21 tubal factor infertility patients (Rodgers *et al.,* 2010).

Host genetic factors are known to modulate the immune defence mechanisms to a *Chlamydia* infection thus determining the occurrence of *Chlamydia*-induced tubal factor infertility. A study by Morre and colleagues (2002) reported that almost 45% of women infected with genital chlamydial infections cleared the infection after one year with no interventional treatments. However, some authors have claimed that this study by Morre *et al.,*. (2002) was methodologically flawed (Risser and Risser, 2007; Simms and Horner, 2008). An increased risk of tubal pathology (as a result of aberrant immune responses) has been reported in 227 sub-fertile women following a *C. trachomatis* infection and carrying two or more single-nucleotide polymorphisms (SNPs) in genes (toll-like receptor (TLR)-9, TLR-4, CD14, and caspase recruitment domain protein 15 (CARD15)/nucleotide-binding oligomerization domain containing 2(NOD2) that encode pattern recognition receptors (PRRs) involved in sensing bacterial components (den Hartog *et al.,* 2006). In a more recent report that investigated 214 infertile women, 42 of whom had tubal pathology, it was found that polymorphisms in the major histocompatibility complex class I chain related A gene (specifically allele 008) correlated with *C. trachomatis* anti-IgG antibodies in infertilewomen (Mei *et al.,* 2009).

4.4.2 Chlamydia and PID

PID is caused by infection of the female genital tract with microorganisms including *C. trachomatis* (Bakken and Ghaderi, 2009) and testing for serum antibody to the chlamydial 60kDa Heat shock protein (i.e.CHSP60 antibody) is an accurate means for predicting *Chlamydia*-associated tubal factor infertility (Claman *et al.,* 1997). A prospective study into serologic parameters of tubal disease reported that antibodies to CHSP60 were also predictive for lower spontaneous conception and pregnancy outcome after a first episode of ectopic pregnancy (Sziller *et al.,* 2008). A retrospective study of follicular fluid from 253 IVF patients for IgG antibodies to CHSP60 reported that antibodies to CHSP60 were found in

74.1% of women without embryo (s) and in 69.5% of women with tubal occlusion (Jakus *et al.,* 2008). In the PID evaluation and clinical health (PEACH) study 443 women with clinical signs of mild to moderate PID were followed for 84 months and assessed for long-term sequelae of chlamydial infections of the genital tract including PID recurrence and time to pregnancy (Ness *et al.,* 2008). It was found that IgG antibody responses to CHSP60 and elementary bodies (the extracellular form) of *C. trachomatis* serovar D were independently associated with reduced pregnancy rates and increased rates of recurrent PID (Ness *et al.,* 2008). In another study of 72 female patients a significant seropositivity to CHSP60 antibodies was detected in patients with secondary infertility from an infertile cohort clinically characterised primary and/or secondary infertility. This indicated that specific antibodies to CHSP60 may aid in the early prognosis of immunopathologic sequelae following genital tract infections with *C. trachomatis* (Dutta *et al.,* 2008). The 10kDa chlamydial heat shock protein 10 (CHSP10) has also been identified as a target of cell-mediated responses in human chlamydial infections. Women with tubal infertility have been shown to recognise CHSP10 more frequently than those women with current active chlamydial infections. Co-expression of both CHSP60 and CHSP10 were subsequently detected at higher levels in the infertile women compared to the fertile women (Jha *et al.,* 2009). CHSP10 and CHSP60 stimulation was reported to increase the cytokine responses of IFN-γ and IL-10 in *Chlamydia*-positive infertile women (Srivastava *et al.,* 2008). Srivastava *et al.,*. (2008) suggested that this could significantly affect the release of these cytokines from the cervical mononuclear cells, thus affecting the mucosal immune function against this pathogen and hence fertility outcomes in these women.

Linhares and Witkin (2010) recently reviewed the immunopathogenic consequences of CHSP60 expression in the female genital tract and they reported that scar formation and tubal occlusion resulted from the induction of pro-inflammatory immune responses following the release of CHSP60 from a *C. trachomatis* infection. They further reported that the production of CHSP60 cross-reacting antibodies and cell-mediated immunity to the human HSP60 was detrimental to subsequent pregnancy outcome in women infected in the upper reproductive tract with this microbial pathogen (Linhares and Witkin 2010).

4.4.3 Chlamydia screening

Screening for, and treatment of, chlamydial infection is aimed at reducing chlamydial transmission and preventing PID and the long-term sequelae of PID including infertility, chronic pain, recurrent episodes of PID and ectopic pregnancy.

For the host to successfully clear infections of the female genital tract caused by *C. trachomatis* an adequate immune response is required following recognition of the pathogen by pattern recognition receptors (PRRs) of the Toll-like receptor (TLR) and nucleotide binding oligomerization domain (NOD) families. If functioning correctly, the host immune response clears the infection but in some females the infection is not cleared and this allows for a persistent infection to manifest in these hosts. Since most infections with *Chlamydia* remain asymptomatic it is difficult to ascertain the risk of potential disease sequelae associated with previous chlamydial infections. There are several methods used to assess the risk of chlamydial infections in women that may lead to tubal factor sub-fertility and these have been reviewed (den Hartog et al., 2006). In particular it has been found that testing for anti-chlamydial IgG antibody in serum can indicate a previous infection but cannot predict a persistent infection. It has been noted that screening for serological markers of persistence (including C-reactive protein) seems useful for identifying infected women at highest risk of tubal pathology. It has been proposed that three screening strategies would be useful for identifying tubal factor sub-fertility in women infected in the genital tract with *C. trachomatis*: (1) *C. trachomatis* IgG antibody testing, (2) high sensitivity CRP testing and (3) hysterosalpingography (den Hartog, 2008). A recent mathematical modelling study has analysed previously published data on the persistence of asymptomatic *C. trachomatis* infection in women, and has estimated the mean duration of the asymptomatic period to be longer (433 days) than previously anticipated. These authors conclude that their study shows that a longer duration of the asymptomatic period results in a more pronounced impact of a screening programme (Althaus *et al.*, 2010).

The incidence of PID in untreated women infected with *C. trachomatis* has been reviewed and widely discussed in the literature in terms of (1) its cost-effectiveness as a screening program and (2) as a predictor of tubal damage in infertile patients (Aghaizu *et al.*, 2008; Althaus et al., 2010; Bakken & Ghaderi 2009; den Hartog *et al.*, 2008; Dietrich *et al.*, 2010; Kalwij *et al.*, 2010; Land *et al.*, 2010; Low *et al.*, 2009; Low & Hocking 2010; Oakeshott *et al.*, 2010; Risser & Risser 2007; Simms & Horner 2008). In a comprehensive study that evaluated all available original research and assessed the incidence of PID following *C. trachomatis* infection, it was concluded that no study could adequately answer the question and that many studies either had inaccuracies, validition problems or only indirect evidence to support their reported incidences (Risser and Risser, 2007). A similar review of the literature was undertaken by Simms and Horner (2008) who stated that a reasonable estimate of PID incidence in untreated women after *C. trachomatis* infection was likely to be in the range of 10-20%. A Norwegian registry-linkage study of 24,947 women who were tested for *C. trachomatis* infection reported a correlation between diagnosed *Chlamydia* infection and subsequent PID. The incidence rate of PID in this study was found to be higher in women with prior *C. trachomatis* infection than among women with negative *C. trachomatis* tests although the rates were notably low in both groups (Bakken & Ghaderi 2009). It has therefore been suggested that the benefits of current *Chlamydia* screening programmes may have been overestimated (Low *et al.*, 2006).

A comprehensive review of seven electronic databases covering 17 years of register-based reports (until 2007) and opportunistic screening programmes for *Chlamydia* found that there was no evidence to support the most commonly recommended approach of opportunistic *Chlamydia* screening in a general population younger than 25 years. Furthermore, it was proposed by these authors that an effective approach when assessing biological outcomes of chlamydial infection currently reuqires multiple rounds of screening in randomized control trials (RCT) (Low *et al.*, 2009). A recent RCT (the POPI-prevention of pelvic infection-trial) was undertaken to determine whether a single screening test and treating a subset of 2529 women for chlamydial infection can in fact reduce the incidence of PID over a 12-month period (Oakeshott et al., 2010). The baseline prevalence of *Chlamydia* was 5.4% in the screened population of 2529 sexually active female students (mean age 20.9 years) and 5.9% in (deferred screening) controls with the incidences of PID found to be 1.3% and 1.9% respectively in these cohorts. It was reported that after 12 months, most episodes of PID occurred in women who tested negative for *Chlamydia* at baseline (9.5%) when compared to the intervention group (1.6%) and these authors concluded that the effectiveness of a single *Chlamydia* test in preventing PID over 12 months may also have been overestimated (Oakeshott et al., 2010).

A Danish randomised trial was conducted with 9-year follow-up testing of 4000 asymptomatic women for the presence of urogenital *Chlamydia trachomatis*. Data were collected on PID, ectopic pregnancy EP, infertility diagnoses, IVF treatment and births in women. Results showed that no differences were found between the intervention group and the control groups of women for PID, ectopic pregnancy, infertility, IVF treatment and births. It was concluded that a population-based offer to be tested for urogenital *C. trachomatis* infection using non-invasive samples and DNA amplification testing did not reduce the long-term risk of reproductive complications such as PID and ectopic pregnancies in asymptomatic women (Anderson *et al.,* 2011). This finding agrees with the conclusions made by authors of an earlier review of 12 databases who reported (from the one study that satisfied inclusion criteria for their review) the absence of valid evidence on the risk of tubal factor infertility following an infection of the genital tract with *C. trachomatis* (Wallace *et al.,* 2008) and is also in agreement with the finding of Oakeshott and colleagues (Oakeshott et al., 2010).

Of note from the Oakeshott study was that a screening intervention at 12 months would not have prevented the 10 reported cases of chlamydia-positive PID among women who were *Chlamydia*-negative at baseline and serves to highlight the ongoing transmission of *Chlamydia* as the elemental problem. The results of the POPI trial suggested that current levels of chlamydial screening are unlikely to have much impact on the overall incidence of PID (Low & Hocking 2010). A recent modelling study based on a comprehensive literature survey on the epidemiology of chlamydial infection and risk-estimates of its late complications has concluded that the risk of developing tubal infertility after a *Chlamydia* lower genital tract is low (at around 4.6%), and these authors stated that high quality RCTs investigating the transition from cervicitis to tubal infertility are needed (Land et al., 2010). It has also been reported in a prospective study evaluating the sensitivity of multiple-site swab testing (cervix, urethra, vagina and Fallopian tubes) in 2,020 fertility patients over 12 months that multiple site sampling does not increase the detection rate of *C. trachomatis* among infertile women and in fact that routine DNA testing for *C. trachomatis* should be confined to cervical sampling (Dietrich et al., 2010). A review from the National *Chlamydia* screening programme in London has highlighted the need for *Chlamydia* testing to be offered routinely to young people (under 25 years) as part of an overall approach to sexual health in the community (Kalwij et al., 2010).

It has been noted recently that no studies have yet published results of the effects of greater than one round of screening or indeed screening for repeat *Chlamydia* infections on reproductive sequelae in women following asymptomatic *C. trachomatis* genital infection (Gottlieb *et al.,* 2010). However two new trials the *Chlamydia* Screening Implementation (CSI) Project (van den Broek *et al.,* 2010) and the Australian *Chlamydia* Control Effectiveness Pilot (ACCEPt) trial (Hocking *et al.,* 2008) are currently underway investigating multiple screening rounds and using *Chlamydia* prevalence (and not PID) as the end point. These trials should provide more conclusive information regarding the effectiveness of chlamydial screening to control morbidity associated with genital chlamydial infection.

4.4.4 Chlamydia and vaccines

Fertility in women is overwhelmingly affected by unresolved or untreated infection of the female reproductive tract with *C. trachomatis.* Since greater than 70% of chlamydial genital infections in women are asymptomatic and sequelae of infection manifest as diseases resulting from severe pathological consequences such as tubal occlusion, a vaccine is likely to be imperative to control infections caused by this sexually transmitted mucosal pathogen. Many animal models of infection-induced immunity including murine and guinea pig models continue to be essential in providing knowledge of the infection processes and immune responses to a variety species found within the Chlamydiaceae. These have recently been reviewed by several groups (Cochrane *et al.*, 2010; Farris & Morrison 2011; Hafner *et al.*, 2008; Hafner 2007; Hafner & McNeilly 2008; Lyons et al., 2006; Miyairi *et al.*, 2010; Rank & Whittum-Hudson 2010). These animal models have proved invaluable in providing knowledge of many novel candidate antigens for a vaccine (Barker *et al.*, 2008; McNeilly *et al.*, 2007; Murthy AK *et al.*, 2011; Murthy et al., 2009) as well as novel delivery vehicles (Xu *et al.*, 2011) and delivery routes such as oral and transcutaneous immunization for protection of genital infections (Hickey *et al.*, 2010; Hickey et al., 2009) and have investigated a myriad of potential adjuvants (reviewed in Cochrane *et al.*, 2010; Farris and Morrison, 2011; Hafner *et al.*, 2008) and immune responses elicited following animal immunization trials (Cunningham *et al.*, 2011; McNeilly et al., 2007; Patton *et al.*, 1983). For example it has recently been reported that a *Vibrio cholerae* ghost (VCG) multisubunit chlamydial vaccine delivered to mice by the intramuscular route stimulated immune memory in these animals (Eko *et al.*, 2011). Protection correlates that have been assessed in these models to determine vaccine efficiency have included reduced shedding of viable chlamydial infectious bodies, reduced duration of infection and reduced tissue pathologies such as hydrosalpinx; a vaccine that can achieve one and/or any of these outcomes will greatly aid in diminishing the pathological sequelae of chlamydial genital infections.

Results of recent studies using animal models have revealed many promising novel candidate antigens for eliciting protection against chlamydial genital tract infections in humans. The fusion protein CTH1 is composed of chlamydial proteins from two highly conserved (>97% homology) immune-dominant antigens CT443 (*omc*B) and CT521 (r116) that are targets both for cell-mediated and for humoral immunity and thus can be expected to allow for cross-protection amongst the various chlamydial serotypes (Olsen AW *et al.*, 2010). In addition, CT 521 has also been found to be a strong and frequent target for T cells during a natural *C. trachomatis* infection in humans (Olsen *et al.*, 2006). In 2009 a study investigating 55 chlamydial ORFs covering all putative type III secretion components and control molecules were expressed as fusion proteins. This study measured the reactivity of these fusion proteins with antibodies from sera collected from patient infected with *C. trachomatis* in the urogenital tract (24 antisera) (Wang *et al.*, 2009). It was reported that immunization of mice with the translocated actin recruiting phosphoprotein (Tarp) induced Th1-dominant immunity that significantly reduced the shedding of live bacteria from the lower genital tract and attenuated inflammatory pathologies in the Fallopian tube tissues (Wang *et al.*, 2009). Using the C3H/HeN murine model the subunit vaccine CtH1 delivered subcutaneously with a Th1-inducing adjuvant (CAF01) induced a protective CD4+T cell response and high levels of CTH1-specific antibodies in both the sera and genital tracts of immunised mice however it failed to provide a CD4 independent protective response needed for complete protection (Olsen et al., 2010). A second promising vaccine candidate that has induced CD4+Th1 cells both in *Chlamydia*-infected mice and in humans diagnosed with chlamydial genital tract infections is CT043 a highly conserved hypothetical protein that could potentially provide cross-serotype protection. DNA priming/protein boost immunization with this protein the bacterial load was also significantly reduced in the murine lung infection model (Meoni *et al.*, 2009). The fact that CTD43 has been shown to reduce (1) chlamydial infectivity in the murine model and (2) to prime a CD4+Th1 response in over 60% of patients infected with genital serovars of *C. trachomatis*, means that this antigen could be a promising vaccine candidate for chlamydial genital tract infections. A third candidate antigen showing great promise particularly for prevention of infertility resulting from repeated infections with *C. trachomatis* is the recombinant chlamydial protease-like activity factor (rCPAF) (Murthy et al., 2011).This antigen has been reviewed as a potential vaccine candidate (Murthy *et al.,* 2009) and has successfully induced a combination of neutralising antibodies and cell-mediated responses against genital chlamydial challenge in a murine model of genital chlamydial infection (Li *et al.,* 2010). More recent studies have reported that mice vaccinated intranasally with rCPAF and the adjuvant CpG were significantly protected against infertility as seen by a reduction in hydrosaplinx in rCPAF+CpG vaccinated mice following a primary genital challenge with *C. muridarum* (Murthy *et al.,,* 2011). This latest finding augurs well for the inclusion of this candidate antigen in a vaccine for use in humans to protect against female infertility.

Recently, a proteomics approach has been used to identify potential vaccine candidates for chlamydial infections. In one study three strains of mice, BALB/c, C3H/HeN and C57BL/6, were inoculated with live and inactivated *C. muridarum* by different routes of immunization. Using a protein microarray, serum samples collected from the mice after immunization were tested for the presence of antibodies against specific chlamydial antigens. This has identified a panel of seven *C. muridarum* dominant antigens (TC0052, TC0189, TC0582, TC0660, TC0726, TC0816 and, TC0828) (Molina, 2010). In a second study by the same group antigen identification was done by constructing a protein chip array by expressing the open reading frames (ORFs) from *C.muridarum* genomic and plasmid DNA and testing it with serum samples from *C.muridarum* immunized mice. This second approach has resulted in the identification of several new immunogens, including 75 hypothetical proteins thus identifying a new group of immunodominant chlamydial proteins that can be tested for their ability to induce protection (Cruz-Fisher *et al.,* 2011).

4.5 *Neisseria gonorrhoeae*

N. gonorrhoeae has been implicated in tubal infections. Both the bacteria themselves or components of the bacterial cell wall, lipopolysaccharide or peptidoglycan reportedly cause cessation of the ciliary activity (Mardh 1979) however, infection of the Fallopian tubes does not always result in ultrastructural damage to the mucosal surface (Woods & McGee 1986). Gonococci only invade the non-ciliated cells of the Fallopian tube mucosa, whereby the neighbouring ciliated cells become sloughy and detached (McGee 1981). *Neisseria* spp. infection of the Fallopian tubes results in a dose-dependent response to bacterial cells. Low numbers of bacterial cells induce secretion of TNF-α and subsequently apoptosis of infected cells, however, when bacterial cell numbers increase, the apoptosis appears to be inhibited, favouring bacterial survival (Dean and Powers, 2001). Studies have suggested that ectopic pregnancy is now more likely to be associated with non-gonococcal rather than *N. gonorrhoeae* upper genital tract infection (Kamwendo *et al.,* 1996).

4.6 Mycoplasma species

M. hominis reportedly causes ciliostasis and swelling of Fallopian tube cilia (Mardh & Westrom 1970). *Mycoplasma* spp. have been isolated from the female upper genital tract and Fallopian tubes (Cohen 2005; Heinonen & Miettinen 1994; Stagey *et al* 1992). Serological testing of women has confirmed an association between mycoplasmas and cases of PID (Moller *et al.,* 1985)and mycoplasma, PID and ectopic pregnancy (Jurstrand *et al.,* 2007). A prospective study of 212 infertile couples was undertaken to investigate the presence of

M.genitalium in women with tubal factor infertility and it was found that antibodies to *M.genitalium* were shown to be independently and significantly associated with tubal factor infertility (Svenstrup *et al.,* 2008).

Recently it has been reported that a genetic polymorphism in one of the components of the inflammasome - a cytoplasmic structure producing interleukin-1 - increases the likelihood of mycoplasma infection-associated female infertility (Witkin *et al.,* 2010).

4.7 *Ureaplasma spp.*

Ureaplasma spp. have been implicated in infections of the lower (bacterial vaginosis) and of the upper genital tracts (PID, endometritis) of women (Kanakas *et al* 1999). Further, tubal infertility has been associated with ureaplasma PID in a small number of cases (Henry-Suchet *et al* 1980. Inoculation of *Ureaplasma* spp. into *in vivo* Fallopian tube organ cultures resulted in replication of the pathogen, suggesting that this genital mycoplasma may also play a role in tubal damage.

4.8 Anaerobic bacteria

Anaerobic species are frequently isolated from the female genital tract and in cases of acute PID (Saini *et al* 2003). The polymicrobial nature of anaerobic infections appears to enhance the pathogenicity of the implicated species implicated (Eschenbach et al 1975). Previous upper genital tract pathology caused by upper genital tract infections, pelvic adhesions, endometriosis or prolonged or continuous menstruation, have been associated with the reactivation of PID. It is likely that the compromised areas of the pelvic cavity promote the establishment of a niche for bacterial survival (El-Shawarby *et al* 2004). Ness *et al.* (2005) reported that the presence of anaerobic bacterial vaginosis-associated microorganisms in the vagina was a significant risk factor for infection of the upper genital tract leading to long-term sequelae and possible PID.

Mobiluncus spp. are frequently isolated from women with bacterial vaginosis. Members of the *Mobiluncus* genera have been shown to produce cytotoxins, resulting in the loss of cilia, and bloating and detachment of the ciliated cells of the Fallopian tube mucosa (Taylor-Robinson *et al* 1993). Another of the genera associated with bacterial vaginosis, the gram-negative *Bacteroides* spp. also releases lipopolysaccharide, resulting in the sloughing of Fallopian tube epithelial cells and loss of ciliary activity within the Fallopian tubes (Fontaine *et al* 1986).

4.9 Aerobic/Microaerophilic bacteria

Gram-positive species, *Enterococcus* spp., *Staphylococcus* spp., and *Streptococcus* spp. have been isolated from Pouch of Douglas aspirates of a polymicrobial microflora in women with symptoms of genital tract infection (Saini et al 2003). Saini *et al.* (2003) proposed that the microflora of the Pouch of Douglas was likely to be more representative of Fallopian tube microorganisms in women with salpingitis than the vaginal flora of those same women.

Members of the Enterbactereaceae have been detected in upper genital tract infections. The Gram-negative bacillus, *Klebsiella* spp. are frequently isolated from women with PID (Saini et al., 2003). Laufer *et al.,.* ((Laufer *et al.,* 1984)) reported that inoculation of the Fallopian tubes with *Escherichia coli* resulted in complete de-ciliation or damage to the cilia. When damage occurred, the cilia were swollen and short. In addition, microvilli were lost from the non-ciliated cells. The oxidative species, *Pseudomonas aeruginosa* is also a causal agent of PID in females (King *et al.,* 2002).

Based on previous studies, it has been concluded that genital tract infections including salpingitis, which causes tubal factor infertility are polymicrobial in nature. Furthermore, a diverse range of microorganisms are capable of colonising and possibly infecting the genital tract tissues. Opportunistic pathogens identified in genital tract infections are frequently members of the normal regional flora and should be further investigated given that 60% of PID is non-gonococcal and non-chlamydial. Infectious causes of salpingitis and tubal factor infertility require further investigation to better establish prevalence and causality. The identification of microorganisms that are particularly detrimental to the Fallopian tubes may result in effective treatment and a reduction in the overall frequency of tubal factor infertility and tubal ectopic pregnancy.

5. Ectopic pregnancy and chlamydia

Infectious agents cause damage to the Fallopian tube mucosa either directly or because of the host inflammatory response aimed at clearing the infection. Alteration to the mucosa can result in poor transport of the embryo and subsequent implantation of the blastocyst outside the endometrial lining of the uterine cavity - an ectopic pregnancy. Tubal ectopic pregnancy is a result not only of impaired transport of the embryo causing the embryo to be maintained in the Fallopian tube but also a result from alterations in the tubal environment that allows early implantation to occur (reviewed in Shaw *et al.*, 2010). A recent review also summarises the results of investigations of the Fallopian tube with respect to the roles of of caspase 1, cannabinoid receptor and Dicer 1 knockout mice and how these contribute to tubal dysfunction and contribute to ectopic pregnancies (Shao 2010).
A recent review highlighted the many risk factors for ectopic pregnancy and these are summarised in Table 1.

Risk Factors for ectopic pregnancy
High risk
Tubal surgery
Tubal Ligation
Previous ectopic pregnancy
In utero exposure to diethylstilbestrol
Use of intrauterine devices
Tubal pathology
Assisted reproduction
Moderate risk
Infertility
Previous genital infections
Multiple sexual partners
Salpingitis isthmica nodosa
Low risk
Previous pelvic infection
Cigarette smoking
Vaginal douching
First intercourse (<18 years)

Table 1. Risk Factors for ectopic preganacy (adapted from Kulp and Barnhart, 2008)

Ectopic pregnancy accounts for up to 11% of all pregnancies and there is serological evidence that links ectopic pregnancies with *C. trachomatis* infection in women (Chow *et al.*, 1990; Swenson & Schachter 1984) It was noted in one study that 19/21 *C. trachomatis* seropositive women with ectopic pregnancies had antibodies to the chlamydial 57kDa antigen and it was suggested that perhaps immune responses to this antigen may be involved in the immunopathogenesis of ectopic pregnancy associated with *C. trachomatis* infections (Brunham *et al.*, 1992). A recent review has reported that one third of ectopic pregnancies could be attributable to chlamydial infection (Bebear and de Barbeyrac, 2009).

The finding of chlamydial RNA in Fallopian tube biopsy samples collected from women with ectopic pregnancies suggested that viable, metabolically active bacteria were present in the Fallopian tubes of these women (Gerard *et al.*, 1998). Chlamydial DNA has also been detected in the Fallopian tube tissue collected from women at the time of ectopic pregnancy (Barlow *et al.*, 2001; Noguchi *et al.*, 2002). A report to the contrary regarding the detection of chlamydial DNA in fresh tissue from the Fallopian tubes of women with ectopic pregnancy has, however, also been published and suggested that persistent chlamydial infection of Fallopian tubes was rare in ectopic pregnancy (Bjartling *et al.*, 2007). A retrospective study looking at births and ectopic pregnancy in 20, 762 women in Norway has reported that the risk of ectopic pregnancy increased in a dose-dependent manner with the increasing number of prior chlamydial infections (Bakken *et al.*, 2007). In a comprehensive review by the same author it has been reported that relatively low risks of ectopic pregnancy are recorded after a positive *C. trachomatis* diagnosis with, in Sweden for example, a cumulative incidence before the age of 35 years of rates of 2.7% *C. trachomatis*-positive and 2% *C. trachomatis*-negative (Bakken 2008).

In a small study of 14 ectopic pregnancy patients who were serologically-positive for *C. trachomatis*, subjective immunohistochemistry techniques were used to show an increase in the expression of inducible nitric oxide synthase (iNOS) (which is related to inflammation and infection and which can generate nitric oxide) and activin A (a member of the transforming growth factor beta family that has been reported to increase inflammation and repair) in Fallopian tubes from these women (Refaat *et al.*, 2009). It was proposed by these authors that tubal activin A and nitric oxide (NO) could perhaps be involved in microbial-mediated damaging immune response within the Fallopian tubes of *Chlamydia*-infected women and that their pathological expression may lead to ectopic pregnancy development (Refaat *et al.*, 2009). Nitric oxide is similarly proposed as the damaging agent of cells in the uterine tubes of female mice in the murine model of chlamydial genital infection. It is proposed that nitric oxide expressed in macrophages in response to a *C. muridarum* infection in mice could perhaps be the cause of damage to oviduct interstitial cells of Cajal (ICC-OVI) that have been identified as oviduct pacemaker cells critical for egg transport along the Fallopian tubes (Dixon *et al.*, 2010). The expression of iNOS by human Fallopian tubes has recently been reported as being cyclical during different stages of the menstrual cycle and the intensity of expression of iNOS was found to be higher in the Fallopian tubes of 15 women bearing an ectopic pregnancy when compared with pseudo-pregnant women (Al-Azemi *et al.*, 2010). These results suggested that increased iNOS levels in response to a microbial infection could lead to an increased expression of nitric oxide which may in turn affect the contraction of muscles and/or the ciliary beat in Fallopian tubes, ultimately leading to retention of the embryo at this site.

A recent report from The Netherlands has presented the finding that a peak incidence of admissions for PID in 1983 preceded a peak incidence of ectopic pregnancy in 1988 mainly

due to a decrease in ectopic pregnancy in women over 35 years of age. The report also states that women born between 1985 and 1990 and less than 25 years of age are now at an increased risk of ectopic pregnancy and this rise has not been preceded by a peak incidence of PID (Mol *et al.,* 2010). These authors further conclude that the significant rise in ectopic pregnancies may in fact be related to an increase in positive tests for chlamydial infection of the genital tracts (Mol *et al.,* 2010).
The management of ectopic pregnancy has recently been addressed (Kulp & Barnhart 2008; Mol *et al.,* 2011).

6. Endometriosis and Fallopian tube function

Women with endometriosis have an increased incidence of tubal ectopic pregnancy, suggesting that endometriosis results in impairment of tubal transport of gametes and embryos. Previous *in vitro* studies have revealed that peritoneal fluid collected from women with endometriosis caused a decrease in the Fallopian tube ciliary beat frequency (Lyons *et al.,* 2006), which supports the increased incidence of implantation of the embryo within the Fallopian tubes of these women. The pelvic inflammation associated with endometriosis can also cause adhesion and scar tissue formation within the Fallopian tubes creating a physical obstruction to embryo transport (Halis & Arici 2004). The pathogenesis of endometriosis involves changes both in cellular and in humoral immunity. Impaired natural killer cell activity results in inadequate removal of debris following retrograde menstruation. Elevated primary inflammatory mediators, which are characterised by increased numbers of macrophages, result in the production of secondary inflammatory mediators such as cytokines, chemokines and growth factors (Harada *et al.,* 2001) However, the secretion of primary inflammatory mediators can also be induced by microbial stimuli (Wira *et al.,* 2005). This highlights the relevance of a non-sterile endometrium in this aetiology. It may be that the retrograde menstruation of colonised or contaminated (by microorganisms) menstrual blood enhances the pathology of endometriosis by recruiting macrophages, which then secrete elevated levels of pro-inflammatory cytokines.
A small study investigating eutopic and ectopic endometrium, identified DNA with a 96% homology to the Gram-negative bacterium *Shigella* spp. in ectopic but not in eutopic endometrium. Therefore, an infection hypothesis was proposed for the pathogenesis of endometriosis (Kodati *et al.,* 2008). Recently, Khan *et al.,*. (Khan *et al.,* 2010) reported a significant increase in the number of colony forming units of *E. coli* recovered from the menstrual blood of women with endometriosis when compared to women without the disease. In their study, the bacterial endotoxin concentration was also higher both in the menstrual blood and in the peritoneal fluid samples from women with endometriosis. The relative level of *E. coli* within the peritoneal fluid of women with endometriosis was likely due to retrograde menstruation through the Fallopian tubes and into the pelvic cavity. The 'open' nature of the female genital tract makes it unlikely that secretions from the uterus, Fallopian tubes and peritoneal cavity remain compartmentalised. Transport of microorganisms within the upper genital tract may well be an area requiring further investigation in the pathogenesis of endometriosis and its increased association with tubal ectopic pregnancy.
Interestingly, *E. coli* has also been cultured from tubo-ovarian abscesses in women with ovarian endometriomas and pelvic endometriosis (Kavoussi *et al.,* 2006; Lin *et al.,* 2010).The fluid-filled ovarian endometrioma may provide an excellent growth medium for

microorganisms, and endometriomas have been identified as a risk factor for tubo-ovarian abscess formation (Kubota *et al.*, 1997; Lin *et al.*, 2010). Women with endometriosis appear to represent a population at increased risk of infection and subsequent tubo-ovarian abscess due to an altered local immune environment (Chen *et al.*, 2004; Lebovic *et al.*, 2001). The risk of endometriosis is also increased in women with shorter menstrual cycles and an increased menstrual flow (Halme *et al.*, 1984). Again, the retrograde menstruation of non-sterile menstrual blood into the peritoneal cavity provides a route for microbial transport. The menstrual debris may also promote continued survival and persistence of these microorganisms in the upper genital tract. Microorganisms have been detected in the endometrium of 83% of women during the post-partum period (Andrews *et al.*, 2005). However, both vaginal and endocervical cultures demonstrated low concordance with endometrial cultures (Cicinelli *et al.*, 2009). This may suggest that tropisms exist in the genital tract that can modulate microbial survival. In studies investigating women with chronic endometritis, Cicinelli *et al.*,. (Cicinelli *et al.*, 2008) reported isolation aerobic bacteria in over 73% of cases in symptomatic women but in only 5% of women without clinical evidence of endometritis. A shortcoming if their study was that they did not screen endometrial samples for the presence of anaerobes, which dominate the genital microflora. Together, these studies suggest that the endometrial cavity is not sterile, and that the presence of microorganisms does not necessarily result on overt inflammation. The possibility exists that in women with endometriosis, who have an impaired genital tract immune response, that (1) these microorganisms may replicate causing increased pathology, including tubal damage and (2) the microflora represent a stimulus for the enhanced chemotaxis of macrophages and the subsequent secretion of secondary inflammatory mediators identified in this condition.

Other chemical mediators have also been investigated in women with endometriosis. Inducible nitric oxide synthase, activated by cytokines and growth factors (Morris and Billiard, 1994; Nussler and Billiar, 1993), regulates embryo transport within the Fallopian tube. What is interesting is that in women with endometriosis and PID, nitric oxide levels are increased (Alpay *et al.*, 2006; Bouyer *et al.*, 2002; Sioutas *et al.*, 2008). Lipopolysaccharide was capable of *in vitro* activation of macrophages in the peritoneal fluid of women with endometriosis, increasing inducible nitric oxide synthase and nitric oxide production in these women but not in women without disease (Osborn *et al.*, 2002). If endometriosis is part of an infectious condition, then these results may be evidence of the activity f polarised macrophages in this population. A macromolecular ovum capture inhibitor, causing formation of a membrane over the fimbrial cilia, has been also detected in the peritoneal fluid from women with endometriosis (Suginami & Yano 1988).

Studies investigating ectopic pregnancy following IVF are limited however, it has been suggested that the hormonal stimulation protocol and the infertility history may also be mechanisms predisposing women to ectopic pregnancy (Chang & Suh 2010).

7. IVF

Hydrosalpinx is associated with decreased IVF success (Wainer *et al.*, 1997). Approximately 30% of women undergoing IVF for tubal factor infertility have hydrosalpinges (Blazar *et al.*, 1997; Murray 1997). The incidence of ectopic pregnancy was significantly higher in patients having IVF treatment for tubal factor infertility than in those diagnosed with infertility die to endometriosis or idiopathic infertility (Dubuisson *et al.*, 1991). It has been reported that

there was no relationship between the ectopic pregnancy rate and the ovarian hyperstimulation protocol used for ovulation induction (Dubuisson *et al.,* 1991). This is despite some studies suggesting that the hormonal protocols used in IVF contribute to ectopic pregnancy possibly by alterations in tubal muscle contractions or ciliary beat.
The ectopic pregnancy rate for women having IVF with natural and stimulated cycles was around 11% (Dubuisson et al., 1991), this is consistent with previous reports (Yovich *et al.,* 1985) indicating that in infertile women undergoing IVF and embryo transfer, the rate of tubal ectopic pregnancy is significantly higher compared to women conceiving naturally.

8. Conclusions

Infectious agents can damage biological functions of the female reproductive tract with devastating consequences. Among the most common microorganisms involved in sexually transmitted infections and interfering with female fertility are *C. trachomatis* and *N. gonorrhoeae*. These two pathogens are involved in damage to the cervix, Fallopian tubes and tubal luminal architecture in infected women. Tubo-peritoneal damage seems to be the leading cause of microbial interference with human fertility. *C. trachomatis* is considered the most important cause of tubal obstruction and PID. Screening for repeat chlamydial infections using randomised control trials and prevalence of *Chlamydia* rather than PID as an end point should provide information useful for controlling morbidity associated with these infections. Infection of the female genital tract with other bacterial organisms including *M. genitalium,* Ureaplasma spp., anaerobes and aerobes/microaerophiles can also affect the precise functioning of components of this site resulting in tubal occlusion and infertility. Bacterial vaginosis is strongly linked to tubal infertility as causative agents can produce ascending infections of the female upper genital tract. The role of bacterial infections particularly those caused by *C. trachomatis* and immune responses to these infections as causes of damage to sperm function require further investigation. Finally, continued efforts in vaccine development to control *C. trachomatis* genital infections would seem prudent to prevent sequelae of unresolved or untreated infections of the female genital tract that can have profound effects on fertility in women.

9. References

Aghaizu A, Atherton H, Mallinson H, Simms I, Kerry S, Oakeshott P, Hay PE. 2008. Incidence of pelvic inflammatory disease in untreated women infected with Chlamydia trachomatis. *Int J STD AIDS* 19:283

Agrawal, T., Gupta, R., Dutta, R. Srivastava, P.,Bhengraj, A. R., Salha, S. and Mittal, A., (2009) Protective or pathogenic immune response to genital chlamydial infection in women--a possible role of cytokine secretion profile of cervical mucosal cells. *Clin Immunol.*, 130 (3): 347-54

Al-Azemi M, Refaat B, Amer S, Ola B, Chapman N, W. L. 2010. The expression of inducible nitric oxide synthase in the human fallopian tube during the menstrual cycle and in ectopic pregnancy. *Fertil Steril.* 94(3):833-40.

Alpay Z, Saed GM, Diamond MP. 2006. Female infertility and free radicals: potential role in adhesions and endometriosis. *J Soc Gynecol Investig* 13:390-8

Althaus CL, Heijne JC, Roellin A, Low N. 2010. Transmission dynamics of Chlamydia trachomatis affect the impact of screening programmes. *Epidemics* 2:123-31

Anderson M, Suh JM, Kim EY, Dryer SE. 2011. Functional NMDA receptors with atypical properties are expressed in podocytes. *Am J Physiol Cell Physiol* 300:C22-32

Andrews WW, Goldenberg RL, Hauth JC, Cliver SP, Conner M, Goepfert AR. 2005. Endometrial microbial colonization and plasma cell endometritis after spontaneous or indicated preterm versus term delivery. *Am J Obstet Gynecol* 193:739-45

Bakken IJ. 2008. Chlamydia trachomatis and ectopic pregnancy: recent epidemiological findings. *Curr Opin Infect Dis* 21:77-82

Bakken IJ, Ghaderi S. 2009. Incidence of pelvic inflammatory disease in a large cohort of women tested for Chlamydia trachomatis: a historical follow-up study. *BMC Infect Dis* 9:130

Bakken IJ, Skjeldestad FE, Lydersen S, Nordbo SA. 2007. Births and ectopic pregnancies in a large cohort of women tested for Chlamydia trachomatis. *Sex Transm Dis* 34:739-43

Barker CJ, Beagley KW, Hafner LM, Timms P. 2008. In silico identification and in vivo analysis of a novel T-cell antigen from Chlamydia, NrdB. *Vaccine* 26:1285-96

Barlow RE, Cooke ID, Odukoya O, Heatley MK, Jenkins J, Narayansingh G, Ramsewak SS, A. E. 2001. The prevalence of Chlamydia trachomatis in fresh tissue specimens from patients with ectopic pregnancy or tubal factor infertility as determined by PCR and in-situ hybridisation. *J Med Microbiol.* 50(10)::902-8

Barron A. L., Pasley, J. N., Rank, R. G., White H. J. and Mrak R.E. (1988) Chlamydial salpingitis in female guinea pigs receiving oral contraceptives *Sex Transm Dis* 15 (3): 169-73.

Bebear C, de Barbeyrac B. 2009. Genital Chlamydia trachomatis infections. *Clin Microbiol Infect* 15:4-10

Biagi E, Vitali B, Pugliese C, Candela M, Donders GG, Brigidi P. 2009. Quantitative variations in the vaginal bacterial population associated with asymptomatic infections: a real-time polymerase chain reaction study. *Eur J Clin Microbiol Infect Dis* 28:281-5

Bjartling C, Osser S, Persson K. 2007. Deoxyribonucleic acid of Chlamydia trachomatis in fresh tissue from the Fallopian tubes of patients with ectopic pregnancy. *Eur J Obstet Gynecol Reprod Biol* 134:95-100

Blandau RJ, Boling JL, Halbert S, Verdugo P. 1975. Methods for studying oviductal physiology. *Gynecol Invest* 6:123-45

Blazar AS, Hogan JW, Seifer DB, Frishman GN, Wheeler CA, Haning RV. 1997. The impact of hydrosalpinx on successful pregnancy in tubal factor infertility treated by in vitro fertilization. *Fertil Steril* 67:517-20

Bouyer J, Coste J, Fernandez H, Pouly JL, Job-Spira N. 2002. Sites of ectopic pregnancy: a 10 year population-based study of 1800 cases. *Hum Reprod* 17:3224-30

Brunham RC, Peeling R, Maclean I, Kosseim ML, M. P. 1992. Chlamydia trachomatis-associated ectopic pregnancy: serologic and histologic correlates. *J Infect Dis.* 165(6):1076-81

Brunham R.C and Peeling, R.W(1994) *Chlamydia trachomatis* antigens: role in immunity and pathogenesis *Infectious Agents & Disease* 3 (5): 218-33

Casari E, Ferrario A, Morenghi E, Montanelli A. 2010. Gardnerella, Trichomonas vaginalis, Candida, Chlamydia trachomatis, Mycoplasma hominis and Ureaplasma urealyticum in the genital discharge of symptomatic fertile and asymptomatic infertile women. *New Microbiol* 33:69-76

Catlin BW. 1992. Gardnerella vaginalis: characteristics, clinical considerations, and controversies. *Clin Microbiol Rev* 5:213-37

Chang HJ, Suh CS. 2010. Ectopic pregnancy after assisted reproductive technology: what are the risk factors? *Curr Opin Obstet Gynecol* 22:202-7

Chen MJ, Yang JH, Yang YS, Ho HN. 2004. Increased occurrence of tubo-ovarian abscesses in women with stage III and IV endometriosis. *Fertil Steril* 82:498-9

Cherpes TL, Wiesenfeld HC, Melan MA, Kant JA, Cosentino LA, Meyn LA, Hillier SL. 2006. The associations between pelvic inflammatory disease, Trichomonas vaginalis infection, and positive herpes simplex virus type 2 serology. *Sex Transm Dis* 33:747-52

Chow JM, Yonekura ML, Richwald GA, Greenland S, Sweet RL, Schachter J. 1990. The association between Chlamydia trachomatis and ectopic pregnancy. A matched-pair, case-control study [see comments]. *JAMA* 263:3164-7

Cicinelli E, De Ziegler D, Nicoletti R, Colafiglio G, Saliani N, Resta L, Rizzi D, De Vito D. 2008. Chronic endometritis: correlation among hysteroscopic, histologic, and bacteriologic findings in a prospective trial with 2190 consecutive office hysteroscopies. *Fertil Steril* 89:677-84

Cicinelli E, De Ziegler D, Nicoletti R, Tinelli R, Saliani N, Resta L, Bellavia M, De Vito D. 2009. Poor reliability of vaginal and endocervical cultures for evaluating microbiology of endometrial cavity in women with chronic endometritis. *Gynecol Obstet Invest* 68:108-15

Claman P, Honey L, Peeling RW, Jessamine P, Toye B. 1997. The presence of serum antibody to the chlamydial heat shock protein (CHSP60) as a diagnostic test for tubal factor infertility. *Fertility & Sterility* 67:501-4

Cochrane M, Armitage CW, O'Meara CP, Beagley KW. 2010. Towards a Chlamydia trachomatis vaccine: how close are we? *Future Microbiol* 5:1833-56

Cohen C, Mugo, N., Astete, S., Odondo, R., Manhart, L., Kiehlbauch, J., Stamm, W., Waiyaki, P., Totten, P. 2005. Detection of Mycoplasma genitalium in women with laparoscopically diagnosed acute salpingitis. *Sex. Transm. Infect* 81:463-6

Critoph FN, Dennis KJ. 1977. Ciliary activity in the human oviduct. *Obstet Gynecol Surv* 32:602-3

Croxatto HB, Diaz S, Fuentealba B, Croxatto HD, Carrillo D, Fabres C. 1972. Studies on the duration of egg transport in the human oviduct. I. The time interval between ovulation and egg recovery from the uterus in normal women. *Fertil Steril* 23:447-58

Croxatto HB, Ortiz ME, Diaz S, Hess R, Balmaceda J, Croxatto HD. 1978. Studies on the duration of egg transport by the human oviduct. II. Ovum location at various intervals following luteinizing hormone peak. *Am J Obstet Gynecol* 132:629-34

Cruz-Fisher MI, Cheng C, Sun G, Pal S, Teng A, Molina DM, Kayala MA, Vigil A, Baldi P, Felgner PL, Liang X, LM. dlM. 2011. Identification of immunodominant antigens by probing a whole Chlamydia trachomatis open reading frame proteome microarray using sera from immunized mice. *Infect Immun.* 79(1): 246-57

Cunningham KA, Carey AJ, Hafner L, Timms P, Beagley KW. 2011. Chlamydia muridarum major outer membrane protein-specific antibodies inhibit in vitro infection but enhance pathology in vivo. *Am J Reprod Immunol* 65:118-26

Darville, T. J. M. O'Neill, J.M., Andrews, Jr., C.W., Nagarajan, U.M., Stahl, L., and Ojcius, D.M. (2003) Toll-like receptor-2, but not Toll-like receptor-4, is essential for development of oviduct pathology in chlamydial genital tract infection *J Immunol.* 171(11): 6187-97

Dean D, and Powers, V. 2001. Persistent *Chlamydia trachomatis* infections resist apoptotic stimuli. *Infect Immun* 69:2442-7

den Hartog JE, Lardenoije CM, Severens JL, Land JA, Evers JL, Kessels AG. 2008. Screening strategies for tubal factor subfertility. *Hum Reprod* 23:1840-8

den Hartog JE, Ouburg S, Land JA, Lyons JM, Ito JI, Pena AS, Morre SA. 2006. Do host genetic traits in the bacterial sensing system play a role in the development of Chlamydia trachomatis-associated tubal pathology in subfertile women? *BMC Infect Dis* 6:122

Derbigny WA, Hong SC, Kerr MS, Temkit M, Johnson RM. 2007. Chlamydia muridarum infection elicits a beta interferon response in murine oviduct epithelial cells dependent on interferon regulatory factor 3 and TRIF. *Infect Immun* 75:1280-90

Diaz S, Ortiz ME, Croxatto HB. 1980. Studies on the duration of ovum transport by the human oviduct. III. Time interval between the luteinizing hormone peak and recovery of ova by transcervical flushing of the uterus in normal women. *Am J Obstet Gynecol* 137:116-21

Dietrich W, Rath M, Stanek G, Apfalter P, Huber JC, Tempfer C. 2010. Multiple site sampling does not increase the sensitivity of Chlamydia trachomatis detection in infertility patients. *Fertil Steril* 93:68-71

Dixon RE, Ramsey KH, Schripsema JH, Sanders KM, SM. W. 2010. Time-dependent disruption of oviduct pacemaker cells by Chlamydia infection in mice. *Biol Reprod.* 83(2)::244-53.

Draper DL, Donegan EA, James JF, Sweet RL, Brooks GF. 1980. Scanning electron microscopy of attachment of Neisseria gonorrhoeae colony phenotypes to surfaces of human genital epithelia. *Am J Obstet Gynecol* 138:818-26

Dubuisson JB, Aubriot FX, Mathieu L, Foulot H, Mandelbrot L, de Joliere JB. 1991. Risk factors for ectopic pregnancy in 556 pregnancies after in vitro fertilization: implications for preventive management. *Fertil Steril* 56:686-90

Dutta, R.,Jha, R.,Salhan S. and Mittal, A.(2008). *Chlamydia trachomatis*-specific heat shock proteins 60 antibodies can serve as prognostic marker in secondary infertile women. *Infection,* 36(4): 374-8

Eko FO, Ekong E, He Q, Black CM, Igietseme JU. 2011. Induction of immune memory by a multisubunit chlamydial vaccine. *Vaccine* 29:1472-80

El-Shawarby S, Margara R, Trew G, Lavery S. 2004. A review of complications following transvaginal oocyte retrieval for in-vitro fertilization. *Hum Fertil (Camb)* 7:127-33

Eschenbach DA, Buchanan TM, Pollock HM, Forsyth PS, Alexander ER, Lin JS, Wang SP, Wentworth BB, MacCormack WM, Holmes KK. 1975. Polymicrobial etiology of acute pelvic inflammatory disease. *N Engl J Med* 293:166-71

Farooki MA. 1967. Epidemiology and pathology of chronic endometritis. *Int Surg* 48:566-73

Farris CM, Morrison RP. 2011. Vaccination against Chlamydia genital infection utilizing the murine C. muridarum model. *Infect Immun* 79:986-96

Feghali J, Bakar J, Mayenga JM, Segard L, Hamou J, Driguez P, Belaisch-Allart J. 2003. [Systematic hysteroscopy prior to in vitro fertilization]. *Gynecol Obstet Fertil* 31:127-31

Fontaine EA, Bryant TN, Taylor-Robinson D, Borriello SP, Davies HA. 1986. A numerical taxonomic study of anaerobic gram-negative bacilli classified as *Bacteroides ureolyticus* isolated from patients with non-gonococcal urethritis. *J Gen Microbiol* 132:3137-46

Franks AL, Beral V, Cates W, Jr., Hogue CJ. 1990. Contraception and ectopic pregnancy risk. *Am J Obstet Gynecol* 163:1120-3

Friberg J, Confino E, Suarez M, Gleicher N. 1987. Chlamydia trachomatis attached to spermatozoa recovered from the peritoneal cavity of patients with salpingitis. *J Reprod Med* 32:120-2

Gaudoin M, Rekha P, Morris A, Lynch J, Acharya U. 1999. Bacterial vaginosis and past chlamydial infection are strongly and independently associated with tubal infertility but do not affect in vitro fertilization success rates. *Fertil Steril* 72:730-2

Gerard HC, Kohler L, Branigan PJ, Zeidler H, Schumacher HR, Hudson AP. 1998. Viability and gene expression in Chlamydia trachomatis during persistent infection of cultured human monocytes. *Med Microbiol Immunol* 187:115-20

Gottlieb SL, Berman SM, Low N. 2010. Screening and treatment to prevent sequelae in women with Chlamydia trachomatis genital infection: how much do we know? *J Infect Dis* 201 Suppl 2:S156-67

Hafner L, Beagley K, Timms P. 2008. Chlamydia trachomatis infection: host immune responses and potential vaccines. *Mucosal Immunol* 1:116-30

Hafner LM. 2007. Reducing the risk of Chlamydia trachomatis transmission: male circumcision or a female vaccine? *Future Microbiol* 2:219-22

Hafner LM, McNeilly C. 2008. Vaccines for Chlamydia infections of the female genital tract. *Future Micro.*3:67-77

Halis G, Arici A. 2004. Endometriosis and inflammation in infertility. *Ann N Y Acad Sci* 1034:300-15

Harada T, Iwabe T, Terakawa N. 2001. Role of cytokines in endometriosis. *Fertil Steril* 76:1-10

Hay PE, Taylor-Robinson D, Lamont RF. 1992. Diagnosis of bacterial vaginosis in a gynaecology clinic. *Br J Obstet Gynaecol* 99:63-6

Heinonen PK, Miettinen A. 1994. Laparoscopic study on the microbiology and severity of acute pelvic inflammatory disease. *European Journal of Obstetrics & Gynecology and Reproductive Biology* 57:85-9

Henry-Suchet J, Catalan F, Loffredo V, Serfaty D, Siboulet A, Perol Y, Sanson MJ, Debache C, Pigeau F, Coppin R, de Brux J, Poynard T. 1980. Microbiology of specimens obtained by laparoscopy from controls and from patients with pelvic inflammatory disease or infertility with tubal obstruction: Chlamydia trachomatis and Ureaplasma urealyticum. *Am J Obstet Gynecol* 138:1022-5

Hickey DK, Aldwell FE, Beagley KW. 2010. Oral immunization with a novel lipid-based adjuvant protects against genital Chlamydia infection. *Vaccine* 28:1668-72

Hickey DK, Aldwell FE, Tan ZY, Bao S, Beagley KW. 2009. Transcutaneous immunization with novel lipid-based adjuvants induces protection against gastric Helicobacter pylori infection. *Vaccine*

Hillier SL. 1993. Diagnostic microbiology of bacterial vaginosis. *Am J Obstet Gynecol* 169:455-9

Hillier SL, Kiviat NB, Hawes SE, Hasselquist MB, Hanssen PW, Eschenbach DA, Holmes KK. 1996. Role of bacterial vaginosis-associated microorganisms in endometritis. *Am J Obstet Gynecol* 175:435-41

Hirano T, Hoshino Y. 2010. Sperm dimorphism in terms of nuclear shape and microtubule accumulation in Cyrtanthus mackenii. *Sex Plant Reprod* 23:153-62

Hocking JS, Parker RM, Pavlin N, Fairley CK, Gunn JM. 2008. What needs to change to increase chlamydia screening in general practice in Australia? The views of general practitioners. *BMC Public Health* 8:425

Holmes KK, Eschenbach DA, Knapp JS. 1980. Salpingitis: overview of etiology and epidemiology. *Am J Obstet Gynecol* 138:893-900

Holmes KK, Sparling, P. F., Mardh, P., Lemon, S. T., Stamm, S. E., Piot, P., Wasserheit, J. N, ed. 2008. *Sexually Transmitted Diseases*. New York: McGraw-Hill

Horne AW, Duncan WC, King AE, Burgess S, Lourenco PC, Cornes P, Ghazal P, Williams AR, Udby L, Critchley HO. 2009. Endometrial cysteine-rich secretory protein 3 is inhibited by human chorionic gonadotrophin, and is increased in the decidua of tubal ectopic pregnancy. *Mol Hum Reprod* 15:287-94

Horne AW, Stock SJ, King AE. 2008. Innate immunity and disorders of the female reproductive tract. *Reproduction* 135:739-49

Hvid,A., Baczynska,A., Deleuran,B. Fedder,J., Knudsen, H.J., Christiansen, G and Birkelund, S., (2007) Interleukin-1 is the initiator of Fallopian tube destruction during *Chlamydia trachomatis* infection *Cell Microbiol* 9(12):2795-803

Jacobsson B, Pernevi P, Chidekel L, Jorgen Platz-Christensen J. 2002. Bacterial vaginosis in early pregnancy may predispose for preterm birth and postpartum endometritis. *Acta Obstet Gynecol Scand* 81:1006-10

James-Holmquest AN, Swanson J, Buchanan TM, Wende RD, Williams RP. 1974. Differential attachment by piliated and nonpiliated Neisseria gonorrhoeae to human sperm. *Infect Immun* 9:897-902

Jha, R., Vardhan, H., Bas, S., Salhan, S. and Mittal, A.(2009) Cervical epithelial cells from *Chlamydia trachomatis*-infected sites coexpress higher levels of chlamydial heat shock proteins 60 and 10 in infertile women than in fertile women *Gynecol Obstet Invest.*, 68 (3): 160-6

Jurstrand M, Jensen JS, Magnuson A, Kamwendo F, Fredlund H. 2007. A serological study of the role of Mycoplasma genitalium in pelvic inflammatory disease and ectopic pregnancy. *Sex TransInfect* 83:319-23

Kalwij S, Macintosh M, Baraitser P. 2010. Screening and treatment of Chlamydia trachomatis infections. *BMJ* 340:c1915

Kamwendo F, Forslin L, Bodin L, Danielsson D. 1996. Decreasing incidences of gonorrhea- and chlamydia-associated acute pelvic inflammatory disease. A 25-year study from an urban area of central Sweden. *Sex Transm Dis* 23:384-91

Kanakas N, Mantzavinos T, Boufidou F, Koumentakou I, Creatsas G. 1999. Ureaplasma urealyticum in semen: is there any effect on in vitro fertilization outcome? *Fertility and Sterility* 71:523-7

Kavoussi SK, Mueller MD, Lebovic DI. 2006. Expression of mannose-binding lectin in the peritoneal fluid of women with and without endometriosis. *Fertil Steril* 85:1526-8

Khan KN, Kitajima M, Hiraki K, Yamaguchi N, Katamine S, Matsuyama T, Nakashima M, Fujishita A, Ishimaru T, Masuzaki H. 2010. Escherichia coli contamination of menstrual blood and effect of bacterial endotoxin on endometriosis. *Fertil Steril* 94:2860-3 e1-3

King JA, Olsen TG, Lim R, Nycum LR. 2002. Pseudomonas aeruginosa-infected IUD associated with pelvic inflammatory disease. A case report. *J Reprod Med* 47:1035-7

Kiviat NB, Wolner-Hanssen P, Eschenbach DA, Wasserheit JN, Paavonen JA, Bell TA, Critchlow CW, Stamm WE, Moore DE, Holmes KK. 1990. Endometrial histopathology in patients with culture-proved upper genital tract infection and laparoscopically diagnosed acute salpingitis. *Am J Surg Pathol* 14:167-75

Kodati VL, Govindan S, Movva S, Ponnala S, Hasan Q. 2008. Role of Shigella infection in endometriosis: a novel hypothesis. *Med Hypotheses* 70:239-43

Kubota T, Ishi K, Takeuchi H. 1997. A study of tubo-ovarian and ovarian abscesses, with a focus on cases with endometrioma. *J Obstet Gynaecol Res* 23:421-6

Kulp JL, Barnhart KT. 2008. Ectopic pregnancy: diagnosis and management. *Womens Health (Lond Engl)* 4:79-87

Land WH, Jr., Margolis D, Gottlieb R, Yang JY, Krupinski EA. 2010. Improving CT prediction of treatment response in patients with metastatic colorectal carcinoma using statistical learning. *Int J Comput Biol Drug Des* 3:15-8

Landers DV, Sweet RL. 1983. Tubo-ovarian abscess: contemporary approach to management. *Rev Inf Dis* 5:876-84

Lara-Torre E, Pinkerton JS. 2002. Viable intrauterine pregnancy with acute salpingitis progressing to septic abortion. A case report. *J Reprod Med* 47:959-61

Laufer N, Sekeles E, Cohen R, Dreizin E, Schenker JG. 1980. The effects of E. coli endotoxin on the tubal mucosa of the rabbit. A scanning electron microscopic study. *Pathol Res Pract* 170:202-10

Laufer N, Simon A, Schenker JG, Sekeles E, Cohen R. 1984. Fallopian tubal mucosal damage induced experimentally by Escherichia coli in the rabbit. A scanning electron microscopic study. *Pathol Res Pract* 178:605-10

Lebovic DI, Mueller MD, Taylor RN. 2001. Immunobiology of endometriosis. *Fertil Steril* 75:1-10

Ledger WL, Sweeting VM, Chatterjee S. 1994. Rapid diagnosis of early ectopic pregnancy in an emergency gynaecology service--are measurements of progesterone, intact and free beta human chorionic gonadotrophin helpful? *Hum Reprod* 9:157-60

Lehner R, Kucera E, Jirecek S, Egarter C, Husslein P. 2000. Ectopic pregnancy. *Arch Gynecol Obstet* 263:87-92

Li W, Murthy AK, Guentzel MN, Chambers JP, Forsthuber TG, Seshu J, Zhong G, BP. A. 2010. Immunization with a combination of integral chlamydial antigens and a defined secreted protein induces robust immunity against genital chlamydial challenge. *Infect Immun* 78(9)::3942-9

Lin JN, Lin HL, Huang CK, Lai CH, Chung HC, Liang SH, Lin HH. 2010. Endometriosis presenting as bloody ascites and shock. *J Emerg Med* 38:30-2

Lindblom B, Andersson A. 1985. Influence of cyclooxygenase inhibitors and arachidonic acid on contractile activity of the human Fallopian tube. *Biol Reprod* 32:475-9

Linhares, I.M.and Witkin, S. S.(2010) Immunopathogenic consequences of *Chlamydia trachomatis* 60 kDa heat shock protein expression in the female reproductive tract. *Cell Stress Chaperones,*15 (5): 467-73

Low N, Bender N, Nartey L, Shang A, Stephenson JM. 2009. Effectiveness of chlamydia screening: systematic review. *Int J Epidemiol* 38:435-48

Low N, Egger M, Sterne JA, Harbord JM, Ibrahim F, Lindblom B. 2006. Incidence of severe reproductive tract complications associated with diagnosed genital chlamydial infection:the Uppsala Women's Cohort Study. *Sex.Trans.Infect.* 82:212-8

Low N, Hocking JS. 2010. The POPI trial: what does it mean for chlamydia control now? *Sex. Transm. Infect.* 86:158-9

Lucisano A, Morandotti G, Marana R, Leone F, Branca G, Dell'Acqua S, Sanna A. 1992. Chlamydial genital infections and laparoscopic findings in infertile women. *Eur J Epidemiol* 8:645-9

Lyons RA, Saridogan E, Djahanbakhch O. 2006. The reproductive significance of human Fallopian tube cilia. *Hum Reprod Update* 12:363-72

Mardh P, Baldetorp, B., Hakansson, C., Fritz, H., Westrom, L. 1979. Studies of ciliated epithelia of the human genital tract. 3. Mucociliary wave activity in organ cultures of human fallopian tubes challenged with Neisseria gonorrhoeae and gonococcal endotoxin. *Br. J Vener. Dis.* 55:256-64

Mardh PA, Westrom L. 1970. Tubal and cervical cultures in acute salpingitis with special reference to Mycoplasma hominis and T-strain mycoplasmas. *Br J Vener Dis* 46:179-86

Mardh, P.A (2004) Tubal factor infertility, with special regard to chlamydial salpingitis. *Curr Opin Infect.Dis.* 17: 49-52

McGee Z, Johnson, A., Taylor-Robinson, D. 1981. Pathogenic mechanisms of Neisseria gonorrhoeae: observations on damage to human fallopian tubes in organ culture by gonococci of colony type 1 or type 4. *J Infect. Dis* 143:413-22

McNeilly CL, Beagley KW, Moore RJ, Haring V, Timms P, Hafner LM. 2007. Expression library immunization confers partial protection against Chlamydia muridarum genital infection. *Vaccine* 25:2643-55

Mei B., Luo, Q.,Du, K.,Huo, Z., Wang, F. and Yu, P.(2009) Association of MICA gene polymorphisms with *Chlamydia trachomatis* infection and related tubal pathology in infertile women *Hum Reprod.*, 24(12): 3090-5

Menard JP, Fenollar F, Henry M, Bretelle F, Raoult D. 2008. Molecular quantification of Gardnerella vaginalis and Atopobium vaginae loads to predict bacterial vaginosis. *Clin Infect Dis* 47:33-43

Meoni E, Faenzi E, Frigimelica E, Zedda L, Skibinski D, Giovinazzi S, Bonci A, Petracca R, Bartolini E, Galli G, Agnusdei M, Nardelli F, Buricchi F, Norais N, Ferlenghi I, Donati M, Cevenini R, Finco O, Grandi G, R. G. 2009. CT043, a protective antigen that induces a CD4+ Th1 response during Chlamydia trachomatis infection in mice and humans. *Infect Immun.* 77(9):. :4168-76

Merki-Feld, G.S., Gosewinkel, A., Imthurn, B., Leeners, B.,(2007) Tubal pathology: the role of hormonal contraception, intrauterine device use and *Chlamydia trachomatis* infection. *Gynecol.Obstet.Invest.*63: 114-120.

Miller HG, Cain VS, Rogers SM, Gribble JN, Turner CF. 1999. Correlates of sexually transmitted bacterial infections among U.S. women in 1995. *Fam Plann Perspect* 31:4-9, 23

Miyairi I, Ramsey KH, Patton DL. 2010. Duration of untreated chlamydial genital infection and factors associated with clearance: review of animal studies. *J Infect Dis* 201 Suppl 2:S96-103

Mol F, van den Boogaard E, van Mello NM, van der Veen F, Mol BW, Ankum WM, van Zonneveld P, Dijkman AB, Verhoeve HR, Mozes A, Goddijn M, Hajenius PJ. 2011. Guideline adherence in ectopic pregnancy management. *Hum Reprod* 26:307-15

Mol F, van Mello NM, Mol BW, van der Veen F, Ankum WM, Hajenius PJ. 2010. Ectopic pregnancy and pelvic inflammatory disease: a renewed epidemic? *Eur J Obstet Gynecol Reprod Biol* 151:163-7

Molina DM PS, Kayala MA, Teng A, Kim PJ, Baldi P, Felgner PL, Liang X, de la Maza LM. 2010. Identification of immunodominant antigens of *C. trachomatis* using proteome microarrays. *Vaccine.* 28(17):3014-24

Moller BR, Taylor-Robinson D, Furr PM, Toft B, Allen J. 1985. Serological evidence that chlamydiae and mycoplasmas are involved in infertility of women. *J Reprod Fertil* 73:237-40

Morikawa H, Okamura H, Takenaka A, Morimoto K, Nishimura T. 1980. Physiological study of the human mesotubarium ovarica. *Obstet Gynecol* 55:493-6

Morre SA, Van den Brule AJ, Rozendaal L, Boeke AJ, Voorhost FJ, De Blok S, Meijer CJ. 2002. The natural course of asymptomatic *Chlamydia trachomatis* infections: 45% clearance and no development of clinical PID after one-year follow-up. . *Int. J. STD AIDS* 13 12-8

Mowa CN, Iwanaga T. 2000. Developmental changes of the oestrogen receptor-alpha and -beta mRNAs in the female reproductive organ of the rat--an analysis by in situ hybridization. *J Endocrinol* 167:363-9

Murray TH. 1997. Money-back guarantees for IVF: an ethical critique. *J Law Med Ethics* 25:292-4, 31

Murthy AK, Li W, Guentzel MN, Zhong G, BP A. 2011. Vaccination with the defined chlamydial secreted protein CPAF induces robust protection against female infertility following repeated genital chlamydial challenge. *Vaccine* 29(14):2519-22

Murthy AK, Chaganty BK, Li W, Guentzel MN, Chambers JP, Seshu J, Zhong G, Arulanandam BP. 2009. A limited role for antibody in protective immunity induced by rCPAF and CpG vaccination against primary genital Chlamydia muridarum challenge. *FEMS Immunol Med Microbiol* 55:271-9

Ness , R.B., Soper, D.E., Richter, H.E., Randall, H., Peipert, J.F., Nelson, D.B., Schubeck, D., McNeely, S.G., Trout, W., Bass, D.C., Hutchison, K., Kip, K and Brunham, R.C. (2008) Chlamydia antibodies, Chlamydia heat shock protein and adverse sequelae after pelvic inflammatory disease: The PID Evaluation and Clinical Health (PEACH) study. *Sex. Trans. Dis.* 35(2): 129-135

Ness, R.B and Brooks-Nelson, D.B. (1999) Pelvic inflammatory disease. In: Goldman, M.B., Hatch, M., Ness, RB et al., Epidemiology of Women's Health, San Diego, CA: Academic Press, 1999

Noguchi Y, Yabushita H, Noguchi M, Fujita M, Asai M, CA. DC. 2002. Detection of Chlamydia trachomatis infection with DNA extracted from formalin-fixed paraffin-embedded tissues. *Diagn Microbiol Infect Dis.* 43(1)::1-6.

Oakeshott P, Kerry S, Aghaizu A, Atherton H, Hay S, Taylor-Robinson D, Simms I, Hay P. 2010. Randomised control trial of screening for Chlamydia trachomatis to prevent pelvic inflammatory disease: the POPI (prevention of pelvic infection) trail. *BMJ* 340

Ohman, H., Tiitnen, A., Haltunen, M., Lehtinen, M., Paavonen, J., and Surcel, H-M (2009) Cytokine polymorphisms and severity of tbal damage in women with Chlamydia-associated infertility. *JID* 199: 1353-9.

Olsen AW, Theisen M, Christensen D, Follmann F, P. A. 2010. Protection against Chlamydia promoted by a subunit vaccine (CTH1) compared with a primary intranasal infection in a mouse genital challenge model. *PLoS One* 5(5):e10768

Olsen AW, Follmann F, Jensen K, Hojrup P, Leah R, Sorensen H, Hoffmann S, Andersen P, Theisen M. 2006. Identification of CT521 as a frequent target of Th1 cells in patients with urogenital Chlamydia trachomatis infection. *J Infect Dis* 194:1258-66

Osborn BH, Haney AF, Misukonis MA, Weinberg JB. 2002. Inducible nitric oxide synthase expression by peritoneal macrophages in endometriosis-associated infertility. *Fertil Steril* 77:46-51

Osborne NG. 1986. Tubo-ovarian abscess: pathogenesis and management. *J Natl Med Assoc* 78:937-51

Paavonen, J and Eggert-Kruse, W (1999) Chlamydia trachomatis: impact on human reproduction. *Hum Reprod Update* 5 (5): 433-47.

Paltieli Y, Eibschitz I, Ziskind G, Ohel G, Silbermann M, Weichselbaum A. 2000. High progesterone levels and ciliary dysfunction--a possible cause of ectopic pregnancy. *J Assist Reprod Genet* 17:103-6

Patten RM, Vincent LM, Wolner-Hanssen P, Thorpe E, Jr. 1990. Pelvic inflammatory disease. Endovaginal sonography with laparoscopic correlation. *J Ultrasound Med* 9:681-9

Patton, D.L., Sweeney, Y.T. and Kuo, C.C. (1994) Oral contraceptives do not alter the course of experimentally induced chlamydial salpingitis in monkeys *Sex Transm Dis.*, 21 (2): 89-92.

Patton D.L., Askienazy-Elbhar, M., Henry-Suchet, J.,Campbell, L. A. Cappuccio, A., Tannous, W. Wang, S. P. and Kuo, C. C. (1994b) Detection of *Chlamydia trachomatis* in fallopian tube tissue in women with postinfectious tubal infertility *Am J Obstet Gynecol.*,171(1): 95-101.

Patton DL, Halbert SA, Kuo CC, Wang SP, Holmes KK. 1983. Host response to primary Chlamydia trachomatis infection of the fallopian tube in pig-tailed monkeys. *Fertil Steril* 40:829-40

Patton, D.L.,Kuo, C.C.,Wang, S.P., and Halbert, S.A.(1987) Distal tubal obstruction induced by repeated *Chlamydia trachomatis* salpingeal infections in pig-tailed macaques. *J Infect Dis*155(6):1292-9.

Phillips D. M., Swenson , C. E. and Schachter J.(1984) Ultrastructure of *Chlamydia trachomatis* infection of the mouse oviduct. *J Ultrastruct Res* 88 (3): 244-56

Pollow K, Inthraphuvasak J, Manz B, Grill HJ, Pollow B. 1981. A comparison of cytoplasmic and nuclear estradiol and progesterone receptors in human fallopian tube and endometrial tissue. *Fertil Steril* 36:615-22

Population Council 2003. *Reproductive Tract Infections: An introductory Overview.* http://www.popcouncil.org/pdfs/RTIFacsheetsRev.pdf

Rank, R.G. and Sanders, M.M.(1992) Pathogenesis of endometritis and salpingitis in a guinea pig model of chlamydial genital infection. *Am J Pathol* 140 (4): 927-36.

Rank RG, Whittum-Hudson JA. 2010. Protective immunity to chlamydial genital infection: evidence from animal studies. *J Infect Dis* 201 Suppl 2:S168-77

Refaat B, Al-Azemi M, Geary I, Eley A, W. L. 2009. Role of activins and inducible nitric oxide in the pathogenesis of ectopic pregnancy in patients with or without Chlamydia trachomatis infection. *Clin Vaccine Immunol.* 16(10):.1493-503

Refaat B, Al-Azemi M, Geary I, Eley A, Ledger W. 2009. Role of activins and inducible nitric oxide in the pathogenesis of ectopic pregnancy in patients with or without Chlamydia trachomatis infection. *Clin Vaccine Immunol* 16:1493-503

Risser WL, Risser JM. 2007. The incidence of pelvic inflammatory disease in untreated women infected with Chlamydia trachomatis: a structured review. *Int J STD AIDS* 18:727-31

Robertson JN, Ward ME, Conway D, Caul EO (1987) Chlamydial and gonococcal antibodies in sera of infertile women with tubal obstruction. *J Clin Pathol.* 40(4):377-83

Rogers, A. K., Wang, J., Zhang, Y. Holden, A.,Berryhill, B., Budrys, N. M. Schenken R. S. and Zhong, G. (2010) Association of tubal factor infertility with elevated antibodies to *Chlamydia trachomatis* caseinolytic protease P. *Am J Obstet Gynecol* 203 (5): 494 e7-494 e14

Saini S, Gupta N, Batra G, Arora DR. 2003. Role of anaerobes in acute pelvic inflammatory disease. *Indian J Med Microbiol* 21:189-92

Sanchez R, Villagran E, Concha M, Cornejo R. 1989. Ultrastructural analysis of the attachment sites of Escherichia coli to the human spermatozoon after in vitro migration through estrogenic cervical mucus. *Int J Fertil* 34:363-7

Shao R. 2010. Understanding the mechanisms of human tubal ectopic pregnancies: new evidence from knockout mouse models. *Hum Reprod* 25:584-7

Sharma S, Mittal S, Aggarwal P. 2009. Management of infertility in low resource countries. *BJOG* 116 Suppl 1:77-83

Shaw JL, Dey SK, Critchley HO, Horne AW. 2010. Current knowledge of the aetiology of human tubal ectopic pregnancy. *Hum Reprod Update* 16:432-44

Simms I, Horner P. 2008. Has the incidence of pelvic inflammatory disease following chlamydial infection been overestimated? *Int J STD AIDS* 19:285-6

Sioutas A, Ehren I, Lundberg JO, Wiklund NP, Gemzell-Danielsson K. 2008. Intrauterine nitric oxide in pelvic inflammatory disease. *Fertil Steril* 89:948-52

Sonnex C. 1998. Influence of ovarian hormones on urogenital infection. *Sex Transm Infect* 74:11-9

Soper DE. 1994. Pelvic inflammatory disease. *Infect Dis Clin North Am* 8:821-40

Soper DE. 2010. Pelvic inflammatory disease. *Obstet Gynecol* 116:419-28

Srivastava P, Gupta R, Jha HC, Jha R, Bhengraj AR, Salhan S, Mittal A. 2008. Serovar-specific immune responses to peptides of variable regions of Chlamydia trachomatis major outer membrane protein in serovar D-infected women. *Clin Exp Med* 8:207-15

Stagey C, Munday P, Taylor-Robinson D, Thomas B, Gilchrist C, Ruck F, Isdn C, Beard R. 1992. A longitudinal study of pelvic inflammatory disease BJOG: An International Journal of Obstetrics and Gynecology 99:994-9

Srivastava, P., Jha, ,R. Bas, S., Salhan, S. and Mittal, A. (2008) In infertile women, cells from *Chlamydia trachomatis* infected sites release higher levels of interferon-gamma, interleukin-10 and tumor necrosis factor-alpha upon heat-shock-protein stimulation than fertile women *Reprod Biol Endocrinol.*,6: 20

Suginami H, Yano K. 1988. An ovum capture inhibitor (OCI) in endometriosis peritoneal fluid: an OCI-related membrane responsible for fimbrial failure of ovum capture. *Fertil Steril* 50:648-53

Svenstrup HF, Fedder J, Kristoffersen SE, Trolle B, Birkelund S, Christiansen G. 2008. Mycoplasma genitalium, Chlamydia trachomatis, and tubal factor infertility--a prospective study. *Fertil Steril* 90:513-20

Swenson, C.E.,Donegan, E., and Schachter, J.(1983) *Chlamydia trachomatis*-induced salpingitis in mice. *J Infect Dis* 148 (6):1101-7

Swenson CE, Schachter J. 1984. Infertility as a consequence of chlamydial infection of the upper genital tract in female mice. *Sex Transm Dis* 11:64-7

Swenson RM, Michaelson TC, Daly MJ, Spalding EH. 1974. Clindamycin in infections of the female genital tract. *Obstet Gynecol* 44:699-702

Sziller I, Fedorcsák P, Csapó Z, Szirmai K, Linhares IM, Papp Z, Witkin SS.(2008). Circulating antibodies to a conserved epitope of the Chlamydia trachomatis 60-kDa heat shock protein is associated with decreased spontaneous fertility rate in ectopic pregnant women treated by salpingectomy. *Am J Reprod Immunol.* , 59 (2): 99-104

Taylor-Robinson AW, Borriello SP, Taylor-Robinson D. 1993. Identification and preliminary characterization of a cytotoxin isolated from Mobiluncus spp. *Int J Exp Pathol* 74:357-66

Taylor S, Frydman R. 1996. [Hysteroscopy and sperm infection]. *Contracept Fertil Sex* 24:549-51

Tibaldi C, Cappello N, Latino MA, Masuelli G, Marini S, Benedetto C. 2009. Vaginal and endocervical microorganisms in symptomatic and asymptomatic non-pregnant females: risk factors and rates of occurrence. *Clin Microbiol Infect* 15:670-9

Toth A, Lesser ML, Labriola D. 1984. The development of infections of the genitourinary tract in the wives of infertile males and the possible role of spermatozoa in the development of salpingitis. *Surg Gynecol Obstet* 159:565-9

van den Broek IV, Hoebe CJ, van Bergen JE, Brouwers EE, de Feijter EM, Fennema JS, Gotz HM, Koekenbier RH, van Ravesteijn SM, de Coul EL. 2010. Evaluation design of a systematic, selective, internet-based, Chlamydia screening implementation in the Netherlands, 2008-2010: implications of first results for the analysis. *BMC Infect Dis* 10:89

Van Voorhis W. C., Barrett, L. K., Sweeney, Y. T. , Kuo C. C. and Patton D. L.(1997) Repeated *Chlamydia trachomatis* infection of Macaca nemestrina fallopian tubes produces a Th1-like cytokine response associated with fibrosis and scarring *Infect Immun* 65 (6): 2175-82

Verteramo R, Pierangeli A, Mancini E, Calzolari E, Bucci M, Osborn J, Nicosia R, Chiarini F, Antonelli G, Degener AM. 2009. Human Papillomaviruses and genital co-infections in gynaecological outpatients. *BMC Infect Dis* 9:16

Wainer R, Camus E, Camier B, Martin C, Vasseur C, Merlet F. 1997. Does hydrosalpinx reduce the pregnancy rate after in vitro fertilization? *Fertil Steril* 68:1022-6

Wallace LA, Scoular A, Hart G, Reid M, Wilson P, Goldberg DJ. 2008. What is the excess risk of infertility in women after genital chlamydia infection? A systematic review of the evidence. *Sex Transm Infect* 84:171-5

Wang J, Chen L, Chen F, Zhang X, Zhang Y, Baseman J, Perdue S, Yeh IT, Shain R, Holland M, Bailey R, Mabey D, Yu P, G. Z. 2009. A chlamydial type III-secreted effector protein (Tarp) is predominantly recognized by antibodies from humans infected with Chlamydia trachomatis and induces protective immunity against upper genital tract pathologies in mice. *Vaccine.* 27(22):2967-80.

Wanggren K, Stavreus-Evers A, Olsson C, Andersson E, Gemzell-Danielsson K. 2008. Regulation of muscular contractions in the human Fallopian tube through prostaglandins and progestagens. *Hum Reprod* 23:2359-68

Westrom L. 1980. Incidence, prevalence, and trends of acute pelvic inflammatory disease and its consequences in industrialized countries. *Am J Obstet Gynecol* 138:880-92

Westrom L, Joesoef R, Reynolds G, Hagdu A, Thompson SE. 1992. Pelvic inflammatory disease and fertility. A cohort study of 1,844 women with laparoscopically verified disease and 657 control women with normal laparoscopic results. *Sex Transm Dis* 19:185-92

Wiesenfeld HC, Hillier SL, Krohn MA, Amortegui AJ, Heine RP, Landers DV, Sweet RL. 2002. Lower genital tract infection and endometritis: insight into subclinical pelvic inflammatory disease. *Obstet Gynecol* 100:456-63

Wiesenfeld HC, Sweet RL. 1993. Progress in the management of tuboovarian abscesses. *Clin Obstet Gynecol* 36:433-44

Wilson JD, Ralph SG, Rutherford AJ. 2002. Rates of bacterial vaginosis in women undergoing in vitro fertilisation for different types of infertility. *BJOG* 109:714-7

Wira CR, Fahey JV, Sentman CL, Pioli PA, Shen L. 2005. Innate and adaptive immunity in female genital tract: cellular responses and interactions. *Immunol Rev* 206:306-35

Witkin SS, Bierhals K, Linhares I, Normand N, Dieterle S, Neuer A. 2010. Genetic polymorphism in an inflammasome component, cervical mycoplasma detection and female infertility in women undergoing in vitro fertilization. *J Reprod Immunol* 84:171-5

Witkin SS, Linhares IM, Giraldo P. 2007a. Bacterial flora of the female genital tract: function and immune regulation. *Best Pract Res Clin Obstet Gynaecol* 21:347-54

Witkin SS, Linhares IM, Giraldo P, Ledger WJ. 2007b. An altered immunity hypothesis for the development of symptomatic bacterial vaginosis. *Clin Infect Dis* 44:554-7

Wolner-Hanssen P, Mardh PA. 1984. In vitro tests of the adherence of Chlamydia trachomatis to human spermatozoa. *Fertil Steril* 42:102-7

Woods ML, 2nd, McGee ZA. 1986. Molecular mechanisms of pathogenicity of gonococcal salpingitis. *Drugs* 31 Suppl 2:1-6

Xu W, Liu J, Gong W, Chen J, Zhu S, Zhang L. 2011. Protective immunity against Chlamydia trachomatis genital infection induced by a vaccine based on the major outer membrane multi-epitope human papillomavirus major capsid protein L1. *Vaccine* 29:2672-8

Yip L, Sweeny PJ, Bock BF. 1993. Acute suppurative salpingitis with concomitant intrauterine pregnancy. *Am J Emerg Med* 11:476-9

Yovich JL, McColm SC, Turner SR, Matson PL. 1985. Heterotopic pregnancy from in vitro fertilization. *J In Vitro Fert Embryo Transf* 2:143-50

Zegers-Hochschild F, Adamson GD, de Mouzon J, Ishihara O, Mansour R, Nygren K, Sullivan E, van der Poel S, on behalf of I, Who. 2009. The International Committee for Monitoring Assisted Reproductive Technology (ICMART) and the World Health Organization (WHO) Revised Glossary on ART Terminology, 2009. *Hum. Reprod.* 24:2683-7

3

Ectopic Pregnancy and Assisted Reproductive Technologies: A Systematic Review

Anastasia Velalopoulou et al.*
Laboratory of Physiology, Faculty of Medicine, University of Ioannina, Ioannina, Greece

1. Introduction

Ectopic pregnancy represents a rare pregnancy complication. In the last 20 years, with the use of IVF, heterotopic pregnancies have become more frequent, while this percentage differs between IVF programs. Many factors contribute to this, like the active management of hydrosalpinx or treatment of Chlamydia infection before starting a cycle. Although, *in vitro* fertilization is an expensive treatment, ectopic complication adds to this cost.

Not a lot of studies exist for ectopic pregnancy after IVF. Most of them are case reports. Not a standard way exists, for dealing with heterotopic pregnancies, even in the era of modern laparoscopy. Not a lot of research has been performed on molecules that involved. Studies have tried to associate certain techniques during IVF, with this entity, but with controversial results. There is no standard form for diagnosing, dealing and presenting heterotopic pregnancies. Most of them are diagnosed when ruptured. Because it is rare event, cost-effectiveness studies could not be performed and this complication is added to the overall IVF. Knowledge, on this field, is taken from the management of ectopic pregnancies in the general population, even if these present at a lower percentage.

The purpose of the study is to systematically evaluate studies on molecular aspects of ectopic pregnancy, the ART techniques that are associated with ectopic pregnancy, the diagnosis of this entity and finally present case reports of heterotopic pregnancies and their management. At the end, cost-effectiveness models from the general population will be presented in parallel with systematic examination of these studies. Finally, new research targets will be pointed.

---

* Dimitrios Peschos[1], Mynbaev Ospan[2], Eliseeva Marina[2], Ioannis Verginadis[1], Yannis Simos[1], Tsirkas Panagiotis[3], Spyridon Karkabounas[1], Vicky Kalfakakou[1], Angelos Evangelou[1] and Ioannis P. Kosmas[1,3]
[1]*Laboratory of Physiology, Faculty of Medicine, University of Ioannina, Ioannina, Greece*
[2]*Centre of Obstetrics, Gynaecology & Perinatology, Moscow State University of Medicine & Dentistry, Moscow, Russia*
[3]*Department of Obstetrics and Gynecology, Ioannina State General Hospital G Chatzikosta, Ioannina, Greece*

2. Methods

2.1 Identification and eligibility of relevant studies

Medline searches (up to March 2011) were performed using various combinations of terms: ectopic pregnancy, heterotopic pregnancy, *In Vitro* Fertilization, Intrauterine Insemination, pelvic inflammatory disease, Chlamydia trachomatis, heterotopic pregnancy, cervical pregnancy, cost-effectiveness.

The search was complemented with perusal of the bibliographies of retrieved papers and review articles. We included studies that evaluated the presence of an ectopic pregnancy after IVF in case reports, although in other chapters information was obtained from studies in the general population.

Number of tested samples was not an exclusion criterion. Only studies including human subjects were included.

2.2 Data extraction

For each study, information was obtained on authors, journal, year of publication, country and years of study enrollment, study design and study target, number of tested samples, tissue and disease tested, searched molecules and pathways involved, clinical outcome and whether biopsy was performed with the site.

Data extraction was performed independently by two investigators, and conflicts were resolved after discussion.

3. Main outcomes

3.1 Statistical methods

Frequencies of all important parameters were performed. Statistical analyses were performed in using the Statistical Package for Social Sciences (SPSS) version 12.0 (SPSS, Chicago, IL, USA).

3.2 Founding source

No sponsor was involved in the study design, report writing, or paper submission.

4. Results

4.1 Studies examining biological factors playing a role to ectopic pregnancy

A total of 42 abstracts were retrieved and further screened. Only studies that performed basic investigations were included in this part. Out of 20 included studies, 3 were performed in USA (15%), 2 in Germany (10%), Israel, Sweden and UK, and from one (5%) in Brazil, Canada, China, Croatia, Denmark, Finland, Hungary, India and Poland. 8 (40%) of them considered themselves clinical, 8 (40%) experimental, 1 (5%) prospective, 1 (5%) as pilot study, 1 (1%) as preliminary report, 1 (5%) as hypothesis testing. The type of study per country initiated can be seen in Fig 1.

All studies selected used human tissue. Five studies used fallopian tubes (25%). From the other studies 1 (5%) used fallopian tube and peripheral blood, 1 used deciduas, placenta, primary first trimester trophoblast cells and peripheral blood, 1 used decidual tissue, 2 endometrial tissue, 1 epithelial tissue and 1 mucosal tissue, 1 cervical specimen and

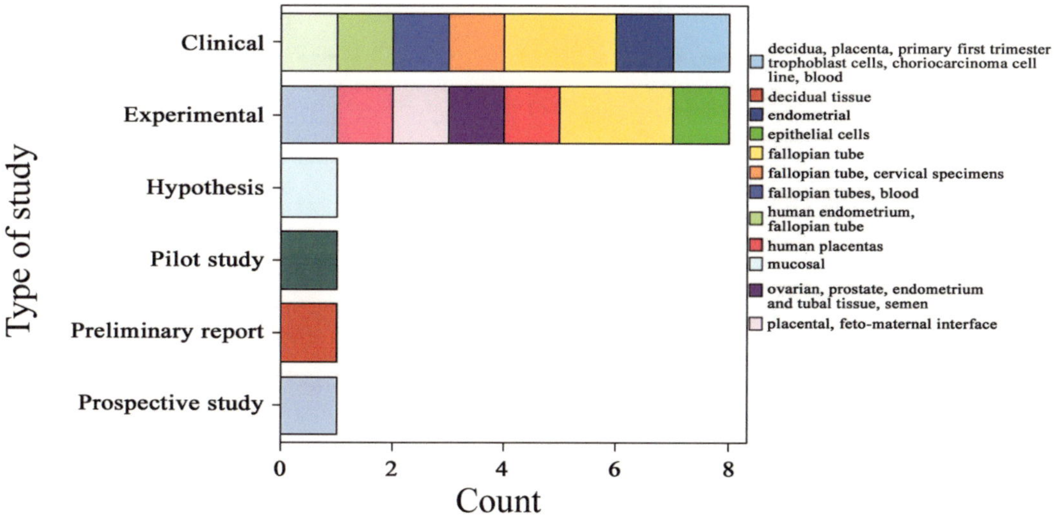

Fig. 2. Type of study per tissue used when examining biological factors in ectopic pregnancy

fallopian tube samples, 1 used human endometrium and fallopian tube, 2 used human placental tissue, 1 used ovarian, prostate, endometrial, tubal and semen, 1 used trophoblast, 2 used serum samples, 1 used transervical specimens and one used stimulated cervical mononuclear cell supernatants. The type of study per tissue used can be seen in Fig 2.

4 (20%) of the studies were published in American Journal of Reproductive Immunology, 2 (10%) in Human Reproduction and from 1 (5%) in Molecular Human Reproduction, Reproduction, Reproductive Biology & Endocrinology, Reproductive Sciences, Biology of Reproduction, Cellular Microbiology, Clinical and Vaccine Immunology, European Journal of Obstetrics & Gynecology, Histochemistry & Cellular Biology, Infection and Immunity, The Journal of Immunology, The Journal of Infectious Diseases ,The Journal of Clinical Endocrinology & Metabolism, The Medical Hypothesis journal. The distribution of type of study per Journal is seen in Fig 3. Eight studies (40%) did not mentioned their controls, four studies (20%) used normal pregnant patients and intrauterine pregnancy, and from one study (5%) used women with no infection and without infertility problem, normal desidual tissue, normal endometrium and normal Fallopian tube, normal pregnant patient peripheral blood, spontaneous abortion,, tissue from women undergoing tubal ligation with segmental resection and women with viable and non-viable intrauterine pregnancy.

Samples size examined ranged from 3 (in each group) to 144. Disease distribution examined presented as: ectopic pregnancy (8/40%), spontaneous abortion and ectopic pregnancy (2/10%), Chlamydia infection (2/10%), Chlamydia infection in patients with no infertility compared with women with Chlamydia and tubal damage, ectopic pregnancy and decidualized endometrium, ectopic pregnancy and blighted ovum, ectopic pregnancy and Chlamydia infection, pelvic inflammatory disease and ectopic pregnancy, post IVF ectopic pregnancy, viable ectopic pregnancy while 1 (5%) did not mentioned disease. Funding source of each study per Journal published is seen on Fig 4.

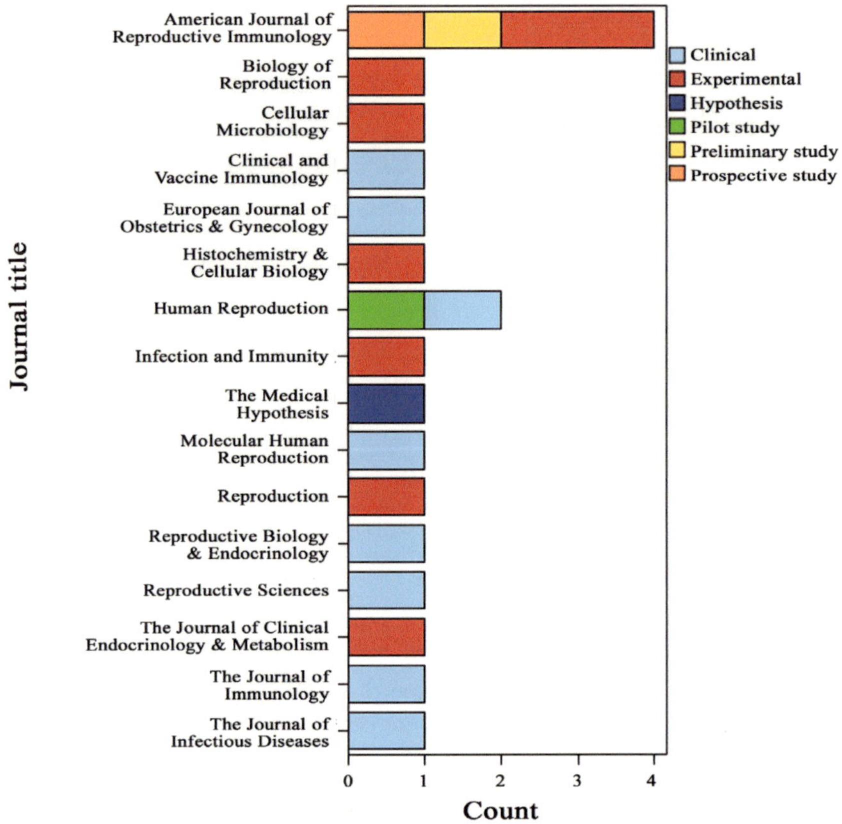

Fig. 3. The distribution of type of study per Journal when examining biological factors in ectopic pregnancy

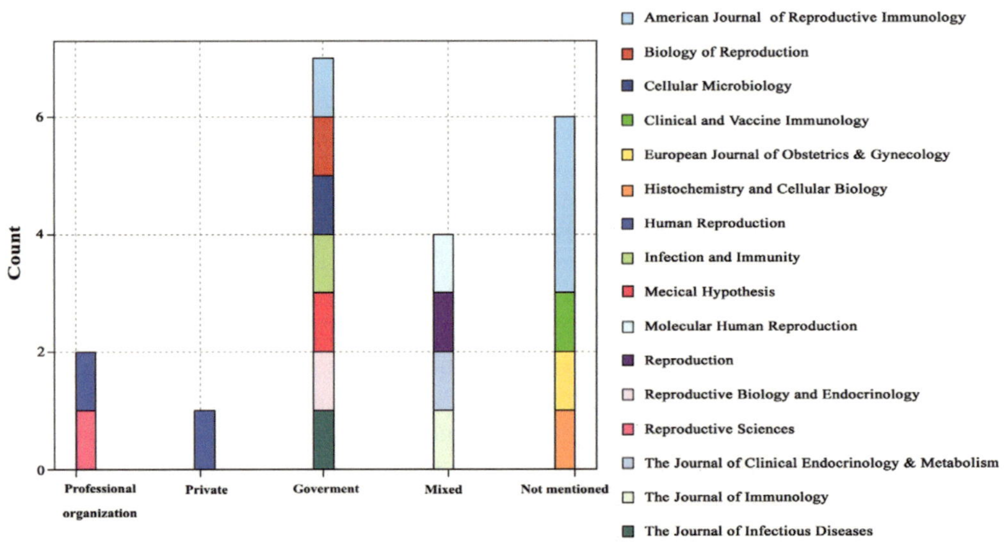

Fig. 4. Funding source of each study per Journal published

4.2 Outcomes

All studies except two (3/15%) mentioned the molecule studied. Two studies (10%) mentioned C Trachomatis DNA, one C Trachomatis serum antibodies, while from one study mentioned CD14B7H4,CHSP-60,E-Cadherin,estrogen receptor, IgG antibodies, IL-1, IL-8, Ki-67, MMP-2, PIGF, SLIT/ROBO proteins, Svcam-1, TAG-72, Treg. Ten studies (50%) did not mentioned a second molecule while the other studies mentioned CT antibodies (1/5%) chlamydial sarkosyl-soluble 57-kDa protein, cHSP 60, Cytokeratin 7, estrogen receptor, hCG, IL-1a, MMP-9, P38 and progesterone. 11 studies (55%) did not mentioned third outcome while the other ones mentioned Chsp 60 (2/10%), bhCG, cHSP 10 (1/5%), ERK, Fibronectin, FOXP 3, IL-10 and MMP-14. Thirteen studies (13/65%) did not mentioned a fourth outcome, while the other mentioned activin (1/5%) IFN-γ, Laminin, MAPK, neurophilin, p38 inhibitor and TIMP-1. Fifth molecule was mentioned in only 6 studies. Only four studies mentioned pathways involved: invasive pathway, p38 MAP-kinasses pathway, ERK-MAPK pathway and SLIT/ROBO pathway. Only two studies (2/5%) mentioned intervention medication.

In terms of bio-analytic techniques, PCR techniques and immunohistochemistry was mainly used. For immunohistochemistry techniques, four studies (20%) did not mentioned it, seven studies (7%) mentioned as immunohistochemistry, 23 (15%) as immunofluorence immunohistochemistry, and from one as electron microscopic immunohistochemistry, immunoblotting, immunoperoxidase staining (IP), immunosorbent assay, microimmuno-fluoresence, microimmunofluorence-immunoblot. For PCR techniques, eleven studies (55%) did not mentioned PCR technique, 4 (20%) studies mention it as quantitative PCR, 2 (10%) studies mention it as PCR, two (10%) as RT-PCR, and 1 (5%) as N-PCR.

When ectopic pregnancy exists, Arias-Stella reaction is observed in endometrium. At that time, B7H4 positive macrophages is significantly lower when compared with secretory endometrium (Wicherek et al., 2009)

Chlamydia trachomatis are highly associated with ectopic pregnancy (Brunham et al., 1992). Chlamydia trachomatis antigens, exist in asymptomatic, culture negative men and women with chronic infection and may act as immunostimulants and re-activate Chlamydia (Toth et al., 2000). After first episode of ectopic pregnancy, antibody response to conserved epitope of cHSP-60 (Chlamydia heat shock protein) is associated with increased probability of adverse pregnancy outcome (Sziller et al., 2007). So this biomarker could be used for counseling women with first episode of ectopic pregnancy: if sensitized to this epitope, *in vitro* fertilization should be offered. Another indication for the significance of this biomarker is that in infertile women, when Chlamydia infected tissue is exposed to Chlamydia heat shock proteins (cHSP-60 and cHSP-10) increased release of IFN-gamma, IL-10 and TNF-alpha (Srivastava et al., 2008) affect mucosal immune function. From the other side, Ct-IgG and c-hsp6 antigens, were not found as an independent predictor of ectopic pregnancy (Bjartling et al., 2006).

In the fallopian tube of serologically positive patients for Chlamydia trachomatis that had ectopic pregnancy, there is an increase in the expression of activin βA subunit, type II receptors, follistatin and iNOS (Refaat et al., 2009).

In infected tubes from Chlamydia trachomatis infection, interleukin -1 production from epithelial cells initiates tissue destruction. By blocking IL-1 with IL-1RA receptor antagonist and/or IL-10, tissue destruction is eliminated. Chlamydia infected cells, also, produce IL-8 by ERK MAPK pathway (Buchholz et al., 2007).

Regulators T cells (Treg) express LH/CG receptor on their surface during pregnancy and are present at the fetal-maternal interface, attracted by high levels of human chorionic gonadotrophin. In ectopic pregnancies, regulatory T cells are not attracted to the same degree by the lower levels of hCG (Schumacher et al., 2009).

Another possible biomarker for ectopic pregnancy after IVF is E-cadherin, because it is highly expressed in cytotrophoblast cells of chorionic villi from these pregnancies, when compared with spontaneous ectopic pregnancy (Revel et al., 2008).

From micro-array studies, Savaris et al, by using the model of ectopic pregnancy, found that the transcriptome of the decidua is influenced by trophoblast products, in endocrine fashion (Savaris et al., 2008).

In close proximity of the tubal implantation site, MUC-1 and TAG-72 are present in the epithelial cells and might contribute to the deeper trophoblast invasion in the tubal wall (von Rango et al., 2003) while a significant reduction in NK-cell numbers at the tubal implantation site, could be seen, induced by local antigen-presenting cells in the presence of mucins (Laskarin et al., 2010).

Viable tubal pregnancies implant at the mesosalpingeal side of the tubal wall show a massively increased invasion of extravillous trophoblast cells (EVT) into the tubal wall, and the proliferation of trophoblast cells extends deeply into the invasive zone in the invasive pathway (Kemp et al., 1999). Tubal pregnancies that will undergo tubal abortion implant at the antimesometrial side which show shallow invasion and poor trophoblast proliferation (Kemp et al., 1999). In extrauterine pregnancy, expression of integrin subunit α3 is nearly exclusively restricted to the basal plasmalemma of the first layer of trophoblast cells while only the first proximal layer of EVT (in direct contact to the basement membrane) expresses integrin α6. The switch to the integrin subunits αv and α5 takes place already in the second layer of trophoblast cells, as soon as the latter detach from the basement membrane (Kemp et al., 2002).

In tubal pregnancies, MMP-9 and TIMP-1, -2 and -3 are produced by all types of extravillous cytotrophoblast (EVCT) cells, while MMP-2 and -14 mainly exist in distal column cytotrophoblast (CCT) cells and invasive EVCT cells (Bai et al., 2005). In parallel, MMP-14 and TIMP-1 and -2 are increased along the invasive pathway toward maternal interstitium. MMP-2, -9 and -14 and TIMP-1, -2 and -3 were all detected in the villous CT (VCT) cells (Bai et al., 2005).

Another promising technique for early detection of an ectopic pregnancy is that trophoblast cells can be reliably obtained and identified among cervical cells in the first trimester and labeled with antibody to HLA-G. The number of trophoblast cells per total cervical cells (trophoblast frequency) is significant lower in ectopic pregnancy when compared to intrauterine pregnancy but not to blighted ovum (Imudia et al., 2009). Using ROC curves the positive predictive value for abnormal pregnancy was 97% and the negative predictive value was 87%. From intrauterine tissue and sera, Horne et al, examined PIGF, localized to the cytotrophoblast cells (Horne et al, 2010). Expression of PIGF mRNA was significantly reduced in trophoblast cells, isolated from women with ectopic pregnancy compared with intrauterine pregnancies. Serum PIGF was undetectable in women with tubal ectopic pregnancies and reduced, or undetectable, in miscarriage compared with viable intrauterine pregnancies.

From the other side, it seems that SLT/ROBO pathway and protein expression in endometrium and fallopian tube, is not implicated in ectopic pregnancy because known factors that contribute to EP (e.g. smoking/cotinine or chlamydial infection) do not alter

protein expression (Duncan et al., 2010). Also serum VCAM-1 was found comparable between the three pregnancy types, normal, ectopic and failed thus making this marker not useful for the diagnosis of ectopic pregnancy (Daniel et al., 2000).
Also a role for ectopic pregnancy formation might exist from ovulation induction regimens. Clomiphene citrate, which used for anovulatory infertility, may indirectly contribute to ectopic pregnancy creation. Chronic treatment with clomiphene activates estrogen receptors, particularly in cilia, and inducing tubal apoptosis of isthmus epithelial cells while slowing oocyte cumulus complex passage from the fallopian tube (Shao et al., 2009). This may contribute to ectopic pregnancy formation.

5. Section 2

5.1 Ectopic pregnancy and IVF

A total of 56 abstracts were retrieved and further screened. Out of 40 included studies, 10 (25%) were performed in USA, 3 (7.5%) in England, India and in Netherlands, 2 (5%) in France, Greece, Israel, Italy and Nepal, while 1 (2.5%) in Australia, Canada, Germany, Japan, Jordan, Korea, Norway, Singapore, Taiwan, Thailand and between USA/Sweden. 17 (42.5%) of them considered themselves retrospective, 11 (27.5%) as case report, and from 1 (2.56%) as cohort study, prospective randomized double blinded cross over study, prospective cohort study, population based cost-effectiveness study, epidemiological study, economical analysis, cost effectiveness analysis, cost benefit analysis, cost analysis, while 3 (7.5%) do not mentioned the type of study. The type of study per country initiated can be seen in Fig 5.

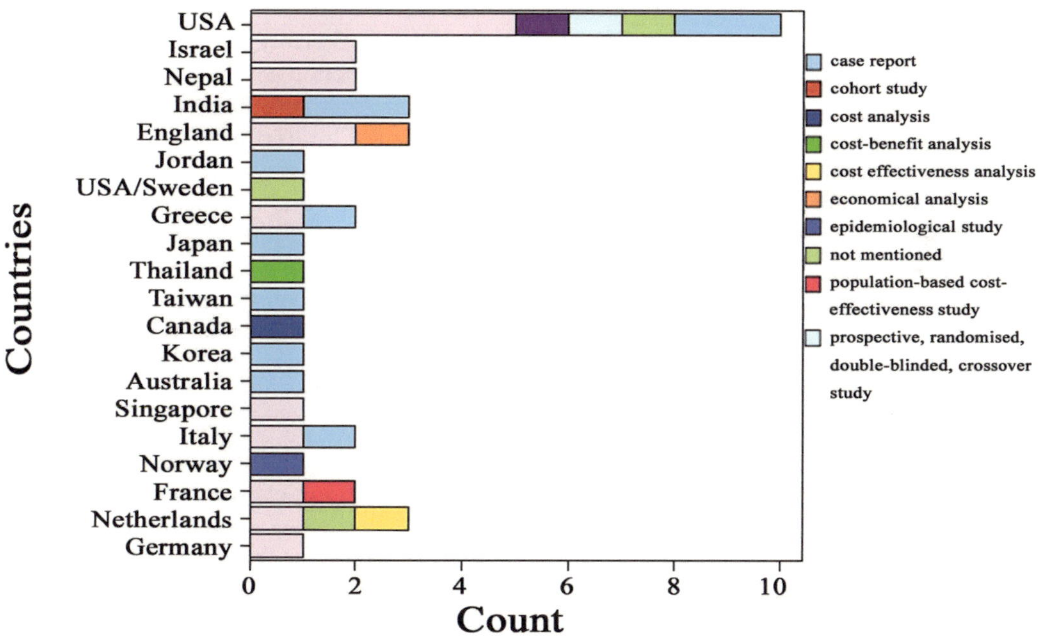

Fig. 5. The type of study per country initiated examining IVF and ectopic pregnancy

All studies selected used human tissue. Fourteen studies mentioned embryo (35%) as tissue examined plus 4 (10%) mentioned especially the blastocyst, 4(10%) used fallopian tube and from 1 (2.5%) used embryos with thickened zona pellucida, fallopian tube ectopic pregnancy and sperm with abnormal characteristics, hydrosalpinx, ovarian tissue and trophoblastic tissue, while one tested newborns for congenital abnormalities after failed emergency contraception while 12 (30%) did not specified the tissue examined. The type of study per tissue used can be seen in Fig 6.

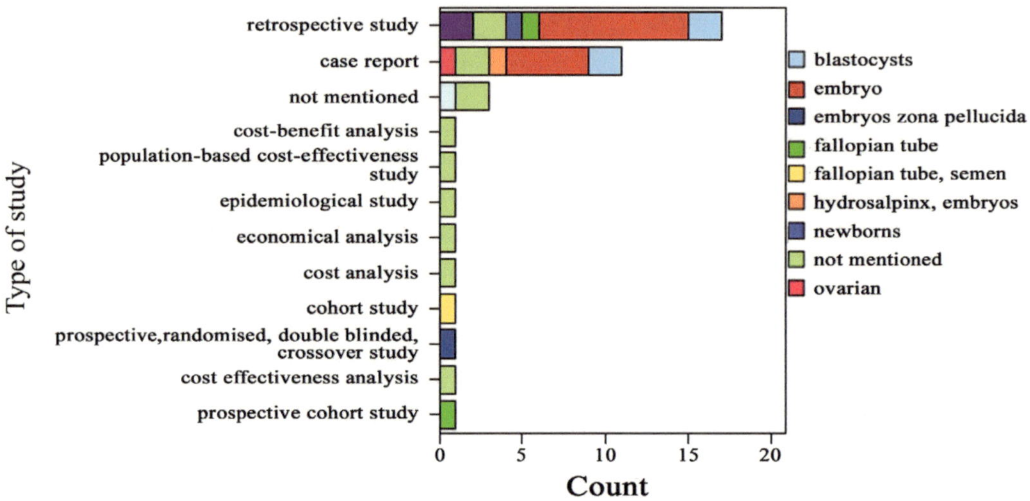

Fig. 6. The type of study per tissue used examining IVF and ectopic pregnancy

12 (30.0%) of the studies were published in Fertility & Sterility,5 (12.5%) in Human Reproduction, 5 (12.5%) in the Journal of Assisted Reproduction & Genetics, and from 1 (2.5%) in Acta Obstetricia et Gynecologica Scandinavica, American Journal of Emergency Medicine, Annals Academy of Medicine, BMC Pregnancy & Childbirth, BMJ, British Journal of General Practice, British Journal of Obstetrics & Gynecology, Clinical Chemistry, Contraception, European Journal of Obstetrics, Gynecology & Reproductive Biology, International Federation of Gynecology & Obstetrics, International Journal of Gynecology & Obstetrics and Journal of Obstetrics & Gynecology, Kathamandu University Medical Journal, Nepal Medical College Journal, Obstetrics & Gynecology, Sex Transmission Infections and The Lancet. The distribution of type of study per Journal is seen in Fig 7. Samples size examined ranged from 1 (case reports) to 44. Disease distribution examined presented as: ectopic pregnancy (17/42.5%), and from 1 (2.5%) bilateral tubal ligation, chlamydial infection-tubal infertility-ectopic pregnancy ,ectopic pregnancy on patients after IVF with abnormal sperm characteristics, ectopic pregnancy after oocyte donation in menopausal patients, ectopic pregnancy after donation surviving even with the absence of exogenous steroids, ectopic pregnancy after embryos with thickened zona pellucida, ectopic pregnancy after empty follicle syndrome, ectopic pregnancy after exposure to levonorgestrel, heterotopic abdominal pregnancy, heterotopic abdominal pregnancy, ectopic pregnancy after hydrosalpinx, menopause and oocyte donation, ovarian heterotopic pregnancy, ectopic pregnancy after pelvic inflammatory disease, pelvic inflammatory disease-ectopic pregnancy and neonatal complications, primary infertility, tubal factor infertility and bilateral ovarian pregnancy, tubal sterilization while 3 (7.5%) did not mentioned disease. Funding source of each study per Journal published is seen on Fig 8.

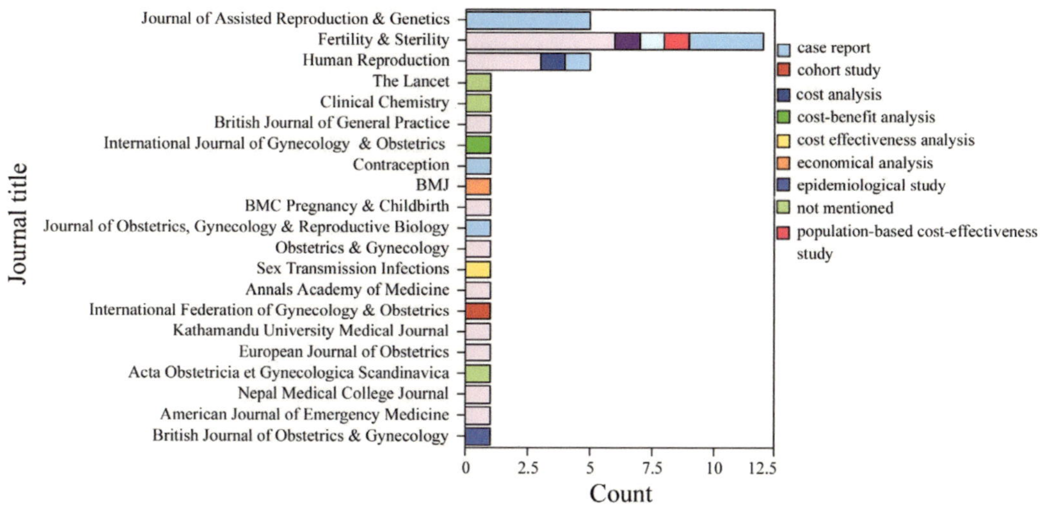

Fig. 7. The distribution of type of study per Journal examining IVF and ectopic pregnancy

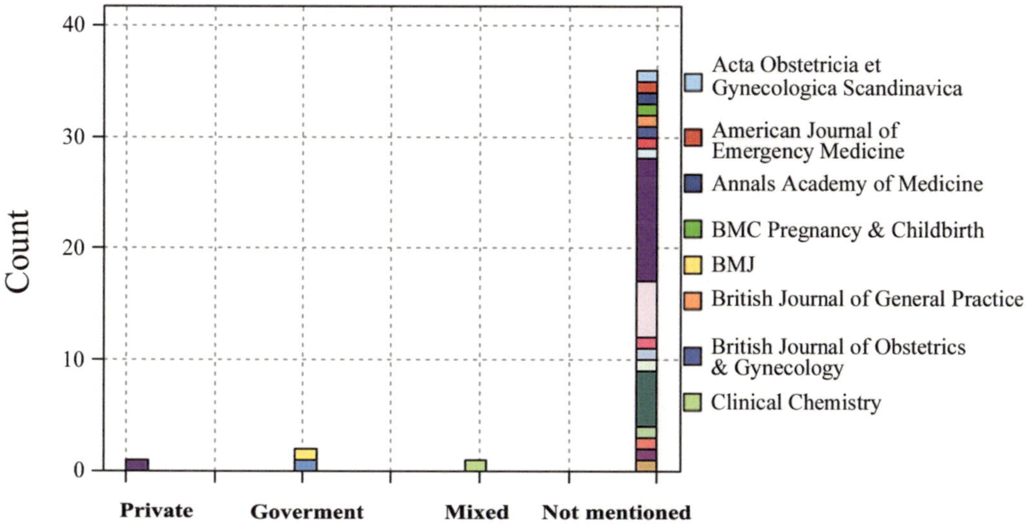

Fig. 8. Funding source of each study per Journal published examining IVF and ectopic pregnancy

5.2 Outcomes

5.2.1 Factors contributing to ectopic pregnancy after IVF

Pyrgiotis et al, retrospectively analyzed a large series of fresh (n=2812) and frozen embryo transfers (n=405) showing a 2.4% and 7.6% EP rate, respectively (Pyrgiotis et al., 1994). Tubal factor presented as 85.7% of all causes of ectopic pregnancies. In a previous study, an EP rate of 3.3% was found (26 patients) and the major contributing factor was a prior ectopic (Karande et al., 1991). Heterotopic pregnancy rates remained low in both studies while the majority of them were tubal. Also cervical pregnancies were low.

Clayton et al, in the largest series of 94.118 pregnancies found an EP rate of 2.2% in fresh non-donor cycles while ZIFT procedures EP rate was 3.6% (Clayton et al., 2006). Tubal factor with or without hydrosalpinx was the main factor of ectopic pregnancy while endometriosis, uterine factor and diminished ovarian reserve was some of the less but important factors. Although all other factors may be well understood, the last factor could be explained from the fact that when higher implantation embryo potential was present, EP rate was minimal. When two or less embryos transferred, then the EP rate was less than when three or more embryos transferred.

To the extent of the previous study, abnormal embryogenesis was a major factor for ectopic pregnancy. From this study it was found that DNA aneuploidy was associated with tubal implantation in 33% (Karikoski et al., 1993). Similar rates (24%) of abnormal amount of DNA content in tubal pregnancies was found also by Toikkanen et al., 1993.

In a recent study Chang et al, found that tubal factor infertility and endometriosis was the main factor (Chang et al., 2010). Tubal surgery and previous ectopic pregnancies was another important factor while risk for EP was seriously decreased with a previous live birth. Donor oocytes do not attribute to more ectopic pregnancies and this apply to higher embryo implantation potential, as mentioned above.

Contradictory to previous results, Bhattacharya et al, found that ectopic pregnancies in IVF are associated with significantly lower percentage of motile sperm (Bhattacharya et al., 2010).

A more detailed approach follows:

5.2.2 Heterotopic pregnancy

It is considered a rare entity of ectopic pregnancy (1/30000) and could be seen especially after IVF(<0. 01) (Dimitry et al, 1990; Molloy et al., 1990). It has been presented in literature in various forms: 1) Triplet heterotopic pregnancy a) in a previous caesarian scar and intrauterine pregnancy b) a tubal singleton and two intrauterine pregnancies and an ovarian abscess c) bilateral tubal and intrauterine pregnancy 2) Cornual pregnancy a) recurrent cornual pregnancy b) cornual pregnancy and twin intrauterine pregnancy 3) heterotopic pregnancy with intrauterine dizygotic twins after blastocyst transfer 4) heterotopic cervical pregnancy a) intrauterine and twin cervical pregnancy b) cervico-istmic pregnancy 5) Heterotopic pregnancy in parallel with ovarian hyperstimulation syndrome 6) heterotopic pregnancy ruptured after spontaneous abortion.

Eventually the presence of an intrauterine gestation sac in a patient without symptoms should not exclude the diagnosis of a concomitant extrauterine pregnancy until the pelvis is carefully visualized (Rizk et al., 1991).

5.2.3 Differences in the prevalence in different countries of the world

EP complicates about 2% of all pregnancies. Although no studies exists that specifically describe the prevalence in different countries, especially after IVF treatment, certain studies present this, as a secondary outcome. In Nigeria (Okohue et al., 2010), prevalence for EP was 7.8% after IVF, while in general population in the same country, EP rate was 1.74% (Musa et al., 2009). The same percentage in Jordan was 0.005% (Obeidat et al., 2010). In Cameroon, this percentage is 0.72% (Leke et al., 2004). In a large follow up study, in Sweden, ectopic pregnancy rates where compared between women from different countries of birth, but small differences were found (Eggert et al., 2008). In New York, ectopic pregnancy rates in black women are 4.78% (Fang et al., 2000).

5.2.4 Contraception as a risk factor

Ghosh et al, described a right ampullary ruptured ectopic pregnancy after the failure of levonorgestrel as emergency contraception (Ghosh et al., 2009), while Fabunmi and Perks, reported a case of Caesarean section scar pregnancy after the same LNG failure (Fabunmi & Perks, 2002). From the other side, opposite to the numerous case reports, De Santis et al, in a retrospective observational cohort study found no association of LNG failure with ectopic pregnancy (De Santis et al., 2005).

5.2.5 Ectopic pregnancy rates in fresh vs. frozen cycles

Controversy exists in this issue. Jun et al, found no difference in ectopic pregnancy rates between fresh and frozen cycles while Yanaihara et al, found a significant difference in ectopic pregnancies when two frozen blastocysts were transferred, than one (Jun et al., 2007; Yanaihara et al., 2008). From the other side, Ishihara et al, in a large registry retrospective study, found that frozen-thawed single blastocyst transfer significantly reduce EP rates (Ishihara et al., 2010). Even when data were stratified for age, EP rates varied, but remained low.

5.2.6 Day 3 versus day 5

Milki et al, found no difference in ectopic pregnancy rates when blastocyst transfer compared with day 3 embryo transfer (Milki et al., 2003). In this study important confounding factors like tubal disease between the two groups, cryopreserved transfers but not number of embryos transferred were checked between the two groups and no significant difference was found.

5.2.7 Blastocyst (single vs. double blastocyst transfer)

Knopman et al, reported a heterotopic abdominal pregnancy after the transfer of two blastocysts (Knopman et al., 2006). Intrauterine pregnancy miscarried first while abdominal pregnancy ruptured two weeks later and ectopic removed by laparoscopy. Ectopic pregnancies are significant lower when single frozen-thawed blastocysts transferred compared with two blastocysts (Yanaihara et al., 2008).

5.2.8 Oocyte donation and ectopic pregnancy rates

Cohen et al, found that hydrosalpinx patients that undergo oocyte donation have higher ectopic pregnancy rates than patients in the same program with no hydrosalpinx (Cohen et al., 1999). Possible explanation for that is the chronic alteration of endometrium rather the direct embryotoxic effect of hydrosalpinx fluid. In case, after oocyte donation, an ectopic takes place, minimal monitoring may allow rupture of ectopic with significant complication (Ledger et al., 1992). Mantzavinos et al, reported three case of ovarian pregnancy after oocyte donation (Mantzavinos et al., 1994). Cases were resolved with laparoscopy and removal of ovarian pregnancy tissue. Pantos et al, in a large series of donation patients found only one ectopic pregnancy (Pantos et al., 1993). Rosman et al, in a large retrospective study (4186 non-donor IVF cycles vs. 884 donor ET cycles found that there is no difference in ectopic pregnancy rates between donor and IVF cycles (Rosman et al., 2009). From the other side, donor patients showed significant lower incidence of tubal disease than standard IVF patients.

5.2.9 The ICSI role

In a large retrospective study, Clayton et al, found that use of ICSI was not associated with EP while male factor infertility was associated more with EP with all other races than white-non-Hispanic (Clayton et al., 2006).

5.2.10 Ultrasound guided embryo transfer

In a meta-analysis of clinical trials (on 5,968 ET cycles), comparing ultrasound guided ET vs. clinical touch ET (Abou-Setta et al., 2007), it was found that ectopic pregnancy rates were no different between the two groups. In a another meta-analysis on 17 studies,(Brown et al., 2010), it was found the same results, although it was stated that EP are relatively rare and study sample sizes limit the ability to detect such differences. Even when a single clinician performs all embryo transfers, (Kosmas et al., 2007), no difference in ectopic pregnancy rates was found.

5.2.11 Assisted hatching

Hagemann et al, found no difference in ectopic pregnancy rates in patients that their embryos had assisted hatching or not (Hagemann et al., 2008). From the other side Milki et al, in a large series of retrospectively examined patients saw that a significant higher ectopic pregnancy rate was found in cases where assisted hatching (AH) was performed when compared with cases that hatching was not preformed (Milki et al., 2004). Possible explanation for that is: 1) assisted hatching may accelerate embryo implantation, 2) a mechanism exists, that prevents embryos that reached fallopian tube to divert back to uterus and 3) the much higher embryo transfer volume that used in certain IVF programs.

5.2.12 Air bubble position after embryo transfer

No difference in ectopic pregnancy rates was observed with different distances of embryo deposition from the uterine fundus (10-15 mm or < 10 mm) (Pacchiarotti et al., 2007).

5.2.13 Reanastomosis

Patients with tubal infertility may undergo microsurgical reconstructive surgery of the fallopian tubes for adhesiolysis, anastomosis, fimbrioplasty, salpingostomy, and refertilization after former sterilization. These patients, if choose the microsurgical approach, show higher ectopic pregnancy rates after a single IVF trial (Schippert et al., 2009). From the other side, in a small series of patients, higher incidence of ectopic pregnancies was observed when previous tubal sterilization was reversed by laparoscopy than open microsurgical reversal (Tan et al, 2010). Even if suture less laparoscopic tubal re-anastomosis was performed (using a serosamuscular fixation/biological glue technique) an ectopic pregnancy rate of 3.9% was observed (Schepens et al., 2011). In a small series of robotic tubal reanastomosis (Dharia Patel et al., 2007) more ectopic pregnancies were observed when compared with open reanastomosis.

5.2.14 Other complications of ectopic pregnancies

Rh immunization could be observed in ruptured ectopic pregnancy.

6. Section 3

6.1 Diagnosis of an ectopic in IVF

Pregnancies of unknown location include viable pregnancies, ectopic pregnancies and miscarriages (Condous et al., 2005). Only a small portion of them are high risk pregnancies

(Condous et al., 2005) and there is difficulty in diagnosis and management. Serial measurements of hCG and progesterone should be performed on a wait and see approach, in parallel with TVS. Serum hCG increase over 48 h of more than 66% - that is,
an hCG ratio of >1.66 - correlates well with a developing intrauterine pregnancy. The use of discriminatory zone technique (Condous et al., 2005), is currently evaluated for prediction of probability of ectopic pregnancy. By this technique, if an intra-uterine sac cannot be seen on ultrasound scan above the threshold value, then steps must be taken to determine whether the pregnancy is abnormal or ectopic. After that a D&C can be safely performed only when a non-viable pregnancy has been documented by either a serum progesterone level of 15.9 nM or the absence of a rise in serum hCG after 2 days; that is, an hCG ratio of <1.50 (Pisarska et al., 1998).

6.2 Transvaginal ultrasound and hCG levels for prediction

With the use of TVS, before 35 days a pregnancy could be considered as a pregnancy of unknown location, from 35 to 41 days a pregnancy of uncertain viability and from 42 days a viable intrauterine pregnancy (Bottomley et al., 2009. Time for diagnosis of ectopic pregnancy was 48 days. In case, previous ectopic pregnancies took place, then diagnosis could be made before this time. Viability scans should be deferred until 49 days of gestation with a minimal benefit delaying after that. The addition of abdominal pain and vaginal bleeding ads to ectopic pregnancy risk. Statistical models have been developed, based on the hCG ratio to predict the outcome of pregnancies of unknown location and especially ectopic pregnancies (Kirk et al., 2006), but this is not easily implemented in clinical practice.

6.3 Newer biomarkers for ectopic pregnancy

Daniel et al, tested for serum sVCAM-1, ectopic and normal pregnancies, but did not found any difference (Daniel et al., 2000).
C. trachomatis antigen and nucleic acid could be found at 33% among ectopic pregnancies tissue even if they are negative for cervical Chlamydia (Toth et al., 2000).
Activin A subunit, type II receptors, follistatin, and iNOS show increased expression within the fallopian tube of ectopic pregnancy patients tested serologically positive for C. trachomatis (Refaat et al., 2009). Especially for iNOS, elevated activity positively correlates with protection from hydrosalpinx formation and prevention of the systemic spread of C. trachomatis. In a clinical setting, Florio et al, found that Activin A levels were significantly lower in spontaneous abortions and intrauterine pregnancies than ectopic ones,and at the cutoff of 0.37ng/ml a sensitivity and a specificity of 100 and 99.6%, respectively, was achieved, for prediction of EP (Florio et al., 2007). From the other side, on a different approach, Kirk et al, found no more discriminatory capacity of Activin A and inhibin than serum hCG levels for ectopic pregnancy in case of a pregnancy of unknown location (Kirk et al., 2009).

7. Section 4

7.1 Management of specific ectopic pregnancies

In this section, a total of 26 abstracts were retrieved and further screened. Only studies that performed clinical interventions for ectopic pregnancy after IVF were included in this part. Out of 16 included studies, 5 (31.25%) were performed in Taiwan, 4 in USA (25%), 2 in Italy

(12.5%), 1 (6.25%) in France, 1 in Germany (6.25%), 1 (6.25%) in Netherlands, 1 in Turkey (6.25%), and one in Serbia and Montenegro. 15 (93. 75%) of them considered themselves case report while 1 (6. 25%) clinical. The type of study per country initiated can be seen in Fig 9.

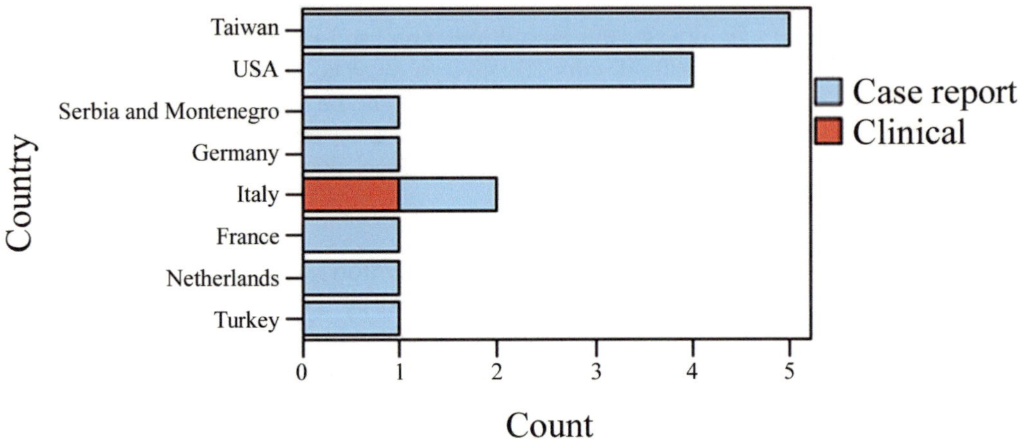

Fig. 9. The type of study per country initiated

All studies selected used human tissue. Thirteen studies did not mention anatomical tissue used (81.25%). From the other studies 1 (6.25%) used fallopian tissue, 1 used endometrium & fallopian tube, and one used cornual pregnancy. The type of study per tissue used can be seen in Fig 10.

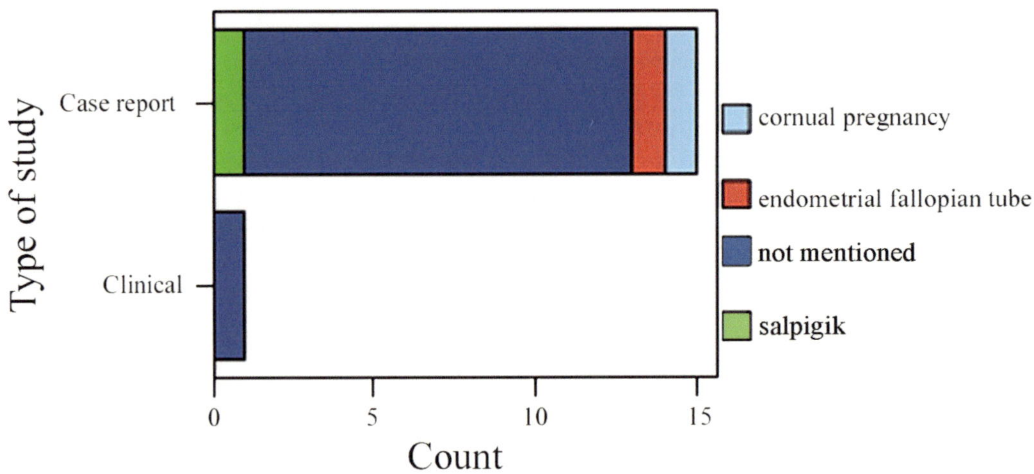

Fig. 10. The type of study per tissue used

10 (62.5%) of the studies were published in Fertility & Sterility, 2 (12.5%) in Human Reproduction and from 1 (6.25%) in Archives Gynecological & Obstetrics, Journal of Obstetrics & Gynecology, Journal of Assisted Reproduction & Genetics and Mayo Clinical Proceedings. The distribution of type of study per Journal is seen in Fig 11. All studies did not mention their controls.

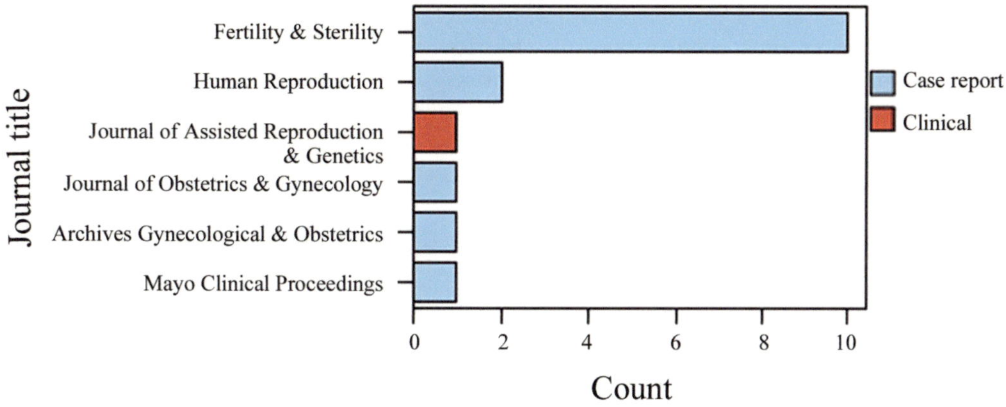

Fig. 11. Type of study per Journal published

Samples size examined ranged from 1 (case report) to 104. Disease distribution examined presented as: heterotopic cesarean scar pregnancy, (5/31.25%) (one study described ectopic twin pregnancy in a Cesarean section scar (1/6.,67%) and a second described a triplet heterotopic cesarean scar pregnancy), heterotopic cervical pregnancy (4/25%), cornual pregnancy (1/6.25%), heterotopic cornual pregnancy, heterotopic triplet pregnancy, Intersitial Heterotopic pregnancy, unilateral ectopic twin pregnancy while one study did not mentioned the type of ectopic pregnancy. Tissue used per disease is seen on Fig12.

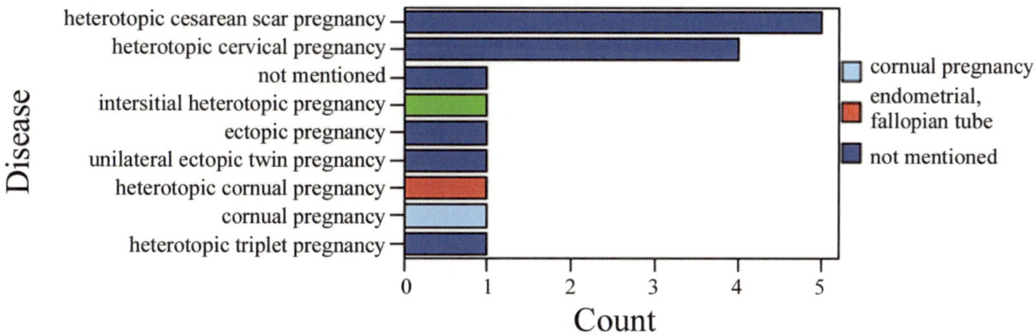

Fig. 12. The type of tissue used per disease

Funding source of each study per Journal published is seen on Fig 13.

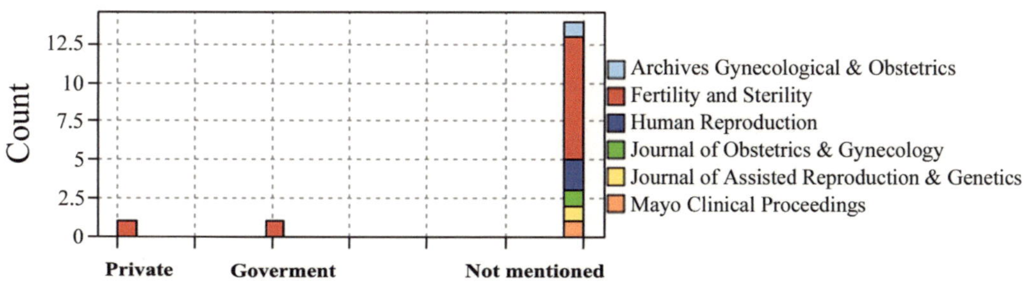

Fig. 13. Funding source of each study per Journal published

Five studies (31.25%) did dot used any pharmacological interventions while the other 11 described it: two studies used potassium chloride, one study used sodium chloride, one used systemic methotrexate, one used vasopressin. The other six studies described the pharmacological interventions from IVF, previously performed.

7.2 Rare cases of ectopic pregnancies

Papers that report ectopic pregnancies after IVF and their clinical picture will be presented in this section. Case studies will be presented according to anatomical location and management.

7.2.1 Ovarian ectopic pregnancies

In a large series of patients, Raziel et al., found that ovarian ectopic pregnancy rate comprises 2.7% of all ectopic pregnancies, is highly associated with the use of intrauterine device and treated with laparoscopic wedge resection (Raziel et al., 2004). The use of ultrasound for diagnosis of hemoperitoneum makes culdocentesis not necessary.
Case reports presenting ovarian ectopic pregnancies present: 1) ovarian heterotopic pregnancy after IVF (Kamath et al., 2010), 2) bilateral ovarian pregnancy after IVF and previous tubal pregnancy after reanastomosis (Han et al., 2004), 3) left ovarian pregnancy after empty follicle syndrome in IVF treatment (Qublan et al., 2008), 4) ovarian pregnancy from cornual fistulae after bilateral salpingectomy and IVF treatment (Hsu et al., 2004).

7.2.2 Management of a late ectopic pregnancy

A case of a cervical intrauterine pregnancy has been reported by Fruscalzo et al., after IVF (Fruscalzo et al., 2007). At the 13th gestational week, a viable intrauterine pregnancy and a non viable cervical pregnancy were diagnosed. The cervical pregnancy was anteriorly confined near a thick cervical blood vessel with low resistance flow at Doppler ultrasound. Due to the proximity to the cervical venous vessel, there was increased hemorrhagic risks associated with a cervical pregnancy expulsion After hospitalization and observation, cervical pregnancy was expulsed at 15th gestational week + 6 days and hemorrhage was managed through cervical curettage and multiple cervical stitches under general anesthesia. Unfortunately, some hours later, intrauterine pregnancy expulsed also, leading to a curettage.
Another case of heterotopic pregnancy at 16 wks gestation after IVF was presented by Hassiakos et al., 2002. It was ruptured and presented with intra-abdominal bleeding and hemorrhagic shock.

7.2.3 Maternal-embryo complications from use of Potassium chloride

A study by Gyamfi et al, described a cervical heterotopic pregnancy (one in the intrauterine cavity and the other in the upper portion of the cervix) treated with KCl (3 mL) injection and aspiration of the gestational sac contents (Gyamfi et al., 2004). A blood supply, separate from that of the remaining pregnancy was seen at 19 wks by color Doppler. Unfortunately remaining trophoblastic tissue did not resolve, leading to obstetric hemorrhage at 31 wks gestation and subsequently to emergency cesarean hysterectomy with a viable infant,while patient waited for an elective Cs at 32 wks. Another possible complication of this technique is that diffuse of KCL in the target amniotic sac, may lead to diffuse to adjacent sac, thus makes harm to the intrauterine embryo.

7.3 Rare ectopic pregnancies

7.3.1 Cervical pregnancies

A heterotopic cervical pregnancy treated with TVS-guided aspiration at day 34 after her embryo transfer, developed of uterine varices at the cervical site, bilateral hypogastric artery occlusion was used while a fundal classic cesarean section at 37 weeks gave birth to an infant (Shah et al., 2008). Uterine varices were diagnosed at 28 weeks gestation, as prominent vessels associated with the empty sac located anteriorly and posteriorly occupying a significant portion of the myometrium of the lower uterine segment and cervical stroma. Venous waveforms were observed on Doppler studies. Fundal C section was planned to avoid entry into the gestational tissue and vasculature that occupied the lower uterine segment. After delivery, the patient went for pelvic angiography and possible embolization to diminish the risk of bleeding.

Prorocic et al. described the treatment of a heterotopic cervical pregnancy with TVS-guided aspiration and instillation of hypertonic solution of sodium chloride and ligation of descending cervical branches of the uterine arteries (Prorocic et al., 2006). The latter took place before TVS guided aspiration. By vagina retraction, two DEXON sutures were placed bilaterally on the cervix, high below the fornix vaginae thus reducing hemorrhage, significantly. Twin pregnancy in the uterine cavity continue to grow till article publication (at 12th week of pregnancy).

A cervical twin ectopic pregnancy has been described by Aboulfoutouh et al. (Aboulfoutouh et al., 2011). Treatment consistent from transvaginal ultrasound-guided aspiration plus systemic single injection of methotrexate.

A 37-year-old woman after IVF developed severe ovarian hyperstimulation syndrome. Transvaginal ultrasound revealed two gestational sacs with one viable fetus located below the internal cervical os at 7 weeks' gestation while Doppler imaging demonstrated a cervical mass containing numerous tortuous and dilated blood vessels and vascular communication beds in the implantation site and established abundant peritrophoblastic arterial flows. 2 days later developed vaginal bleeding and Intracervical Foley catheter tamponade was performed. Persistently active gestatinal tissue and bleeding leads to hysteroscopic endocervical resection (12-degree resectoscope with an outer diameter of 8 mm) in combination with temporary balloon occlusion of bilateral common iliac arteries (CIA). After complete removal of gestational tissue, electrocoagulation was done using the rollerball for homeostasis. After that, a 24-Fr Foley balloon catheter was placed at the cervical canal to achieve homeostasis while methotrexate 50 mg im was injected on the following day, and the 24-Fr Foley balloon catheter was removed 3 days after surgery (Yang et al., 2010). Same method of treatment was used by Peleg et al. (Peleg et al., 1994).

A 45-year-old woman, diagnosed by ultrasound with a triplet gestation 7 weeks following IVF. Transvaginal ultrasound showed a triplet heterotopic pregnancy consisting of two gestational sacs in the cervix and one in the uterine cavity. Termination of pregnancy was decided for future fertility preservation with catheterization and methotrexate treatment. The right femoral artery was catheterized with catheter and the uterine arteries were cannulated. 42 mg of methotrexate were injected into the right and left uterine arteries (total dose of 84 mg (50 mg/m_2)). Pledgets of Gelfoam were then used to embolize the arteries. Follow-up ultrasound scan (after 48 hours) revealed an absence of cardiac activity in both embryos. A gradual shrinkage of the cervical and intrauterine sacs was seen later (Nitke et al., 2007).

A 37-year-old woman undergone ICSI, due to severe oligoasthenoteratospermia, diagnosed with transvaginal ultrasound two gestational sacs with embryonic heartbeats, one in the cervical region and the second intrauterine. Hysteroscopic removal of the cervical gestational sac was chosen, to preserve the intrauterine pregnancy. The gestational sac was observed on the left side of the endocervical canal 2 cm away from the internal cervical ostium The tip of the resectoscope did not go beyond the internal cervical os during the operation, and the uterine cavity was not touched. By roller ball electrocatery was used for the conception products. Cautery settings were 100 W for cutting, and the coagulation current blend was 1. The entire procedure was performed under continuous ultrasound guidance with an abdominal probe (Jozwiak et al., 2003).

A viable intrauterine and cervical pregnancy was diagnosed in a 34-year-old woman in her 4 IVF attempts. With transabdominal scanning, needle was inserted transcervically and maneuvered into the embryo fetal heart that ceased. After that KCl injected. Then 3 cm^3 of saline were injected for better visualization of the cervical fetus, and to confirm absence of heart beat. The intrauterine pregnancy delivered art 36,5 wks (Carreno et al., 2000).

A heterotopic cervical pregnancy diagnosed 25 days after ET because the patient reported some mild vaginal bleeding. Transvaginal ultrasound and Doppler vascular blood flow confirmed the suspected heterotopic cervical pregnancy that was treated with transvaginal ultrasound-guided aspiration and KCL injection in the heterotopic pregnancy cavity. Sixteen days after the procedure, and under epidural anesthesia, hemostatic synthetic absorbable sutures were placed high on the cervix at 1, 3, 9, and 10 o'clock, ultimately circumferentially tying the cervix. Cervical-stay sutures dissolved by the 18th–20th weeks of gestation while no cervical incompetence was observed. At 38 weeks of gestation, via cesarean section an infant was delivered. For safety precautions, during the procedure, interventional radiologists were on standby to perform uterine artery embolization if necessary (Chen et al., 2001).

7.3.2 Ectopic pregnancies developed in a scar

7.3.2.1 Previous myomectomy scar

Although pre-IVF myomectomy is not a necessity to achieve an ongoing pregnancy (Vimercati et al., 2007), other authors prefer to perform it, especially when repeated implantation failures takes place (Margalioth et al., 2006) or uterine cavity involvement exists (Klatsky et al., 2007). In a retrospective study for laparoscopic myomectomy outcomes, Paul et al, mentioned a 5.2% EP rate (Paul et al., 2006). In the same year, Seracchioli et al., reported an EP rate of 2.6% (Seracchioli et al, 2006). From the other side Campo et al, found no ectopic in their series after laparoscopic myomectomy (Campo et al., 2003). None of the ectopic pregnancies developed in the scar of the previous myomectomy.

7.3.2.2 Previous Caesarean scar (CSP)

Cesarean scar pregnancy carry the high risk of uncontrollable bleeding requiring hysterectomy, so management has to include this risk in its treatment options.

Wang et al, described a heterotopic pregnancy combined with intrauterine pregnancy after IVF (Wang et al., 2007). Embryo reduction was performed with transvaginal ultrasound guided KCL injection (0.2ml) at 10 wks gestation. A mass 3x3 cm remained till 32 wks gestation A male was delivered at 35 weeks delivered by CS. Remaining gestational tissue leads to massive blood loss after CS, blood transfusion and bilateral internal iliac arteries ligation.

Another author (Wang et al., 2010) found a Cesarean Scar pregnancy (within the isthmic area of the lower anterior wall of the uterus) and an intrauterine pregnancy after IVF. At this time, management was performed by hysteroscopy evacuation at 7 wks gestation and coagulation of the implantation vessel site. Cervix was dilated to 11 mm, not beyond the endocervical canal and gestational sac was pulled out, under sonographic guidance. Suction curettage was used to clear the residual gestational tissue and a hysteroscopic rolling ball was used to stop the bleeding point. A healthy infant delivered by Cs at 39 wks gestation.

From the other side two different cases was presented by Chueh et al., 2008. Both cases were a twin cesarean scar pregnancy. Ectopic pregnancies were treated either by laparotomy excision of the scar twin pregnancy (first case) and hysterosocpic resection (second case) with resectoscopic coagulation of placenta bed vessels. In both cases, no fluid was seen in the cul-de-sac.

More pregnancies could be observed in cesarean scar. Litwicka et al, described a triplet heterotopic cesarean scar pregnancy after IVF, a twin pregnancy in the anterior isthmic wall close to the CS scar (separated from the bladder wall by a thin myometrial layer) and one intrauterine gestational sac (Litwicka et al., 2010). Caesarian scar gestation sacs have been diagnosed,one week later than the intrauterine sac. Transvaginal ultrasound-guided potassium chloride (2 ml) and methotrexate (15 mg) was injected in the ectopic gestational sacs while the intrauterine pregnancy continue to ongoing pregnancy.

In another case, described by Hsieh et al, a heterotopic triplet pregnancy was evident after IVF treatment, two intrauterine pregnancies and one cesarean scar pregnancy (Hsieh et al., 2004). Color Doppler sonography revealed proliferated peritrophoblastic vessels around the Caesarean scar pregnancy and the intrauterine twin pregnancy. CSP was treated with embryo aspiration under vaginal ultrasonography with preservation of intrauterine twin pregnancy. Due to preterm labour, two infants delivered at 32 wks gestation.

Rare CSP may exist at different forms after IVF treatments and previous CS. The management of these pregnancies may be performed with laparotomy or hysteroscopic resection of CS ectopic tissue after KCL lethal injection to embryo. Also MTX may be used for the second case. Complications of the second treatment include spontaneous abortion and congenital abnormality of MTX or diffuse of KCL in the target amniotic sac that may lead to diffuse to adjacent sac.

7.3.3 Live twin pregnancy in the same fallopian tube

A left fallopian tube twin pregnancy was presented by Atabekoğlu et al., an isthmic pregnancy and another ampullary sac in the same tube (Atabekoğlu et al., 2009). Both treated with a left laparoscopic salpingectomy.

7.3.4 Cul-de-sac pregnancy

A case of a cul-de-sac ectopic pregnancy after IVF, was described by Shih et al. (Shih et al., 2007). After 4 weeks from ET it was found an ectopic gestational sac with fetal heart beat in the left adnexa. It was revealed, by laparoscopy, an ectopic mass in the congenital blind pouch that was connected to the posterior cul-de-sac. Laparotomy was used for removal of conceptus and homeostasis.

7.3.5 Hepatic pregnancy

Although a lot of case reports exist for a hepatic pregnancy in the literature (Chin et al., 2010; Moores et al., 2010), none of them is reported after IVF, so they mentioned as primary hepatic pregnancy. Chlamydia infections may involved also in this type of ectopic because adhesions between and liver the diaphragm (Fitz-Hugh-Curtis Syndrome) were demonstrated in 34% of those with EP (Picaud et al., 1991). Treatment of this type of pregnancy included direct methotrexate injection (Nichols et al., 1995), laparoscopic suctioning and homeostasis (Chin et al., 2010) or laparotomy. In case an advanced week's live pregnancy is diagnosed, then laparotomy with intact placenta may be performed (Shukla et al., 1995).

7.3.6 Intrauterine and twin bilateral tubal pregnancy

Pan et al, report a case of bilateral tubal pregnancy and intrauterine pregnancy (Pan et al., 2002). After right tubal embryo transfer (due to cervical stenosis) of four embryos, in 5th week, a laparotomy showed a ruptured right tubal pregnancy, hemoperitoneum and a dilated left tube. Bilateral salpingectomy was performed with preservation of intrauterine pregnancy and deliver of a male at term.

7.3.7 Intrauterine and interstitial heterotopic pregnancy after bilateral salpingectomy

Patient had two previous unsuccessful IVF cycles and removed both tubes for bilateral hydrosalpinges. After that she preformed a third IVF cycle. She developed an intrauterine pregnancy and an interstitial pregnancy that ruptured at the left salpingectomy site by its lateral position to the insertion of the ipsilateral round ligment. After laparotomy and left cornual resection, intrauterine pregnancy survived two more weeks and miscarried. Trisomy 21 was revealed, in aborted fetus (Dumesic et al., 2001).

7.3.8 Cornual pregnancy

Two studies exist that describe cornual pregnancy after IVF. First case was a heterotopic triplet pregnancy after in utero transfer of three embryos (Divry et al., 2006). Cornual pregnancy was treated with resection by laparotomy. A special technique was presented in this patient. A Vicryl string with a tight knot was inserted at the base of the implantation site of the corneal pregnancy and the base of the uterine wall above this string was sectioned. Cornual scar was closed with same stitches in X form while a base knot left in place. Intrauterine twin pregnancy continue uneventfully till 31 wks gestation, where the patient delivered two girls with Csection. The site of the corneal pregnancy was well vascularrized and not ruptured.
The second case was a recurrent spontaneous cornual pregnancy 2 years after a heterotopic cornual pregnancy occurred after IVF cycle (van der Weiden et al., 2005). Previous cornual heterotopic pregnancy was treated with injection of 0.5 ml of 15% potassium chloride into the fetal heart while normal pregnancy was delivered at 39 weeks of gestation by elective caesarean section. Spontaneous cornual pregnancy was treated by injection of 40 mg methotrexate in the gestational sac and systemic methotrexate (1.0 mg/kg orally alternated with 15 mg folinic acid).

7.3.9 Interstitial pregnancy

Berkes et al., reported a unilateral triplet ectopic pregnancy, on a woman with a history of right salpingectomy (Berkes et al., 2008). After IVF, in the left fallopian tube, a triplet pregnancy was found (two pregnancies at interstitial and one at ampullary location). Color flow Doppler sonography revealed intensive perithrophoblastic blood flow around the two gestational sacs with live embryos while TVS showed threegestational sacs,in the left

interstitial area,in the isthmic part of the fallopian tube and in the ampullar part next to the left ovary. After multiple dose of methotrexate, hCG levels were lowered but pregnancies were ruptured, so a laparotomy was performed with the removal of the left tube and cornual part of the uterus. Another case of previous bilateral salpingectomy and IVF was reported by Chang et al. (Chang et al., 2003). An intrauterine monozygotic twin and an interstitial monozygotic twin pregnancy were reported. By laparotomy, interstitial pregnancy was removed and intrauterine pregnancy allowed delivering at 38 wks gestation. Another intrauterine monochorionic diamniotic twin pregnancy and an interstitial pregnancy were reported by Nikolaou et al. (Nikolaou et al., 2002). Also after bilateral salpingectomy and IVF, interstitial heterotopic pregnancy was developed that ruptured (Dumesic et al., 2001). A recurrent interstitial pregnancy in uterine horn was seen after IVF (Muzikova et al., 2003).
Laparoscopic loop ligature was used by Qin et al, for heterotopic interstitial pregnancy (Qin et al., 2008). Perez et al., reported medical therapy in two cases of interstitial pregnancy, one with transvaginal ultrasound guided injection of methotrexate and second with potassium chloride into the ectopic sac of the heterotopic twins (Perez et al., 1993).
Overall, interstitial pregnancies are always possible after tubal occlusion.

7.3.10 Rare cases of mild ovarian hyperstimulation and ectopic pregnancy

Korkontzelos et al., reported the co-existence of ovarian hyperstimulation with ascetic fluid accumulation, enlarged ovaries after IVF and a right tubal ectopic pregnancy (Korkontzelos et al., 2006). Right salpingectomy was performed. Same case was presented by Fujii et al., which ended in a bilateral salpingectomy and continuation of intrauterine pregnancy till 32 wks of gestation (Fujii et al., 1996).

7.3.11 Consecutive recurrent ectopic pregnancies

Three consecutive recurrent pregnancies have been reported in the same patient with pelvic inflammatory disease, two in the right fallopian tube and one in the left. Laparotomy was performed in all three cases, to preserve the tubes while removing conceptus (Adelusi et al., 2003). Another case of two consecutive ectopic pregnancies after IVF, was presented by Abu-Musa et al. (Abu-Musa et al., 2002). Three consecutive cases of ectopic pregnancy on the same patient was presented by Oki et al., 1998. The first involved simultaneous intrauterine and left tubal pregnancy, the second was a right tubal pregnancy, and the third was a right interstitial pregnancy. Another case of two ectopic pregnancies in consecutive menstrual cycles was presented by Irvine et al. (Irvine et al., 1999). Left distal ectopic pregnancy was seen and treated with left partial salpingectomy while in the next cycle a right distal ectopic pregnancy was observed which treated with right partial salpingectomy. Except the second case, the other two patients conceived by coitus, so cases are presented in this review because they are rare. Another report of recurrent cornual ectopic pregnancy has been presented (MacRae et al., 2009) but presentation is beyond the scope of this manuscript.

8. Section 5

8.1 Cost effectiveness

8.1.1 Chlamydia trachomatis -ectopic pregnancy-cost effectiveness

Eight studies described cost-effectiveness of Chlamydia screening for pregnancy complications, including ectopic pregnancy. For most of them, proactive screening of

Chlamydia is not cost-effective when tested in general population (Buhaug et al., 1989; Roberts et al., 2007; van Valkengoed et al., 2001) and that only when women aged 18 to 24 years old tested or prevalence of Chlamydia is over 3% (Postma et al., 2000) or 2% (Trachtenberg et al., 1988), cost-effectiveness exist for prevention of ectopic pregnancy. Hu et al, pointed out that annual screening for Chlamydia is indicated for women 15 to 29 years of age and selective targeting with semiannual screening of those women with a history of infection (Hu et al., 2004). Partner treatment should be provided (Postma et al., 1999) to avoid re-infection. Another author (Schiøtz et al., 1991) found that routine post-treatment control of non- systematic genital Chlamydia infection is not cost-beneficial.

8.1.2 Ultrasound for diagnosis of ectopic pregnancy-cost-effectiveness

In an emergency department, to rule out the possibility of ectopic pregnancy, the most cost effective strategy is to screen all patients with first trimester bleeding and lower abdominal cramping with ultrasound (Durston et al., 1999), even if the scan is performed by an emergency doctor. Obviously this technique is not cost-effective in symptoms free women (Mol et al., 2002).

8.1.3 Laparoscopic treatment for Ectopic pregnancy-cost effectiveness

When laparoscopy is compared with methotrexate for its cost savings, methotrexate saves about 1000, Canadian dollars (Yao et al, 1996). In a decision and cost-effectiveness analysis, Seror et al., found that first line treatment with methotrexate is more cost-effective than conservative laparoscopy and radical laparoscopy in sub-acute ectopic pregnancy (Seror et al., 2006). Conservative laparoscopy was more cost-effective than radical laparoscopy in this group of patients, in terms of fertility preservation. Methotrexate treatment effectiveness was increased when diagnostic ultrasound accuracy is increased. If patient after an IVF ectopic pregnancy treated with methotrexate, then, in the next cycle, similar ovarian stimulation characteristics could be obtained (Orvieto et al., 2007).

9. Conclusion

In this systematic review we presented the most important studies dealing with ectopic pregnancy after *in vitro* fertilization. Also, important biological factors that play a role for EP has been presented. Case reports of ectopic pregnancies their position in the uterus, and the steps undertaken to preserve intrauterine pregnancy has been described. Complications of these treatments, where available, have been mentioned. Practices during *in vitro* fertilization treatment and their controversial role for this pregnancy complication have been described. Overall, cost-effectiveness studies in the ectopic pregnancy prediction and management has been described. New research directions have been pointed out.

Although ectopic pregnancies and more specific heterotopic pregnancies are rare, these increase due to infertility treatment. Active and aggressive management of hydrosalpinx has been proposed for heterotopic pregnancy minimization after IVF.

All combinations of heterotopic pregnancies have been described. The major complication was bleeding and rupture of pregnancy. Care was taken for intrauterine pregnancy continuation but many cases miscarried after some time. Laparoscopy and hysteroscopy were methods of choice but laparotomy was chosen when threat of major bleeding was expected. Another method of treatment was vaginal aspiration of embryo sac after a lethal injection with a pharmacological agent. Most cases have not recognized till rupture of ectopic pregnancy.

The majority of studies were case report and retrospective studies. Even if more studies exist in a specific issue (e. g. ectopic pregnancy rates in fresh and frozen IVF cycles) these are not, homogenously designed, and no data synthesis could be made. Also in the management of heterotopic pregnancies, a single methodology was not used, so no best practices outcome could be formed. Screening for ectopic pregnancy show better cost-effectiveness only when we expect increased prevalence of this entity (Roberts et al., 2007; van Valkengoed et al., 2001) or women age from 18 to 24 years old (Buhaug et al., 1990). Also general population screening program for C. Trachomatis, show that costs exceeds the benefits to avoid ectopic pregnancy. The method of choice for treatment is laparoscopy, because show similar cost-effectiveness but less invasiveness (Gray et al., 1995) than laparotomy. Combination therapies, like uterine artery embolization and laparoscopy has been used for complications like hemorrhage. Although these therapies are expensive, the rare cases do not allow a cost-effectiveness analysis to be performed.

Many heterotopic pregnancies were identified after EP rupture, thus leading to a laparoscopy or laparotomy and possible complications while an early identification may lead to MTX therapy, that is by far a more cost-effective treatment strategy. From the other side, close ultrasound monitoring has revealed heterotopic pregnancies developed in previous Caesarean scar pregnancy, cervical pregnancies etc. So for IVF patients, more intense ultrasound and b-hCG monitoring is required. It is not known yet whether this applies to all patients that had an ET or only in the subgroup of patients with risk factors for EP undergoing ET.

Many ectopic pregnancies remained unidentified with viable pregnancies till second trimester. It is important, for these cases, to improve our detection capabilities with new approaches. Heterotopic pregnancy may present with different combinations and uterine locations, at various gestational ages, even when the intrauterine pregnancy aborts. Eventually the presence of an intrauterine gestation sac in a patient without symptoms should not exclude the diagnosis of a concomitant extrauterine pregnancy until the pelvis is carefully visualized (Rizk et al., 1991). Currently, no biomarker could early identify an ectopic pregnancy, especially a heterotopic one. A promising non invasive marker could be developed from the use of cervical trophoblastic cells and special markers on them.

Regarding the IVF procedure, infertility medication should be used cautiously from non-specialists and ovulation induction has to be preformed always under close monitoring. In case of altered tubal motility, close monitoring of pregnancy as evolves, should be performed.

Chlamydia infections and tubal factor infertility still remain the major factor for EP after IVF. Active management for hydrosalpinx seems to lower EP rates, but still no minimal invasive test exists. No other IVF technique could be accounted for increased ectopic pregnancy rates except the transfer of multiple embryos, especially more than two. Where indications exist for increased EPs after specific techniques (e. g. assisted hatching), more clinical trials should be performed, controlled also for EP factors. Tubal transfer techniques (ZIFT) have been abandoned through years, so they could not account for EP in the modern era. Tubal reanastomosis also is not practiced in all IVF clinics, and only where it is practiced it has to be considered as a factor of tubal pregnancy.

Another issue that needs to be checked is the association of ectopic pregnancy and the abnormal embryogenesis. This is important for male factor infertility and increased age. It is not clear yet whether more intense pregnancy monitoring should apply in these patients.

As a general policy, individual IVF practices should evaluate their EP rate in an attempt to identify factors that may increase or decrease the rate compared to national statistics (Keegan et al., 2007).
It is not clear yet, whether a single biological pathway should account for ectopic pregnancy. Although TB implantation mechanism is different from normal uterine mechanism, tubal pregnancies should be used to study embryo implantation. Invasive pathway, as described in ectopic pregnancy seems to be important. Another pathway that may be involved is the NO pathway that is altered through the Chlamydia infection altered immune response.
Researchers performing RCTs in ectopic pregnancies need to consider certain issues in their design. Patients differ in age and the infertility factor. A trial has to control for the number of embryos transferred, the quality of them and patients demography because a common underlying risk factor might exist. A clear measure of complications has to be developed, especially for cost effectiveness studies. Because ectopic pregnancies after IVF always need intervention, no placebo trials could be performed. Length of follow up and follow up plan need to be decided before hand, so pregnant women need to have standardized care. Level of training for the providers of IVF services seems to be important.
Ruptured ectopic pregnancies may present with severe complications, due to hemorrhage. Currently, no single treatment plan is chosen and different groups perform different approaches. Although these treatments are life saving, they are not cost effective. It is important for hospitals with large IVF groups to undertake such studies, so knowledge to be transferred to smaller groups. In case of heterotopic pregnancy, it is important to know how to protect the intrauterine embryo (as valuable pregnancy), so research should direct to this also.

10. References

Aboulfoutouh, I. I.; Youssef, M. A.; Zakaria, A. E.; Mady, A. A. & Khattab, S. M. (2011). Cervical twin ectopic pregnancy after *In Vitro* fertilization-Embryo transfer (IVF-ET): case report. *Gynecol Endocrinol*, (April 2011), [Epub ahead of print]

Abou-Setta, A. M.; Mansour, R. T.; Al-Inany, H. G.; Aboulghar, M. M.; Aboulghar, M. A. & Serour, G. I. (2007). Among women undergoing embryo transfer, is the probability of pregnancy and live birth improved with ultrasound guidance over clinical touch alone? A systemic review and meta-analysis of prospective randomized trials. *Fertil Steril*, Vol. 88, No. 2, (August 2007), pp. 333-341, ISSN 1556-5653

Abu-Musa, A.; Nassar, A.; Sakhel, K. & Usta, I. (2002). Two consecutive ectopic pregnancies after in-vitro fertilization and embryo transfer. Case report. *Clin Exp Obstet Gynecol*, Vol. 29, No. 4, (2002), pp. 302-303, ISSN 0390-6663

Adelusi, B.; al-Meshari, A.; Akande, E. O. & Chowdhury, N. (1993). Three consecutive recurrent ectopic pregnancies. *East Afr Med J*, Vol. 70, No. 9 (September 1993), pp. 592-594, ISSN 0012-835X

Atabekoğlu, C. S.; Gözükuçük, M.; Ozkavukçu, S. & Sönmezer, M. (2009). Rare presentation of ectopic pregnancy following IVF-ET: live twin gestation in the same fallopian tube. *Hum Fertil (Camb)*, Vol. 12, No. 2, (June 2009), pp. 122-124, ISSN 1742-8149

Bai, S. X.; Wang, Y. L.; Qin, L.; Xiao, Z. J.; Herva, R. & Piao, Y. S. (2005). Dynamic expression of matrix metalloproteinases (MMP-2, -9 and -14) and the tissue inhibitors of MMPs (TIMP-1, -2 and -3) at the implantation site during tubal pregnancy. *Reproduction*, Vol. 129, No. 1, (January 2005), pp. 103-113, ISSN 1741-7899

Berkes, E.; Szendei, G.; Csabay, L.; Sipos, Z.; Joo, J. G. & Rigo, J. Jr. (2003). Unilateral triplet ectopic pregnancy after *in vitro* fertilization and embryo transfer. *Fertil Steril,* Vol. 90, No. 5, (November 2008), pp. 0003. e17-20, ISSN 1556-5653

Bhattacharya, S. M. & Ghosh, M. (2010). Abnormal sperm characteristics and risk of ectopic pregnancy. *Int J Gynaecol Obstet,* Vol. 110, No. 2, (August 2010), pp. 161-162, ISSN 1879-3479

Bjartling, C.; Osser, S. & Persson., K. (2007). Deoxyribonucleic acid of Chlamydia trachomatis in fresh tissue from the Fallopian tubes of patients with ectopic pregnancy. *European Journal of Obstetrics & Gynecology and Reproductive Biology,* Vol. 134, No. 1, (September 2007), pp. 95-100, ISSN 1872-7654

Bottomley, C.; Van Belle, V.; Mukri, F.; Kirk, E.; Van Huffel, S.; Timmerman, D. & Bourne, T. (2009). The optimal timing of an ultrasound scan to assess the location and viability of an early pregnancy. *Hum Reprod,* Vol. 24, No. 8, (August 2009), pp. 1811-1817, ISSN 1460-2350

Brown, J.; Buckingham K.; Abou-Setta, A. M. & Buckett, W. (2010). Ultrasound versus 'clinical touch' for catheter guidance during embryo transfer in women. *Cochrane Database Syst Rev,* Vol. 20, No. 1, (January 2010), pp. CD006107, ISSN 1469-493X

Brunham, R. C.; Peeling, R.; Maclean, I.; Kosseim, M. L. & Paraskevas, M. (1992). Chlamydia trachomatis-Associated Ectopic Pregnancy: Serologic and Histologic Correlates. *The Journal of Infectious Diseases,* Vol. 165, No. 6 (June 1992), pp. 1076-1081, ISSN 1537-6613

Buchholz, K. R. & Stephens, R. S. (2007). The Extracellular Signal-Regulated Kinase/Mitogen-Activated Protein Kinase Pathway Induces the Inflammatory Factor Interleukin-8 following Chlamydia trachomatis Infection. *Infection and Immunity,* Vol. 75, No. 12, (December 2007), pp. 5924-5929, ISSN 1098-5522

Buhaug, H.; Skjeldestad, F. E.; Backe, B. & Dalen, A. (1989). Cost effectiveness of testing for chlamydial infections in asymptomatic women. *Med Care,* Vol. 27, No. 8, (August 1989), pp. 833-841, ISSN 1537-1948

Buhaug, H.; Skjeldestad, F. E.; Halvorsen, L. E. & Dalen, A. (1990). Should asymptomatic patients be tested for Chlamydia trachomatis in general practice? Br J Gen Pract. Vol. 40, No. 333, (April 1990), pp. 142-145, ISSN 1478-5242

Campo, S.; Campo, V. & Gambadauro, P. (2003). Reproductive outcome before and after laparoscopic or abdominal myomectomy for subserous or intramural myomas. *Eur J Obstet Gynecol Reprod Biol,* Vol. 110, No. 2, (October 2003), pp. 215-219, ISSN 1872-7654

Carreno, C. A.; King, M.; Johnson, M. P.; Yaron, Y.; Diamond, M. P.; Bush, D. & Evans, M. I. (2000). Treatment of heterotopic cervical and intrauterine pregnancy. *Fetal Diagn Ther,* Vol. 15, No. 1, (Jan-Feb 2000), pp. 1-3, ISSN 1421-9964

Chang, H. J. & Suh, C. S., (2010). Ectopic pregnancy after assisted reproductive technology: what are the risk factors? *Curr Opin Obstet Gynecol,* Vol. 22, No. 3, (June 2010), pp. 202-207, ISSN 1473-656X

Chang, Y.; Lee, J. N.; Yang, C. H.; Hsu, S. C. & Tsai, E. M. (2003). An unexpected quadruplet heterotopic pregnancy after bilateral salpingectomy and replacement of three embryos. *Fertil Steril,* Vol. 80, No. 1, (July 2003), pp. 218-220, ISSN 1556-5653

Chen, D.; Kligman, I. & Rosenwaks, Z. (2001). Heterotopic cervical pregnancy successfully treated with transvaginal ultrasound-guided aspiration and cervical-stay sutures. *Fertil. Steril,* Vol. 75, No. 5, (May 2001), pp. 1030-1033, ISSN 1556-5653

Chin, P. S.; Wee, H. Y. & Chern, B. S. (2010). Laparoscopic management of primary hepatic pregnancy. *Aust N Z J Obstet Gynaecol,* Vol. 50, No. 1, (February 2010), pp. 95-98, ISSN 1479-828X

Chueh, H. Y.; Cheng, P. J.; Wang, C. W.; Shaw, S. W.; Lee, C. L. & Soong, Y. K. (2009). Ectopic twin pregnancy in cesarean scar after *in vitro* fertilization/embryo transfer: case report. *Fertil. Steril,* Vol. 90, No. 5, (November 2009), pp. 19-21, ISSN 1556-5653

Clayton, H. B.; Schieve, L. A.; Peterson, H. B.; Jamieson, D. J.; Reynolds, M. A. & Wright, V. C. (2006). Ectopic pregnancy risk with assisted reproductive technology procedures. *Obstet Gynecol,* Vol. 107, No. 3, (March 2006), pp. 595-604, ISSN 1873-233X

Cohen, M. A.; Lindheim, S. R. & Sauer, M. V. (1999). Hydrosalpinges adversely affect implantation in donor oocyte cycles. *Hum Reprod,* Vol. 14, No. 4, (April 1999), pp. 1087-1089, ISSN 1460-2350

Condous, G.; Okaro, E. & Bourne, T. (2005). Pregnancies of unknown location: diagnostic dilemmas and management. *Curr Opin Obstet Gynecol,* Vol. 17, No. 6, (December 2005), pp. 568-573, ISSN 1473-656X

Daniel, Y.; Geva, E.; Eshed-Englender, T.; Gamzu, R.; Lessing, B. J.; Bar-Am, A. & Amit, A. (2000). Vascular Cell Adhesion Molecule-1 in Normal, Failed, and Ectopic Pregnancy. *Am J Reprod Immunol, Vol.* 43, No. 2, (February 2000), pp. 92-97, ISSN 1600-0897

De Santis, M.; Cavaliere, A. F.; Straface, G.; Carducci, B. & Caruso, A. (2005). Failure of the emergency contraceptive levonorgestrel and the risk of adverse effects in pregnancy and on fetal development: an observational cohort study. *Fertil Steril,* Vol. 84, No. 2, (August 2005), pp. 296-299, ISSN 1556-5653

Dharia Patel, S. P.; Steinkampf, M. P.; Whitten, S. J. & Malizia, BA. (2007). Robotic tubal anastomosis: surgical technique and cost effectiveness. *Fertil Steril* Vol. 90, No. 4, (October 2008), pp. 1175-1179, ISSN 2008 1556-5653

Dimitry, E. S.; Oskarsson, T.; Margara, R. & Winston, R. M. (1990). Heterotopic pregnancy associated with assisted reproductive technology. *Am J Obstet Gynecol,* Vol. 163, No. 1Pt1, (July 1990), pp. 244-245, ISSN 1097-6868

Divry, V.; Hadj, S.; Bordes, A.; Genod, A. & Salle, B. (2007). Case of progressive intrauterine twin pregnancy after surgical treatment of cornual pregnancy. *Fertil. Steril,* Vol. 87, No. 1, (January 2007), pp. 190. e1-3, ISSN 1556-5653

Dumesic, D. A.; Damario, M. A. & Session, D. R. (2001). Interstitial heterotopic pregnancy in a woman conceiving by *in vitro* fertilization after bilateral salpingectomy. *Mayo Clin Proc,* Vol. 76, No. 1, (January 2001), pp. 90-92, ISSN 1942-5546

Duncan, W. C.; McDonald, S. E.; Dickinson, R. E.; Shaw, J. V. L.; Lourenco, P. C.; Wheelhouse, N.; Lee, K. F.; Critchley, H. O. D. & Horne, A. W. (2010). Expression of the repulsive SLIT/ROBO pathway in the human endometrium and Fallopian tube. *Molecular Human Reproduction,* Vol. 16, No. 12, (December 2010), pp. 950-959, ISSN 1460-2407

Durston, W. E.; Carl, M. L.; Guerra, W.; Eaton, A. & Ackerson, L. M. (2000). Ultrasound availability in the evaluation of ectopic pregnancy in the ED: comparison of quality and cost-effectiveness with different approaches. *Am J Emerg Med,* Vol. 18, No. 4, (July 2000), pp. 408-417, ISSN 1532-8171

Eggert, J.; Li, X. & Sundquist, K. (2008). Country of birth and hospitalization for pelvic inflammatory disease, ectopic pregnancy, endometriosis, and infertility: a nationwide study of 2 million women in Sweden. *Fertil Steril,* Vol. 90, No. 4, (October 2008), pp. 1019-1025, ISSN 1556-5653

Fabunmi, L. & Perks, N. (2002). Caesarean section scar ectopic pregnancy following postcoital contraception. *J Fam Plann Reprod Health Care,* Vol. 28, No. 3, (July 2002), pp. 155-156, ISSN 1471-1893

Fang, J.; Madhavan, S. & Alderman, M. H. (2000). Maternal mortality in New York City: excess mortality of black women. *J Urban Health,* Vol. 77, No. 4, (December 2000), pp. 735-744, ISSN 1468-2869

Florio, P.; Severi, F. M.; Bocchi, C.; Luisi, S.; Mazzini, M.; Danero, S.; Torricelli, M. & Petraglia, F. (2007). Single serum activin a testing to predict ectopic pregnancy. *J Clin Endocrinol Metab,* Vol. 92, No. 5, (May 2007), pp. 1748-1753, ISSN 1945-7197

Fruscalzo, A.; Mai, M.; Löbbeke, K.; Marchesoni, D. & Klockenbusch, W. (2008). A combined intrauterine and cervical pregnancy diagnosed in the 13th gestational week: which type of management is more feasible and successful? *Fertil. Steril,* Vol. 89, No. 2, (February 2008), pp. 456. e13-6, ISSN 1556-5653

Fujii, M.; Mori, S.; Goto, T.; Kiya, T.; Yamamoto, H.; Ito, E. & Kudo, R. (1996). Simultaneous intra- and extra-uterine pregnancy with ovarian hyperstimulation syndrome after induction of ovulation: a case report. *J Obstet Gynaecol Res,* Vol. 22, No. 6, (December 1996), pp. 589-594, ISSN 1341-8076

Ghosh, B.; Dadhwal, V.; Deka, D.; Ramesan, C. K. & Mittal, S. (2008). Ectopic pregnancy following levonorgestrel emergency contraception: a case report. *Contraception,* Vol. 79, No. 2, (February 2008), pp. 155-157, ISSN 1879-0518

Gray, D. T.; Thorburn, J.; Lundorff, P.; Strandell, A. & Lindblom, B. (1995). A cost-effectiveness study of a randomised trial of laparoscopy versus laparotomy for ectopic pregnancy. *Lancet,* Vol. 345, No. 8958, (May 1995), pp. 1139-1143, ISSN 1474-547X

Gyamfi, C.; Cohen, S.; Stone, J. L.; (2004). Maternal complication of cervical heterotopic pregnancy after successful potassium chloride fetal reduction. *Fertil. Steril,* Vol. 82, No. 4, (October 2004), pp. 940-943, ISSN 1556-5653

Hagemann, A. R.; Lanzendorf, S. E.; Jungheim, E. S.; Chang, A. S.; Ratts, V. S. & Odem, RR. (2009). A prospective, randomized, double-blinded study of assisted hatching in women younger than 38 years undergoing *in vitro* fertilization. *Fertil Steril,*Vol. 93, No. 2, (February 2009), pp. 586-591, ISSN 1556-5653

Han, M.; Kim, J.; Kim, H.; Je, G. & Hwang, T. (2004). Bilateral ovarian pregnancy after *in vitro* fertilization and embryo transfer in a patient with tubal factor infertility. *J Assist Reprod Genet,* Vol. 21, No. 5, (May 2004), pp. 181-183, ISSN 1573-7330

Hassiakos, D.; Bakas, P.; Pistofidis, G. & Creatsas, G. (2002). Heterotopic pregnancy at 16 weeks of gestation after in-vitro fertilization and embryo transfer. *Arch Gynecol Obstet,* Vol. 266, No. 3, (July 2002), pp. 124-125, ISSN 1432-0711

Horne, A. W.; Shaw, J. L. V.; Murdoch, A.; McDonald, S. E.; Williams, A. R.; Jabbour, H. N.; Duncan, W. C. & Critchley, H. O. D. (2011). Placental Growth Factor: A Promising

Diagnostic Biomarker for Tubal Ectopic Pregnancy. *J Clin Endocrinol Metab,* Vol. 96, No. 1, (January 2011), pp. E104–E108, ISSN 1945-7197

Hsieh, B. C.; Hwang, J. L.; Pan, H. S.; Huang, S. C.; Chen, C. Y. & Chen, P. H. (2004). Heterotopic Caesarean scar pregnancy combined with intrauterine pregnancy successfully treated with embryo aspiration for selective embryo reduction: case report. *Hum. Reprod,* Vol. 19, No. 2, (February 2004), pp. 285-287, ISSN 1460-2350

Hsu, C. C.; Yang, T. T. & Hsu, CT. (2005). Ovarian pregnancy resulting from cornual fistulae in a woman who had undergone bilateral salpingectomy. *Fertil Steril,* Vol. 83, No. 1, (January 2005), pp. 205-207, ISSN 1556-5653

Hu, D.; Hook, E. W. & Goldie, S. J. (2004). Screening for Chlamydia trachomatis in women 15 to 29 years of age: a cost-effectiveness analysis. *Ann Intern Med,* Vol. 141, No. 7, (October 2004), pp. 501-513, ISSN 1539-3704

Imudia, A. N.; Suzuki, Y.; Kilburn, B. A.; Yelian, F. D.; Diamond, M. P.; Romero, R. & Armant, D. R. (2009). Retrieval of trophoblast cells from the cervical canal for prediction of abnormal pregnancy: a pilot study. *Human Reproduction,* Vol. 24, No. 9, (September 2009), pp. 2086-2092, ISSN 1460-2350

Irvine, L. M.; Evans, D. G. & Setchell, M. E. (1999). Ectopic pregnancies in two consecutive menstrual cycles. *J R Soc Med,* Vol. 92, No. 8, (August 1999), pp. 413-414, ISSN 1758-1095

Ishihara, O.; Kuwahara, A. & Saitoh H. (2011). Frozen-thawed blastocyst transfer reduces ectopic pregnancy risk: an analysis of single embryo transfer cycles in Japan. *Fertil Steril,* Vol. 95, No. 6, (May 2011), pp. 1966-1969, ISSN 1556-5653

Jozwiak, E. A.; Ulug, U.; Akman, M. A. & Bahceci, M. (2003). Successful resection of a heterotopic cervical pregnancy resulting from intracytoplasmic sperm injection. *Fertil Steril,* Vol. 79, No. 2, (February 2003), pp. 428-430, ISSN 1556-5653

Jun, S. H. & Milki, AA. (2007). Ectopic pregnancy rates with frozen compared with fresh blastocyst transfer. *Fertil Steril,* Vol. 88, No. 3, (September 2007), pp. 629-631, ISSN 1556-5653

Kamath, M. S.; Aleyamma, T. K.; Muthukumar, K.; Kumar, R. M. & George, K. (2010). A rare case report: ovarian heterotopic pregnancy after *in vitro* fertilization. *Fertil Steril,* Vol. 94, No. 5, (October 2010), pp. 1910. e9-11, ISSN 1556-5653

Karande, V. C.; Flood, J. T.; Heard, N.; Veeck, L. & Muasher, S. J. (1991). Analysis of ectopic pregnancies resulting from in-vitro fertilization and embryo transfer. *Hum Reprod,* Vol. 6, No. 3, (March 1991), pp. 446-449, ISSN 1460-2350

Karikoski, R.; Aine, R. & Heinonen, P. K. (1993). Abnormal embryogenesis in the etiology of ectopic pregnancy. *Gynecol Obstet Invest,* Vol. 36, No. 3, (1993), pp. 158-162, ISSN 1423-002X

Keegan, D. A.; Morelli, S. S.; Noyes, N.; Flisser, E. D.; Berkeley, A. S. & Grifo, J. A. (2007). Low ectopic pregnancy rates after *in vitro* fertilization: do practice habits matter? *Fertil Steril,* Vol. 88, No. 3, (September 2007), pp. 734-736, ISSN 1556-5653

Kemp, B.; Kertschanska, S.; Handt, S.; Funk, A.; Kaufmann, P. & Rath, W. (1999). Different placentation patterns in viable compared with nonviable tubal pregnancy suggest a divergent clinical management. *Am J Obstet Gynecol,* Vol. 181, No. 3, (September 1999), pp. 615-620, ISSN 1097-6868

Kemp, B.; Kertschanska, S.; Kadyrov, M.; Rath, W.; Kaufmann, P. & Huppertz, B. (2002). Invasive depth of extravillous trophoblast correlates with cellular phenotype: a comparison of intraand extrauterine implantation sites. *Histochem Cell Biol*, Vol. 117, No. 5, (May 2002), pp. 401-414, ISSN 1432-119X

Kirk, E.; Condous, G.; Haider, Z.; Lu, C.; Van Huffel, S.; Timmerman, D. & Bourne, T. (2006). The practical application of a mathematical model to predict the outcome of pregnancies of unknown location. *Ultrasound Obstet Gynecol*, Vol. 27, No. 3, (March 2006), pp. 311-315, ISSN 1469-0705

Kirk, E.; Papageorghiou A. T.; Van Calster, B.; Condous, G.; Cowans, N.; Van Huffel, S.; Timmerman, D.; Spencer, K. & Bourne, T. (2009). The use of serum inhibin A and activin A levels in predicting the outcome of 'pregnancies of unknown location'. *Hum Reprod*, Vol. 24, No. 10, (October 2009), pp. 2451-2456, ISSN 1460-2350

Klatsky, P. C.; Lane, D. E.; Ryan, I. P. & Fujimoto, V. Y. (2007). The effect of fibroids without cavity involvement on ART outcomes independent of ovarian age. *Hum Reprod*, Vol. 22, No. 2, (February 2007), pp. 521-526, ISSN 1460-2350

Knopman, J. M.; Talebian, S.; Keegan, D. A. & Grifo, J. A. (2007). Heterotopic abdominal pregnancy following two-blastocyst embryo transfer. *Fertil Steril*, Vol. 88, No. 5, (November 2007), pp. 1437. e13-5, ISSN 1556-5653

Korkontzelos, I.; Tsirkas, P.; Antoniou, N.; Akrivis, C.; Tsirka, A. & Hadjopoulos, G. (2006). Mild ovarian hyperstimulation syndrome coexisting with ectopic pregnancy after *in vitro* fertilization. *Clin Exp Obstet Gynecol*, Vol. 33, No. 3, (2006), pp. 148-150, ISSN 0390-6663

Kosmas, I. P.; Janssens, R.; De Munck, L.; Al Turki, H.; Van der Elst, J.; Tournaye, H. & Devroey, P. (2007). Ultrasound-guided embryo transfer does not offer any benefit in clinical outcome: a randomized controlled trial. *Hum Reprod*, Vol. 22, No. 5, (May 2007), pp. 1327-1334, ISSN 1460-2350

Laskarin, G.; Redzovic, A.; Srsen Medancic, S. & Rukavina, D. (2010). Regulation of NK-cell functions by mucins via antigen-presenting cells. *Medical Hypotheses*, Vol. 75, No. 6, (December 2010), pp. 541-543, ISSN 1532-2777

Ledger, W.; Clark, A.; Olesnicky, G. & Norman, R. (1992). Life-threatening rupture of an interstitial ectopic pregnancy arising from oocyte donation: failure of early detection by quantitive human chorionic gonadotropin (hCG) and progesterone estimation. *J Assist Reprod Genet*, Vol. 9, No. 3, (June 1992), pp. 289-291, ISSN 1573-7330

Leke, R. J.; Goyaux, N.; Matsuda, T. & Thonneau, P. F. (2004). Ectopic pregnancy in Africa: a population-based study. *Obstet Gynecol*, Vol. 103, No. 4, (April 2004), pp. 692-697, ISSN 1873-233X

Litwicka, K.; Greco, E.; Prefumo, F.; Fratelli, N.; Scarselli, F.; Ferrero, S.; Iammarrone, E. & Frusca, T. (2011). Successful management of a triplet heterotopic caesarean scar pregnancy after *in vitro* fertilization-embryo transfer. *Fertil. Steril*, Vol. 95, No. 1, (January 2011), pp. 291. e1-3, ISSN 1556-5653

MacRae, R.; Olowu, O.; Rizzuto, M. I. & Odejinmi, F. (2009). Diagnosis and laparoscopic management of 11 consecutive cases of cornual ectopic pregnancy. *Arch Gynecol Obstet*, Vol. 280, No. 1, (July 2009), pp. 59-64, ISSN 1432-0711

Mantzavinos, T.; Kanakas, N. & Mavrelos, K. (1994). Ovarian pregnancies after oocyte donation in three menopausal patients treated by laparoscopy. *J Assist Reprod Genet*, Vol. 11, No. 6, (July 1994), pp. 319-320, ISSN 1573-7330

Margalioth, E. J.; Ben-Chetrit, A.; Gal, M. & Eldar-Geva, T. (2006). Investigation and treatment of repeated implantation failure following IVF-ET. *Hum Reprod,* Vol. 21, No. 12, (December 2006), pp. 3036-3043, ISSN 1460-2350

Milki, A. A. & Jun, S. H. (2003). Ectopic pregnancy rates with day 3 versus day 5 embryo transfer: a retrospective analysis. *BMC Pregnancy Childbirth,* Vol. 3, No. 1, (November 2003), pp. 7, ISSN 1471-2393

Mol, B. W.; van der Veen, F. & Bossuyt, P. M. (2002). Symptom-free women at increased risk of ectopic pregnancy: should we screen? Acta Obstet Gynecol *Scand,* Vol. 81, No. 7, (July 2002), pp. 661-672, ISSN 1600-0412

Molloy, D.; Deambrosis, W.; Keeping, D.; Hynes, J.; Harrison, K. & Hennessey, J. (1990). Multiple-sited (heterotopic) pregnancy after *in vitro* fertilization and gamete intrafallopian transfer. *Fertil Steril,* Vol. 53, No. 6, (June 1990), pp. 1068-1071, ISSN 1556-5653

Moores, K. L.; Keriakos, R. H.; Anumba, D. O.; Connor, M. E., & Lashen, H. (2010). Management challenges of a live 12-week sub-hepatic intra-abdominal pregnancy Picaud. *BJOG,* Vol. 117, No. 3, (February 2010), pp. 365-368, ISSN 1471-0528

Musa, J.; Daru, P. H.; Mutihir, J. T. & Ujah, I. A. (2009). Ectopic pregnancy in Jos Northern Nigeria: prevalence and impact on subsequent fertility. *Niger J Med,* Vol. 18, No. 1, (January-March 2009), pp. 35-38, ISSN 1115-2613

Muzíková, D.; Visnová, H.; Ventruba, P. & Juránková, E. (2003). Recurrent interstitial pregnancy in uterine horn after IVF/ET. *Ceska Gynekol,* Vol. 68, No. 3, (May 2003), pp. 201-203, ISSN 1210-7832

Nichols, C.; Koong, D.; Faulkner, K. & Thompson, G. (1995). A hepatic ectopic pregnancy treated with direct methotrexate injection. *Aust N Z J Obstet Gynaecol,* Vol. 35, No. 2, (May 1995), pp. 221-223, ISSN 1479-828X

Nikolaou, D. S.; Lavery, S.; Bevan, R.; Margara, R. & Trew, G. (2002). Triplet heterotopic pregnancy with an intrauterine monochorionic diamniotic twin pregnancy and an interstitial pregnancy following *in vitro* fertilisation and transfer of two embryos. *J Obstet Gynaecol,* Vol. 22, No. 1, (January 2002), pp. 94-95, ISSN 1364-6893

Nitke, S.; Horowitz, E.; Farhi, J.; Krissi, H. & Shalev, J. (2007). Combined intrauterine and twin cervical pregnancy managed by a new conservative modality. *Fertil Steril,* Vol. 88, No. 3, (September 2007), pp. 706. e1-3, ISSN 1556-5653

Obeidat, B.; Zayed, F.; Amarin, Z.; Obeidat, N. & El-Jallad, M. F. (2010). Tubal ectopic pregnancy in the north of Jordan: presentation and management. Clin Exp *Obstet Gynecol,* Vol. 37, No. 2, (2010), pp. 138-140, ISSN 0390-6663

Oki, T.; Douchi, T.; Nakamura, S.; Maruta, K.; Ijuin, H. & Nagata, Y. (1998). A woman with three ectopic pregnancies after in-vitro fertilization and embryo transfer. *Hum Reprod,* Vol. 13, No. 2, (February 1998), pp. 468-470, ISSN 1460-2350

Okohue, J. E.; Ikimalo, J. I. & Omoregie, O. B. (2010). Ectopic pregnancy following *in vitro* fertilisation and embryo transfer. *West Afr J Med,* Vol. 29, No. 5, (September-October 2010), pp. 349-351, ISSN 0189-160X

Orvieto, R.; Kruchkovich, J.; Zohav, E.; Rabinson, J.; Anteby, E. Y. & Meltcer, S. (2007). Does methotrexate treatment for ectopic pregnancy influence the patient's performance during a subsequent *in vitro* fertilization/embryo transfer cycle? *Fertil Steril,* Vol. 88, No. 6, (December 2007), pp. 1685-1686, ISSN 1556-5653

Pacchiarotti, A.; Mohamed, M. A.; Micara, G.; Tranquilli, D.; Linari, A.; Espinola, S. M. & Aragona, C. (2007). The impact of the depth of embryo replacement on IVF outcome. *J. Assist. Reprod. Genet*, Vol. 24, No. 5, (May 2007), pp. 189-193, ISSN 1573-7330

Pan, H. S.; Chuang, J.; Chiu, S. F.; Hsieh, B. C.; Lin, Y. H.; Tsai, Y. L.; Huang, S. C.; Hsieh, M. L.; Chen, C. Y. & Hwang, J. L. (2002). Heterotopic triplet pregnancy: report of a case with bilateral tubal pregnancy and an intrauterine pregnancy. *Hum. Reprod*, Vol. 17, No. 5, (May 2002), pp. 1363-1366, ISSN 1460-2350

Pantos, K.; Meimeti-Damianaki, T.; Vaxevanoglou, T. & Kapetanakis, E. (1993). Oocyte donation in menopausal women aged over 40 years. *Hum Reprod*, Vol. 8, No. 3, (March 1993), pp. 488-491, ISSN 1460-2350

Paul, P. G.; Koshy, A. K. & Thomas, T. (2006). Hum Reprod. Pregnancy outcomes following laparoscopic myomectomy and single-layer myometrial closure. Vol. 21, No. 12, (December 2006), pp. 3278-3781, ISSN 1460-2350

Peleg, D.; Bar-Hava, I.; Neuman-Levin, M.; Ashkenazi, J. & Ben-Rafael, Z. (1994). Early diagnosis and successful nonsurgical treatment of viable combined intrauterine and cervical pregnancy. *Fertil Steril*, Vol. 62, No. 2, (August 1994), pp. 405-458, ISSN 1556-5653

Pérez, J. A.; Sadek, M. M.; Savale, M.; Boyer, P. & Zorn, J. R. (1993). Local medical treatment of interstitial pregnancy after in-vitro fertilization and embryo transfer (IVF-ET): two case reports. *Hum Reprod*, Vol. 8, No. 4, (April 1993), pp. 631-634, ISSN 1460-2350

Picaud, A.; Berthonneau, J. P.; Nlome-Nze, A. R.; Ogowet-Igumu, N.; Engongah-Beka, T. & Faye, A. (1991). Serology of Chlamydia and ectopic pregnancies. Incidence of Fitz-Hugh-Curtis syndrome. *J Gynecol Obstet Biol Reprod (Paris)*, Vol. 20, No. 2, (1991), pp. 209-215, ISSN 0150-9918

Pisarska, M. D.; Casson, P. R.; Moise K. J. Jr.; DiMaio D. J; Buster J. E. & Carson S. A., (1998). Heterotopic abdominal pregnancy treated at laparoscopy. *Fertil Steril*, Vol. 70, No. 1, (July 1998), pp. 159-160, ISSN 1556-5653

Postma, M. J.; Bakker, A.; Welte, R.; van Bergen, J. E.; van den Hoek, J. A.; de Jong-van den Berg, L. T. & Jager, J. C. (2000). Screening for asymptomatic Chlamydia trachomatis infection in pregnancy; cost-effectiveness favorable at a minimum prevalence rate of 3% or more. *Ned Tijdschr Geneeskd*, Vol. 144, No. 49, (December 2000), pp. 2350-2354, ISSN 1876-8784

Postma, M. J.; Welte, R.; van den Hoek, J. A.; van Doornum, G. J.; Coutinho, R. A. & Jager, JC. (1999). Opportunistic screening for genital infections with Chlamydia trachomatis in sexually active population of Amsterdam. II. Cost-effectiveness analysis of screening women. *Ned Tijdschr Geneeskd*, Vol. 143, No. 13, (March 1999), pp. 677-681, ISSN 1876-8784

Prorocic, M. & Vasiljevic, M. (2007). Treatment of heterotopic cervical pregnancy after *in vitro* fertilization-embryo transfer by using transvaginal ultrasound-guided aspiration and instillation of hypertonic solution of sodium chloride. *Fertil. Steril*, Vol. 88, No. 4, (October 2007), pp. 969. e3-5, ISSN 1556-5653

Pyrgiotis, E.; Sultan, K. M.; Neal, G. S.; Liu, H. C.; Grifo, J. A. & Rosenwaks, Z. (1994). Ectopic pregnancies after *in vitro* fertilization and embryo transfer. *J Assist Reprod Genet*, Vol. 11, No. 2, (February 1994), pp. 79-84, ISSN 1573-7330

Qin, L.; Li, S. & Tan, S. (2008). Laparoscopic loop ligature for selective therapy in heterotopic interstitial and intrauterine pregnancy following in-vitro fertilization and embryo transfer. *Int J Gynaecol Obstet*, Vol. 101, No. 1, (April 2008), pp. 80-81, ISSN 1879-3479

Qublan, H.; Tahat, Y. & Al-Masri, A. (2008). Primary ovarian pregnancy after the empty follicle syndrome: a case report. *J Obstet Gynaecol Res*, Vol. 34, No. 3, (June 2008), pp. 422-424, ISSN 1341-8076

Raziel, A.; Schachter, M.; Mordechai, E.; Friedler, S.; Panski, M. & Ron-El, R. (2004). Ovarian pregnancy-a 12-year experience of 19 cases in one institution. *Eur J Obstet Gynecol Reprod Biol*, Vol. 114, No. 1, (May 2004), pp. 92-96, ISSN 1872-7654

Refaat, B.; Al-Azemi, M.; Geary, I.; Eley, A. & Ledger, W. (2009). Role of Activins and Inducible Nitric Oxide in the Pathogenesis of Ectopic Pregnancy in Patients with or without Chlamydia trachomatis Infection. Clinical and Vaccine *Immunology*, Vol. 16, No. 10, (October 2009), pp. 1493-1503, ISSN 1556-679X

Revel, A.; Ophir, I.; Koler, M.; Achache, H. & Prus, D. (2008). Changing etiology of tubal pregnancy following IVF. *Hum Reprod*, Vol. 23, No. 6, (June 2008), pp. 1372-1376, ISSN 1460-2350

Rizk, B.; Tan, S. L.; Morcos, S.; Riddle, A.; Brinsden, P.; Mason, B. A. & Edwards, R. G. (1991). Heterotopic pregnancies after *in vitro* fertilization and embryo transfer. *Am J Obstet Gynecol*, Vol. 164, No. 1 Pt 1, (January 1991), pp. 161-164, ISSN 1097-6868

Roberts, T. E.; Robinson, S.; Barton, P. M.; Bryan, S.; McCarthy, A.; Macleod, J.; Egger, M. & Low, N. (2007). Cost effectiveness of home based population screening for Chlamydia trachomatis in the UK: economic evaluation of chlamydia screening studies (ClaSS) project. *BMJ*, Vol. 335, No. 7614, (August 2007), pp. 291, ISSN 1468-5833

Rosman, ER.; Keegan, D. A.; Krey, L.; Liu, M.; Licciardi, F. & Grifo, J. A., (2009). Ectopic pregnancy rates after *in vitro* fertilization: a look at the donor egg population. *Fertil Steril*, Vol. 92, No. 5, (November 2009), pp. 1791-1793, ISSN 1556-5653

Savaris, R. F.; Hamilton, A. E.; Lessey, B. A. & Giudice, L. C. (2008). Endometrial Gene Expression in Early Pregnancy: Lessons from Human Ectopic Pregnancy. *Reprod Sci*, Vol. 15, No. 8, (October 2008), pp. 797-816, ISSN 1933-7205

Schepens, J. J.; Mol, B. W.; Wiegerinck, M. A.; Houterman, S. & Koks, C. A. (2010). Pregnancy outcomes and prognostic factors from tubal sterilization reversal by sutureless laparoscopical re-anastomosis: a retrospective cohort study. *Hum Reprod*, Vol. 26, No. 2, (February 2010), pp. 354-359, ISSN 1460-2350

Schiøtz, H. A. & Csángó, P. A. (1991). Asymptomatic genital infection by Chlamydia trachomatis in women. A cost analysis of control check-ups. *Tidsskr Nor Laegeforen*, Vol. 111, No. 7, (March 1991), pp. 848-850, ISSN 0807-7096

Schippert, C.; Bassler, C.; Soergel, P.; Hille, U.; Hollwitz, B. & Garcia-Rocha, G. J. (2010). Reconstructive, organ-preserving microsurgery in tubal infertility: still an alternative to *in vitro* fertilization. *Fertil Steril*, Vol. 93, No. 4, (March 2010), pp. 1359-1361, ISSN 1556-5653

Schumacher, A.; Brachwitz, N.; Sohr, S.; Engeland, K.; Langwisch, S.; Dolaptchieva, M.; Alexander, T.; Taran, A.; Malfertheiner, S. F.; Dan Costa, S.; Zimmermann, G.; Nitschke, C.; Volk, H. D.; Alexander, H.; Gunzer, M. & Zenclussen, A. C. (2009). Human Chorionic Gonadotropin Attracts Regulatory T-Cells into the Fetal-

Maternal Interface during Early Human Pregnancy. *J Immunol*, Vol. 182, No. 9, (May 2009), pp. 5488-5497, ISSN 1550-6606

Seracchioli, R.; Manuzzi, L.; Vianello, F.; Gualerzi, B.; Savelli, L.; Paradisi, R. & Venturoli, S. (2006). Obstetric and delivery outcome of pregnancies achieved after laparoscopic myomectomy. *Fertil Steril*, Vol. 86, No. 1 (July 2006), pp. 159-165, ISSN 1556-5653

Seror, V.; Gelfucci, F.; Gerbaud, L.; Pouly, J. L.; Fernandez, H.; Job-Spira, N.; Bouyer, J. & Coste, J. (2007). Care pathways for ectopic pregnancy: a population-based cost-effectiveness analysis. *Fertil Steril*, Vol. 87, No. 4, (April 2007), pp. 737-748, ISSN 1556-5653

Shah, A. A.; Grotegut, C. A.; Likes, C. E; Miller, M. J. & Walmer, D. K. (2009). Heterotopic cervical pregnancy treated with transvaginal ultrasound-guided aspiration resulting in cervical site varices within the myometrium. *Fertil Steril*, Vol. 91, No. 3, (March 2009), pp. 934. e19-22, ISSN 1556-5653

Shao, R.; Nutu, M.; Weijdegard, B.; Egecioglu, E.; Fernandez-Rodriguez, J.; Karlsson-Lindah, L.; Gemzell-Danielsson, K.; Bergh, C. & Billig, H. (2009). Clomiphene Citrate Causes Aberrant Tubal Apoptosis and Estrogen Receptor Activation in Rat Fallopian Tube: Implications for Tubal Ectopic Pregnancy. *Biol Reprod*, Vol. 80, No. 6, (June 2009), pp. 1262-1271, ISSN 1529-7268

Shih, C. C.; Lee, R. K. & Hwu, Y. M. (2007). Cul-de-sac pregnancy following *in vitro* fertilization and embryo transfer. *Taiwan J Obstet Gynecol*, Vol. 46, No. 2, (June 2007), pp. 171-173, ISSN 1875-6263

Shukla, V. K.; Pandey, S.; Pandey, L. K.; Roy, S. K. & Vaidya, M. P. (1985). Primary hepatic pregnancy. *Postgrad Med J*, Vol. 61, No. 719, (September 1985), pp. 831-832, ISSN 1469-0756

Srivastava, P.; Jha, R.; Bas, S.; Salhan S. & Mitta, A. (2008). In infertile women, cells from Chlamydia trachomatis infected site release higher levels of interferon-gamma, interleukin-10 and tumor necrosis factor-alpha upon heat shock protein stimulation than fertile women. *Reprod Biol Endocrinol*, Vol. 6, No. 20, (May 2008), ISSN 1477-7827

Sziller, I.; Fedorcsak, P.; Csapo, Z.; Szirmai, K.; Linhares, I. M.; Papp, Z. & Witkin, S. S. (2008). Circulating Antibodies to a Conserved Epitope of the Chlamydia Trachomatis 60-kDa Heat Shock Protein is Associated with Decreased Spontaneous Fertility Rate in Ectopic Pregnant Women Treated by Salpingectomy. *Am J Reprod Immunol*, Vol. 59, No. 2, (February 2008), pp. 99-104, ISSN 1600-0897

Tan, H. H. & Loh, S. F. (2010). Microsurgical reversal of sterilisation - is this still clinically relevant today? *Ann Acad Med Singapore*, Vol. 39, No. 1 (January 2010), pp. 22-26, ISSN 0304-4602

Toikkanen, S., Joensuu, H. & Erkkola, R. (1993). DNA aneuploidy in ectopic pregnancy and spontaneous abortions. *Eur J Obstet Gynecol Reprod Biol*, Vol. 51, No. 1, (September 1993), pp. 9-13, ISSN 1872-7654

Toth, M.; Patton, D. L.; Campbell, L. A.; Carretta, E. I.; Mouradian, J.; Toth, A.; Shevchuk, M.; Baergen, R. & Ledger. W. (2000). Detection of Chlamydial Antigenic Material in Ovarian, Prostatic, Ectopic Pregnancy and Semen Samples of Culture-Negative Subjects. *Am J Reprod Immunol*, Vol. 43, No. 4, (April 2000), pp. 218-222, ISSN 1600-0897

Trachtenberg, A. I.; Washington, A. E. & Halldorson, S. (1988). A cost-based decision analysis for Chlamydia screening in California family planning clinics. *Obstet Gynecol*, Vol. 71, No. 1 (January 1988), pp. 101-108, ISSN 1873-233X

van der Weiden, R. M. & Karsdorp, V. H. (2005). Recurrent cornual pregnancy after heterotopic cornual pregnancy successfully treated with systemic methotrexate. *Arch Gynecol Obstet*, Vol. 273, No. 3, (December 2005), pp. 180-181, ISSN 1432-0711

van Valkengoed, I. G.; Postma, M. J.; Morré, S. A.; van den Brule, A. J.; Meijer, C. J.; Bouter, L. M. & Boeke, A. J. (2001). Cost effectiveness analysis of a population based screening programme for asymptomatic Chlamydia trachomatis infections in women by means of home obtained urine specimens. *Sex Transm Infect*, Vol. 77, No. 4, (August 2001), pp. 276-282, ISSN 1472-3263

Vimercati, A.; Scioscia, M.; Lorusso, F.; Laera, A. F.; Lamanna, G.; Coluccia, A.; Bettocchi, S.; Selvaggi, L. & Depalo, R. (2007). Do uterine fibroids affect IVF outcomes? *Reprod Biomed Online*, Vol. 15, No. 6, (December 2007), pp. 686-691, ISSN 1472-6491

von Rango, U.; Classen-Linke, I.; Raven, G.; Bocken, F. & Beier, H. M. (2003). Cytokine microenvironments in human first trimester decidua are dependent on trophoblast cells. *Fertil Steril*, Vol. 79, No. 5, (May 2003), pp. 1176-1186, ISSN 1556-5653

Wang, C. J.; Tsai, F.; Chen, C. & Chao, A. (2010). Hysteroscopic management of heterotopic cesarean scar pregnancy. *Fertil Steril*, Vol. 94, No. 4, (September 2010), pp. 1529. e15-8, ISSN 1556-5653

Wang, C. N.; Chen, C. K.; Wang, H. S.; Chiueh, H. Y. & Soong, Y. K. (2007). Successful management of heterotopic cesarean scar pregnancy combined with intrauterine pregnancy after *in vitro* fertilization-embryo transfer. *Fertil Steril*, Vol. 88, No. 3, (September 2007), pp. 706. e13-6, ISSN 1556-5653

Wicherek, L.; Basta, P.; Pitynski, K.; Marianowski, P.; Kijowski, J.; Wiatr, J. & Majka, M. (2009). The Characterization of the Subpopulation of Suppressive $B7H4^+$ Macrophages and the Subpopulation of $CD25^+$ $CD4^+$ and $FOXP3^+$ Regulatory T-cells in Decidua during the Secretory Cycle Phase, Arias Stella Reaction, and Spontaneous Abortion - A Preliminary Report. *Am J Reprod Immunol*, Vol. 61, No. 4, (April 2009), pp. 303-312, ISSN 1600-0897

Yanaihara, A.; Yorimitsu, T.; Motoyama, H.; Ohara, M. & Kawamura, T. (2008). Clinical outcome of frozen blastocyst transfer; single vs. double transfer. *J Assist Reprod Genet*, Vol. 25, No. 11-12, (November-December 2008), pp. 531-534, ISSN 1573-7330

Yang, X. Y.; Yu, H.; Li, K. M.; Chu, Y. X. & Zheng, A. (2010). Uterine artery embolisation combined with local methotrexate for treatment of caesarean scar pregnancy. *BJOG*, Vol. 117, No. 8, (July 2010), pp. 990-996, ISSN 1471-0528

Yao, M.; Tulandi, T.; Kaplow, M. & Smith, A. P. (1996). A comparison of methotrexate versus laparoscopic surgery for the treatment of ectopic pregnancy: a cost analysis. *Hum Reprod*, Vol. 11, No. 12, (December 1996), pp. 2762-2766, ISSN 1460-2350

4

Hysteroscopic Endometrial Embryo Delivery (HEED)

M.M. Kamrava, L. Tran and J.L. Hall
[1]*West Coast IVF Clinic*
[2]*LA Center for Embryo Implantation*
[3]*UCLA, the Geffen School of Medicine*
USA

1. Introduction

It has been over 30 years since the first successful pregnancy using in vitro fertilization (IVF). There have been major advancements in the different components of IVF such as ovulation induction protocols, oocyte retrieval techniques, and culture medium tailored to improving embryo quality (Gardner 1998). However, the discrepancy between women undergoing IVF with normal embryo development and live pregnancy rates continues to exist. It is estimated that up to 85% of replaced embryos fail to implant despite the selection of apparently normal embryos for transfer (Sallam 2002). This failure rate suggests that the embryo transfer stage is a key step to successful live pregnancy rates in assisted reproductive technology (ART) (Meldrum 1987).

Embryo transfer is traditionally performed by "blindly" replacing the embryos into the uterine cavity utilizing a transcervical catheter at approximately 2-5 days of development. This technique relies highly on the skill and tactile senses of the clinician. Many clinicians will transfer the embryos at a fixed distance (6 cm) from the external os; however, with varying cervical lengths and uterine anatomy, this often does not ensure optimal placement (Brown 2007). Recently, there have been many studies proposing potential embryo transfer related factors to the low success rate in pregnancy outcomes such as uterine contractions, expulsion of embryos, blood or mucus on the catheter tip, bacterial contamination of the catheter, and retained embryos (Schoolcraft 2001). Ultrasound guided embryo transfer (UGET) is currently suggested as the standard clinical practice and appears to improve the chances of live/ongoing and clinical pregnancies compared with clinical touch methods (Brown 2007). However, controversies still remain regarding the actual benefit of UGET in successful clinical pregnancy rates (Kosmas 1999). The subendometrial embryo delivery (SEED) technique has been previously reported to increase pregnancy rates and eliminate ectopic pregnancies associated with ART (KAMRAVA 2010). In this study, we set out to use a similar technique which utilized a mini-hysteroscope with a flexible catheter for direct delivery of embryo(s) at the 4-12 cell stage onto the endometrium under direct visualization. The hysteroscopic visual guidance ensures more precise and reliable placement at the desired location of the endometrium.

2. Materials and methods

Patients. 35 patients between 22and 46 years of age undergoing IVF were included in this report. Informed consent was obtained prior to the start of the cycle. Controlled ovarian hyperstimulation was initiated with Follitropin β (Follistim®, Organon Pharmaceuticals, Inc.). Endogenous gonadotropins surge (i.e., the prevention of an LH surge) was controlled with ganirelix acetate (Antagon™, Organon Pharmaceuticals, Inc.). Oocyte retrieval was carried out in an office setting under local anesthesia and mild sedation. Oocytes were fertilized and cultured in a human tubal fluid formulated medium at 37 degrees C and 5% CO_2 in air". Embryos were transferred at 48-72 hours post fertilization (Figure 1a). All women received some type of luteal support, be it progesterone or hCG (3000 IU of hCG at 3 and 6 days post retrieval) (Figure 1b, c). Serum hCG was quantified at 10 days after the last hCG; a concentration of 5 IU/ml with a delayed menses was used as confirmation of pregnancy.

Description of Hysteroscopic Endometrial Embryo Delivery (HEED):

A transvaginal ultrasound of the uterus is performed and the direction and thickness of the endometrial lining is ascertained. With patient in dorsolithotomy position, a bivalved speculum is placed in the vagina and the cervix exposed. Vagina and cervix are washed with modified HAM's solution. Subsequently, 10 cc of 1% xylocaine is injected bilaterally in the utero-sacral nerve endings.

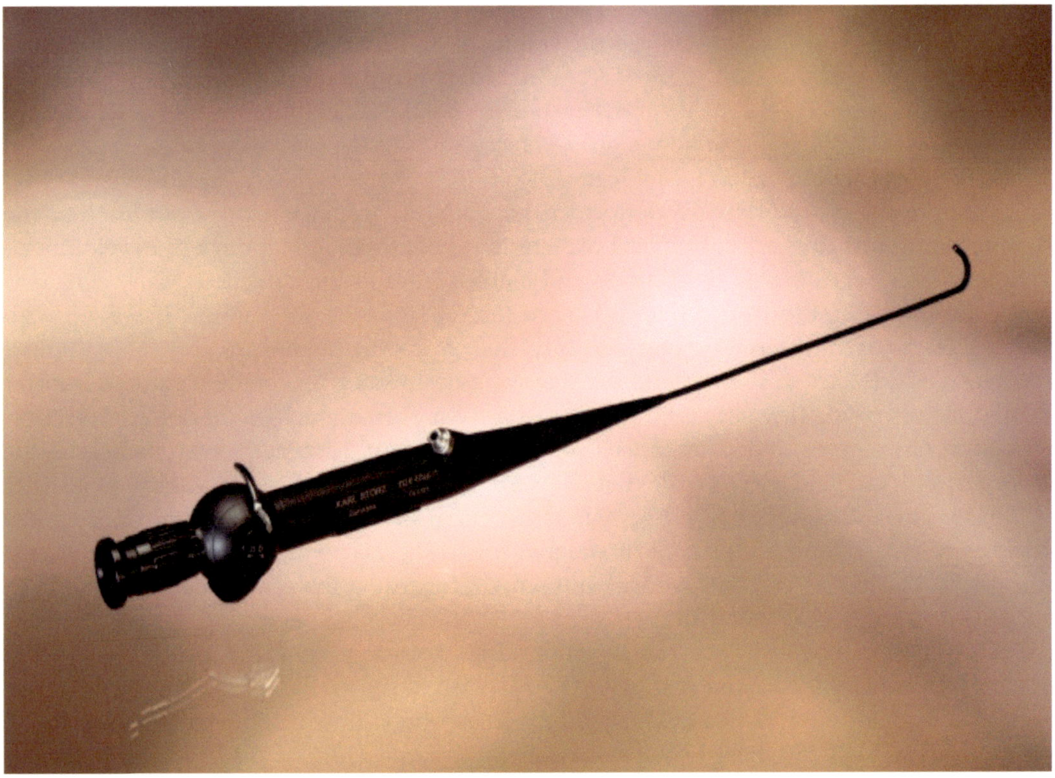

Fig. 1. Mini flexible hysteroscope (Storz®, LA, CA USA)

The cervix is grasped with an allis clamp and stabilized. Nitrogen gas is used as the distention media throughout the procedure via a hysteroscopic insufflator. A 3 mm flexible hysteroscope (Figure 1) loaded with embryo catheter containing the embryos (Figure 2) is then gently inserted through the cervical os under direct visualization of the cervical canal into the uterine cavity. Once the cavity is visualized, it is then further advanced to the fundus of the uterus. The loaded embryo transfer catheter (Precision Reproduction, LA, CA USA) is then advanced to 1.5 cm from the tip of the hysteroscope and placed over the point of embryo deposition, half way between the lowest point of the fundus in the midline and the tubal opening into the uterus (Figure 3). The embryos are then gently released by the embryologist. Our results show that hysteroscopic guided early embryo transfer results in a high pregnancy outcome, 2-3x greater than "blind" transfer technique rates. Direct visualization provides an objective, visually confirmed, replicable technique for embryo transfer. The end result is less operator dependent and in contrast to routine ET techniques in which operator experience may account for the variable overall pregnancy rates (Garcia 2002). Hysteroscopic direct embryo delivery may circumvent many of the known and previously reported embryo transfer related factors associated with poor outcomes. Many of our patients had failed prior IVF-ET attempts due to multiple etiologies.

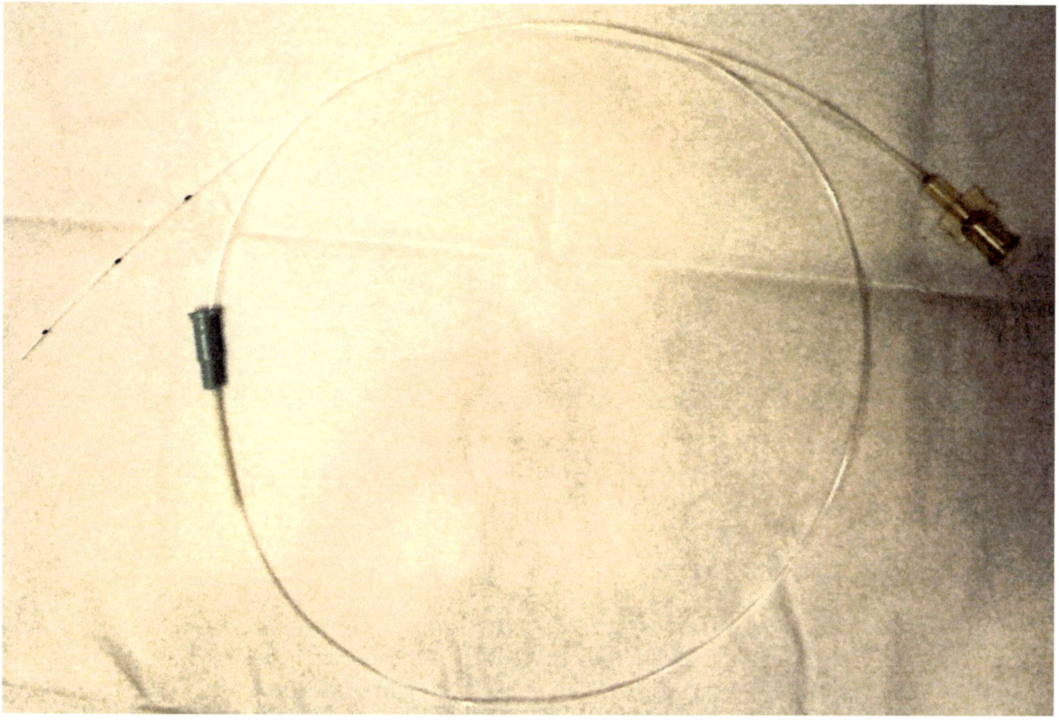

Fig. 2. The flexible catheter for embryo delivery (Precision Reproduction, LLC. LA, CA USA)

A light weight flexible minihysteroscope was used for visualization of the endometrial cavity (Figure 1d) (Storz®, LA, CA USA). The scope incorporates a flexible distal end of 3mm in diameter with a straight through operating channel. In addition, the optic filter is directly connected to a light source, decreasing the weight of the scope and giving a better "feel" for the scope. The transfer catheter (Precision Reproduction, LLC, LA, CA USA) is polycarbonate based with a tapered tip (to 500 μm), beveled to 60°.

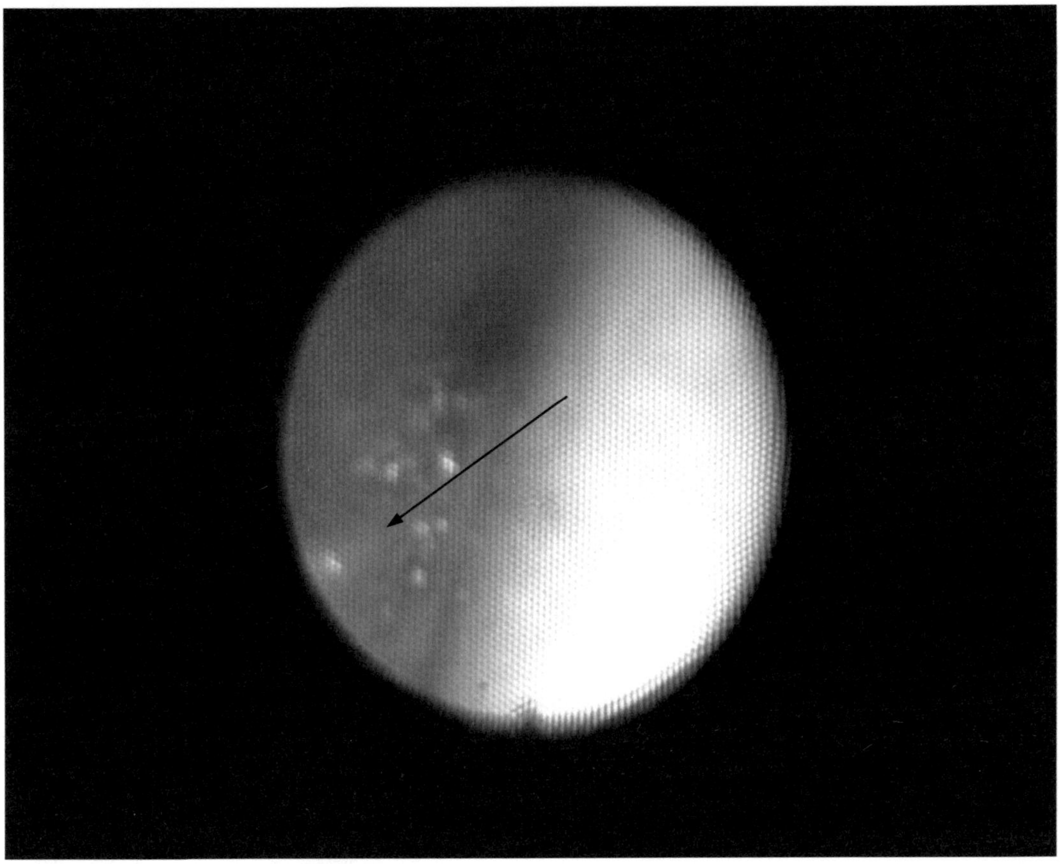

Fig. 3. Placement of embryo(s) under hysteroscopic guidance; arrow points to the tip of the catheter; catheter entry at 8 o'clock position.

3. Results

35 cycles were started and all had retrievals. 22 cycles involved use of intra-cytoplasmic sperm injection (ICSI) due to male factor problems. Endometrial thickness varied between 7 and 16 mm. 22 cycles had transfers on day 2 and 13 cycles had transfers on day 3. There were 16 positive β hCG's greater than 5 IU/ml twelve days after embryo transfer. Of these, 2 had biochemical pregnancies, and 12 had clinical pregnancies as evidenced by presence of gestational sac by ultrasound examination at five weeks of gestation and presence of the fetus and a heart beat at six weeks of gestation. There were 5 first trimester spontaneous abortions at 7-8 weeks of gestation. Seven(7) patients have delivered healthy babies at term; there were 2 ectopic pregnancies (Table 1).

	Day 2 Transfer	Day 3 Transfer
	average age 3835	average age 38
Total Start	22	13
Cancelled	0	0
Retrievals	22	13
Transfers	22	13
Total + Beta	9	7
Chemical Preg	2	0
Spotaneous ab	3	2
Multiple Preg	3	1
Ectopic preg	1	1
LiveBorn	3(13%)	4(30%)

Table 1. Results from HEED on day2 and day 3 transfers

4. Discussion

As may have been expected, the average age of patients for transfers on day 3 versus day 2 was lower (35 vs. 38 years of age), as they had better quality embryos which made it more feasible to continue embryo culture 1 day longer. Interestingly enough, the live pregnancy rate was also higher in day 3 transfers (31% vs. 15%).

Advantages of hysteroscopic guided direct embryo delivery include objectivity and replicability of the procedure. This unique and significant aspect of the procedure increases the reliability of correct entry into the uterine cavity with direct visual confirmation. Furthermore, placement and subsequent implantation at a precise location, with minimal volume of transfer media, provides an obvious benefit to patients with distorted uterine cavities, myomas, and adenomyosis and uterine adhesions. Visualization also provides the advantage of maneuvering along the contours of the uterus, thus decreasing the rate of trauma to the endometrial lining. In addition, performing gas distension of the uterus by an inert gas (N_2), the catheter tip is less likely to come into contact with the uterine fundus which has been associated with

stimulating uterine contractions and creating an unfavorable environment for implantation (Kovacs 1999, Lesny 1998). It has been reported that high frequency uterine contractions are associated with a lower ongoing clinical pregnancy rate and complete expulsion of the embryo (Fanchin 1998). It has also been postulated that the expulsion of the embryo into the lower uterine segment may result in higher rates of cervical ectopic pregnancy and placenta previas (Romundstad 2006; Schoolcraft 2001).

Witnessing uterine contractions hysteroscopically can also guide the clinician to abort and defer the procedure, thus decreasing costs, multiple failed attempts of ET, embryo loss, and risk of cervical ectopics and placenta previas. Direct visualization of the catheter tip ensures that the embryos are not retained in the catheter or lost. Viser et al. found a lower pregnancy rate when retained embryos were present (3% vs. 20.3%). In addition, catheter tip visualization allowed us to deliver smaller aliquot volumes for ET (5μl) as opposed to routine volumes (30μl). Smaller volume allows better handling of the embryo for proper orientation to the uterine lining, stabilizing the position and has been reported to increase pregnancy and implantation rates (Meldrum 1987). It may also contribute to the reduced

ectopic pregnancy rates, as larger volumes have been associated with increased ectopic pregnancy risk (Marcus 1995). Expulsion of this low volume of transfer media, carrying the embryo(s), from the tip of the catheter can only now be verified under direct visualization. In the "blind" procedure there is a real concern that this tiny droplet can be dragged into the lower uterine segment or into the cervical canal or out of the uterus along with the catheter during the final withdrawal of the catheter after embryo transfer.
The potential disadvantage and risk of this technique is disruption of the uterine lining, however the risk is postulated to be less than "blind" and ultrasound guided transfers due to the advantage of direct visualization of the uterine lining and not requiring movement of the catheter to facilitate identification during ultrasound (Garcıa-Velasco 2002). In addition, visualization allows one to place the embryo at a different location if trauma ensues. The major drawback to its acceptance is that hysteroscopy is an invasive procedure. However, as opposed to rigid endoscopes which may cause trauma to the uterus, the hysteroscope used in this study is a mini hysteroscope with a 3 mm diameter and flexible tip that allows one to easily follow the curvature of the uterus. The catheter used is semi-rigid to prevent kinkage as it passes through the endoscope yet with flexibility to bend with the endoscope. In our study, no disruption to the uterine lining or uterine bleeding occurred. Increased cost is another drawback, however utilizing a hysteroscope will decrease the costs from multiple failed IVF-ET attempts and improve patient satisfaction.

5. Conclusion

Hysteroscopic endometrial embryo delivery (HEED) is a beneficial technique in increasing clinical pregnancy rates, especially in patients with repeated failed IVF-ET attempts. Due to the objective and replicable nature of the hysteroscopic procedure along with increased accuracy of placement of embryo(s), efforts in reducing multiple pregnancies should now be more focused on increasing our knowledge of selecting embryo(s) with high survival potential for embryo transfer. Ectopic pregnancies from IVF will be minimized by using lower transfer volumes of 5 μl and visually confirmed positional placement of embryos away from the uterine cornu. Ectopics are almost eliminated when using the SEED technique for blastocyst embryo transfer.

6. Acknowledgment

Supported by: West Coast IVF Clinic, Inc. and LA IVF LAB, LLC. LA, CA USA

7. References

Baba K, Ishihara O, Hayashi N, Saitoh M, Taya J, Kinoshita K. Where does the embryo implant after embryo transfer in humans? Fertil Steril 2001;73:123–5

Brown JA, Buckingham K, Abou-Setta A, Buckett W. Ultrasound versus 'clinical touch' for catheter guidance during embryo transfer in women. Cochrane Database of Systematic Reviews 2007, Issue 1. Art. No.: CD006107. DOI: 10.1002/14651858.CD006107.pub2.

Coroleu et al., 2002 Increased risk of placenta previa in pregnancies following IVF/ICSI; a comparison of ART and non-ART pregnancies in the same mother. Romundstad

LB, Romundstad PR, Sunde A, von Düring V, Skjaerven R, Vatten LJ. Hum Reprod. 2006 Sep;21(9):2353-8. Epub 2006 May 25.

Fanchin R, Righini C, Olivennes F, Taylor S, de Ziegler D, Frydman R. Uterine contractions at the time of embryo transfer alter pregnancy rates after in-vitro fertilization. Hum Reprod 1998;13:1968–74.

Garcia-Velasco J, Isaza V, Martinez-Salazar J, Landazabal A, RequenaA, Remohi J, PellicerA, SimonC.Transabdominal ultrasoundguided embryo transfer does not increase pregnancy rates in oocyte recipients. Fertility and Sterility 2002;78(3):534–539

Gardner DK, Lane M. Culture of viable human blastocysts in defined sequential serum-free media. Hum Reprod 1998;13(suppl 3):148–59

Ghazzawi IM, Al-Hasani S, Karaki R, Souso S. Transfer technique and catheter choice influence the incidence of transcervical embryo expulsion and the outcome of IVF. Hum Reprod 1999;14:677-82.

Kamrava M, Yin M. Hysteroscopic Subendometrial Embryo Delivery (SEED), Mechanical Embryo Implantation. IJFS, Vol 4, No 1, Apr-Jun 2010

Knutzen.V., Scoto-Albors,C.E., Fuller,D., Sher.G., Shynock.K. and Behr,B. (1989) Mock embryo transfer (MET) in early luteal phase, the cycle prior to in-vitro fertilisation and embryo transfer. Presented at the 45th Annual Meeting of the American Fertility Society, San Francisco, California, 13-16 November 1989. Published by the American Fertility Society in the program supplement, p. S152 (Abstract P. 229).

Kosmas IP, R.Janssens R, De Munck L, Al Turki H, Van der Elst J, Tournaye H and Devroey P. Ultrasound-guided embryo transfer does not offer any benefit in clinical outcome: a randomized controlled trial. Human Reproduction Vol.22, No.5 pp. 1327–1334, 2007

Kovacs GT.What factors are important for successful embryo transfer after in-vitro fertilization?. Human Reproduction 1999;14:590–592.

Marcus S, Brinsden P. Analysis of the incidence and risk factors associated with ectopic pregnancy following in-vitro fertilization and embryo transfer. Hum Reprod 1995;10:199 -203.

Meldrum DR, Chetkowski R, Steingold KA, de Ziegler D, Cedars MI, Hamilton M. Evolution of a highly successful in vitro fertilization embryo transfer program. Fertil Steril 1987;48:86–93

Liv Bente Romundstad, Pal R.Romundstad, Arne Sunde, Vidar von Düring, Rolv Skjærven and Lars J.Vatten. Increased risk of placenta previa in pregnancies following IVF/ICSI; a comparison of ART and non-ART pregnancies in the same mother. Human Reproduction Vol.21, No.9 pp. 2353–2358, 2006

Sallam HN, Saad-el-Din S. Performing embryo transfer under ultrasound guidance- A meta analysis of randomized trials. Fertility and Sterility. 2002; Vol. 78, issue 3 (Suppl 1):S46

Schoolcraft WB, Surrey ES, Gardner DK. Embryo transfer: techniques and variables affecting success. Fertil Steril 2001;76:863-70.

Sieck UV, Jaroudi KA, Hollanders JM, Hamilton CJ. Ultrasound guided embryo transfer does not prevent ectopic pregnancies after in-vitro fertilization. Hum Reprod 1997;12:2081–2

Strandell, J. Thorburn and L. Hamberger, Risk factors for ectopic pregnancy in assisted reproduction, Fertil Steril 71 (1999), pp. 282–286.

Visser DS, Fourie FL, Kruger HF. Multiple attempts at embryo transfer: effects on pregnancy outcome in an in vitro fertilization and embryo transfer program. J Assist Reprod Genetics 1993;10:37–43.

5

Ectopic Pregnancy Following Reconstructive, Organ-Preserving Microsurgery in Tubal Infertility

Cordula Schippert, Philipp Soergel and Guillermo-José Garcia-Rocha
Medical School of Hannover, Department of Gynecology and Obstetrics Division of Reproductive Medicine; Carl-Neuberg-Str. 1, 30625 Hannover, Germany

1. Introduction

Disease or damage of the fallopian tubes accounts for 25% to 35% of reported cases of infertility (Pandian at al., 2008). Decreased fecundity may be caused by tubal occlusion, fimbrial damage, and/or peritubal adhesions, usually related to previous pelvic inflammatory disease, endometriosis, pelvic surgery, salpingitis isthmica nodosa or otherwise unknown causes. A special group of women affected by tubal infertility are those who have undergone intentional sterilization; 5% to 25% of these women (Neuhaus et al.; 1995; Kim et al.; 1997; Schippert et al., 2004) later regret having undergone this surgery. Some of them desire an operation to restore fertility, the most frequent reason for this is the desire to have a child with a new partner. The diagnosis of "tubal infertility" is a serious and burdensome diagnosis for the affected woman.

In the presence of a functional impairment of the fallopian tubes, the desire to have a child is (if at all) only possible through complicated, risky and cost-intensive therapies: on the one hand through reconstructive surgery or – on the other hand - by means of assisted reproductive technology procedures (ART). The limitations of surgical repair in many cases have been the driving force behind the rising numbers of ART. However, the success of either treatment - even when attempted multiple times - cannot be guaranteed. Outpatient in-vitro fertilization (IVF) can be repeated several times which results in an overall higher success rate. Unfortunately, a large number of couples is not be able to afford multiple IVF cycles. An IVF therapy also is not without risks and is associated with physical and mental stresses which not infrequently lead to a discontinuation of therapy.

Problems of IVF therapy in many countries, e.g. in Germany, are found in the low birth rates of at most 21% despite a clinical pregnancy rate of approximately 28-30% per embryo transfer, but it is the large number of multiple pregnancies at approximately 20% with occasionally significant maternal and child morbidity and mortality rates. The overall average pregnancy rate in Germany for all IVF cycles in 2009 was 29.5%, compared with a rate of 28.6% for the ICSI cycles (Bühler et al., 2010). Because of German legal restrictions, no embryo selection is permitted and the German Embryo Protection Act, passed in 1991, permits no more than three embryos to be transferred. Oocyte donation as well as surrogate motherhood is illegal.

Microsurgery of the fallopian tubes to restore functioning in the presence of tubal infertility is a therapeutic standard that has been established for decades. In contrast to IVF therapy, reconstructive surgeries of the fallopian tubes are curative measures. They are performed with the intention of permanently restoring the physiological ability of a woman to have a chance to conceive in every ovulating cycle. After successful surgery, additional spontaneous conceptions are, therefore, possible without renewed therapy. The course of pregnancy and the manner of birth in patients who underwent microsurgery do not differ from childbirth in a normal population. Also with respect to premature births, the rate of cesarean section and multiple births there are no differences versus healthy women who have not undergone surgery.

1.1 Ectopic pregnancy

Ectopic pregnancy (EP) is a serious and also nowadays a cause of maternal mortality in early pregnancy. The risk factors for EP in general population are pelvic infection, tubal disease, endometriosis, previous tubal surgery, age >35 years and smoking (Thornburn et al., 1986; Tuomovaara & Kauppila, 1988; Dubuisson et al., 1996; Strandell et al., 1999; Bouyer et al., 2003; Clayton et al., 2006; Practice Committee of American Society for Reproductive Medicine, 2008; Gelbaya, 2010). The incidence of EP in general population is approximately 2% (Strandell et al., 1999).

The first pregnancy conceived after ART and embryo transfer was ectopic (Steptoe & Edwards, 1976). The risk factors for ectopic pregnancy following ART with an incidence of 2.1% to 9.4% (Lesny et al., 1999) in all ART patients and up to 11% in patients with tubal infertility (Dubuisson et al., 1991) are reported to be tubal disease, history of pelvic infection (Marcus & Brinsden, 1995; Strandell et al., 1999) and tubal infertility as it is considered to be the indication for ART (Herman et al., 1990; Dubuisson et al., 1991, Verhulst et al., 1993).

In Germany, the overall rate of EP in women undergoing ART procedures from 1999 to 2009 was 2.0% (95% confidence interval [CI] 1.9-2.1) related to all pregnancies with a maximum of 2.2% in the group of women >39 years of age (95% CI 1.8-2.5). 19.9% of all cycles which lead to a pregnancy are done in couples who had an infertility diagnosis of "tubal factor" or "tubal disease". The incidence of EP according to the presence or absence of tubal pathology ranges from 2.3% to 3.7% in the presence of tubal pathology and from 1.7% to 2.1% in women without documented tubal disease. The highest EP rate was detected to be 4.5% (95% CI: 3.0-6.0) related to all pregnancies in young women <30 years who firstly had a tubal pathology, who secondly had been treated with IVF, and who thirdly smoked (original data from the German IVF-Registry, D.I.R. committee´s office, Bismarckallee 8-12, 23795 Bad Segeberg, Germany).

Tubal EP is also a known adverse effect of tubal reconstructive surgery; however the incidence varies widely between 0% and up to 40% depending on the type, location and severity of the tubal disease and the surgical procedure. The success of infertility surgery and the risk for EP depend on the careful selection of appropriate patients.

When compared with the macrosurgical approach, the use of a microsurgical technique has significantly improved the outcome of tubal anastomosis with reduced EP rates (Lavy et al., 1987).

The reconstructive microsurgical techniques should include the following elements (Gauwerky, 1999, Schippert et al., 2010): Atraumatic surgical technique, complete removal of diseased tissue, careful hemostasis, preparation layer by layer and exact adaptation of the tissue structures, complete peritonealization, and continuous irrigation of exposed peritoneal tissue surfaces.

In the presence of only mild or moderate tubal pathology, term pregnancy rates of 65% to 80% for salpingneostomy, adhesiolysis and reversal of sterilization have been reported (Marana et al., 2003, 2008; Practice Committee of American Society for Reproductive Medicine, 2008). The ectopic rate for mild disease is reported to be 1%-10% (Boer-Meisel et al., 1986; Winston & Margara, 1991; Nackley & Muasher, 1998), in contrast, EP rates can increase up to 20% to 40% in the presence of intrinsic tubal damage, salpingitis isthmica nodosa and severe tubal pathology (Posaci et al., 1999; Taylor et al., 2001; Pandian et al., 2008).

2. Methods of microsurgical reconstruction of the fallopian tubes

2.1 Reversal of sterilization

Microsurgical reversal of sterilization leads to a cumulative pregnancy rate ranging from 40% to 84% and monthly fecundability of 8%-10% (Kim et al., 1997; Land & Evers, 2002), the overall risk of EP appears to be less than 10% (Posaci et al., 1999; Practice Committee of American Society for Reproductive Medicine, 2008). Possible prognostic factors include the type of performed sterilization procedure, the site of anastomosis and the postoperative tubal length (Posaci et al., 1999). Tubal occlusion with rings or clips, isthmic-isthmic anastomosis and a tubal length >5 cm are associated with a greater likelihood of successful pregnancy after resterilization (Practice Committee of American Society for Reproductive Medicine, 2008).

During a retrospective study time of eleven years, 127 women (median age 35.4 years [26-42]) were refertilized in our clinic after a sterilization was performed before (Figure 1; Figure 2a and 2b).

The follow-up data of 89 patients could be collected for analysis. The EP rate following the microsurgical reversal of sterilization was 6.7% (6/89 patients), and the intrauterine pregnancy rate was 73.0% respectively (65/89 patients) (Table 1).

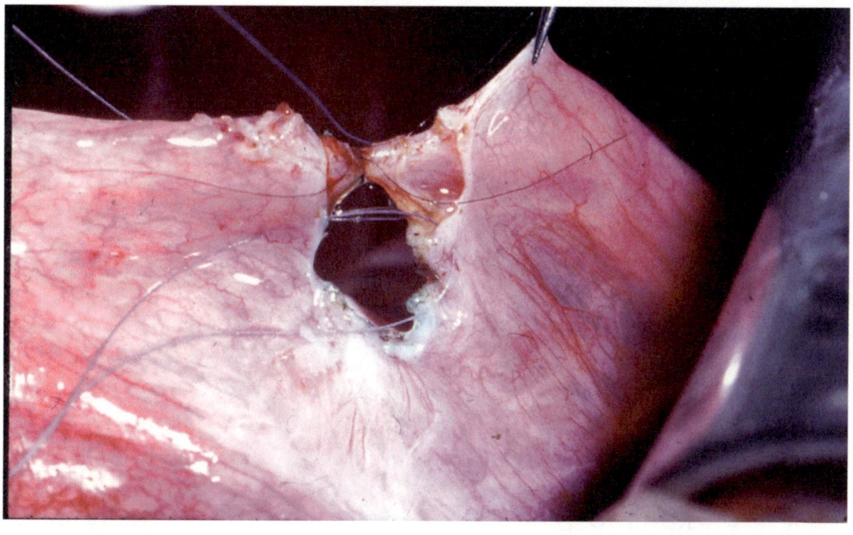

Fig. 1. Isthmic-isthmic reanastomosis of the fallopian tube after sterilization (refertilization) using sutures 8-0 and 6-0 vicryl

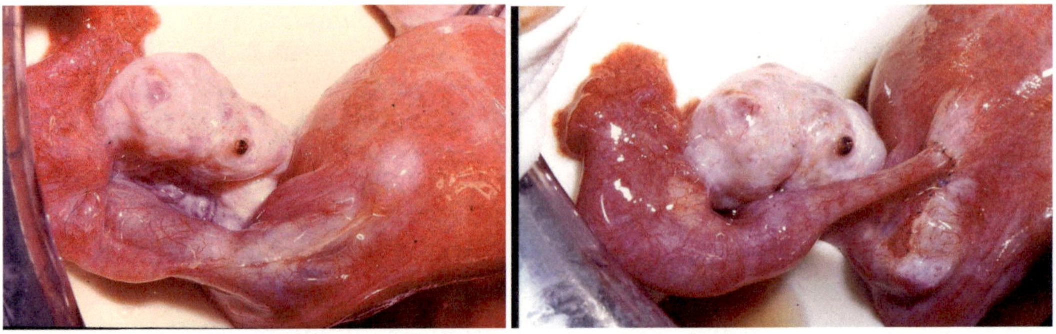

Fig. 2. (a) status after sterilization by bipolar coagulation of the fallopian tube; (b) isthmic-cornual refertilization of the fallopian tube

Method of surgery (microsurgery)	Number of patiens (percent)	Pregnancy rate	Ectopic pregnancy rate	Abortion rate	Birth rate
Refertilization after previous sterilization	89 (100%)	65 (73.0%)	6 (6.7%)	14 (15.7%)	45 (50.6%)

Table 1. Results of reversal of sterilization (refertilization): All types of anastomosis and length of fallopian tubes; 127 patients contacted, 89 patients answered; median age 35.4 years (26-42). Medical School of Hannover, Germany, 1990-2001, analysis 2004; percentages are related to all patients. The analysis considered only the first pregnancy that followed the operation, even if an EP or abortion was followed by a normal pregnancy with subsequent childbirth.

2.2 Microsurgery due to acquired tubal damages

In our study, 426 women (median age 31 years [21-42]) underwent tubal microsurgery after hysteroscopic and laparoscopic diagnosis of acquired tubal sterility and the prior exclusion of serious ovarian and andrological disorders: Adhesiolysis, anastomosis due to an acquired damage of the fallopian tubes, fimbrioplasty and salpingsotomy had been performed. Several of these surgical procedures were occasionally combined in a single procedure, e.g. a fimbrioplasty on one tube and an anastomosis on the other tube. It was finally possible to contact 287 patients and proceed with the analysis (Table 2).

2.2.1 Peritubal adhesiolysis

Overall intrauterine pregnancy rates following adhesiolysis by microsurgery vary widely - from 21% to 80% (Feinberg et al., 2008; Lok et al., 2003; Posaci et al.; 1999), mainly because of bias in case selection and the absence of standardized assessment of the extent of tubal damage, especially the mucosal state. In an analysis including nine studies with 456 patiens, an EP rate of 0% to 16% following adhesiolysis by microsurgery, and a rate of intrauterine pregnancy (IUP) of 21% to 68% respectively is reported (Posaci et al., 1999). High pregnancy rates of about 60% with EP rates of 6% have been reported in cases of the absence of peritoneal damage of serosa after the surgical procedure and a complete removal of adhesions with a good anatomical reconstruction of ovaries and fallopian tubes. EP rates

increased up to 20% if at least one of these criteria was not fulfilled (Posaci et al., 1999; Lundroff et al., 1991) or if the tubal damage was severe (Lok et al., 2003; Boer-Meisel et al., 1986; Schlaff et al., 1990). For this reason, patients with dense adhesions and a severe tubal pathology are best referred to IVF.
In our study, the rate of EP following microsurgical adhesiolysis was 7.8% (9/116 patients), and the IUP rate was 42.2% (49/116) respectively (Table 2).

Method of surgery (microsurgery due to acquired tubal damages)	Number of patiens	Pregnancy rate	Ectopic pregnancy rate	Abortion rate	Birth rate
Adhesiolysis 12,8%	116	49 (42.2%)	9 (7.8%)	3 (2.6%)	37 (31.9%)
Fimbrioplasty 17,3%	55	30 (54.6%)	3 (5.5%)	6 (10.9%)	21 (38.2%)
Salpingostomy 49,7%	153	53 (34.6%)	12 (7.8%)	7 (4.6%)	34 (22.2%)
Anastomosis 20,2 %	68	38 (55.9%)	7 (10.3%)	9 (13.2%)	22 (32.4%)
Total 100 %	392 interventions (287 pat.)	170 (43.4%) related to total number of surgery	31 (7.9%)	25 (6.4%)	114 (29.2%) related to total number of surgery

Table 2. Results of reconstructive tubal surgery due to acquired tubal damages: 426 patients contacted, 287 patients answered; median age 31.0 years (21-42), multiple methods of surgeries during one intervention possible, total rates are related to total number of interventions. Medical School of Hannover, Germany, 1990-2001, analysis 2004. The analysis considered only the first pregnancy that followed the operation, even if an EP or abortion was followed by a normal pregnancy with subsequent childbirth.

2.2.2 Distal tubal surgery: fimbrioplasty and salpingostomy / salpingotomy

Pregnancy outcome after distal tubal microsurgery has been related to several factors such as preexisting tubal disease, the extent of adnexal or even dense adhesions, the ampullary dilatation, the wall thickness, and the lack of normal mucosa (Posaci et al., 1999). In general, salpingostomy has the lowest success rate among the tubal microsurgeries. Pregnancy rates following fimbrioplasty are higher than those after salpingostomy (60% vs. 31%) (Donnez & Casanas-Roux, 1986). The term pregnancy rates following distal tubal surgery varied from 3% to 59% when patients had only few and non-fixed adhesions, a thin tubal wall, and normal mucosal appearance of the endosalpinx (Boer-Meisel et al., 1986). A meta-analysis including eight studies with 399 patients showed EP rates from 3% to 23% with an IUP rate of 0% to 51% (Posaci et al., 1999) following salpingostomy, salpingoneostomy and fimbrioplasty.
Another analysis with a total of 1,514 patients showed an IUP rate and recurrent EP rate following salpingostomy for the treatment of EP of 61% and 15%, respectively (Yao & Tulandi, 1997). A large review of ten case series in women who underwent salpingoneostomy due to distal tubal occlusion (n=1,128) reported a cumulative EP rate per pregnancy of 23% (Marana & Quagliarello, 1988b) and an EP rate of 8% in women who underwent tubocornual anastomosis for proximal tubal occlusion (n=118) (Marana & Quagliarello 1988a).
In our own patient database (Table 2), the EP rates had been 7.8% (12/153 patients) when salpingotomy was performed and 5.5% (3/55 patients) (Figures 3a and 3b), respectively, when fimbrioplasty was done (Figure 4a and 4b). The pregnancy rates had been 34.6% (53/153 salpingotomy), and 54.6% (30/55 fimbioplasty) respectively.

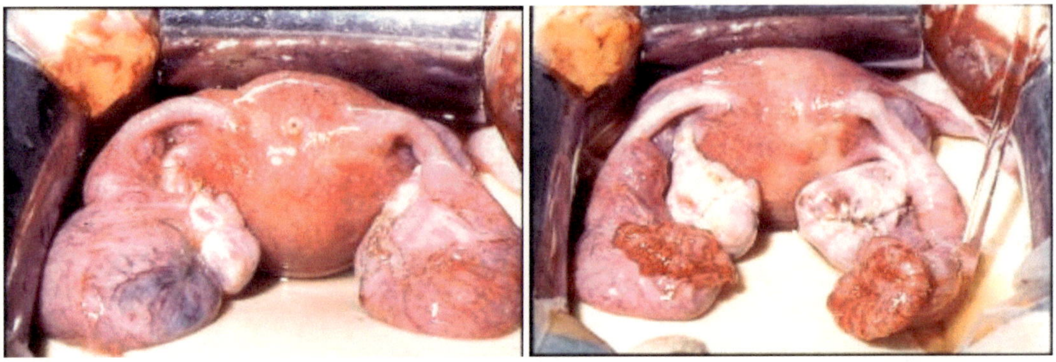

Fig. 3. (a) hydrosalpinges and peritubal adhesions; (b) salpingotomy on both sides and adhesiolysis

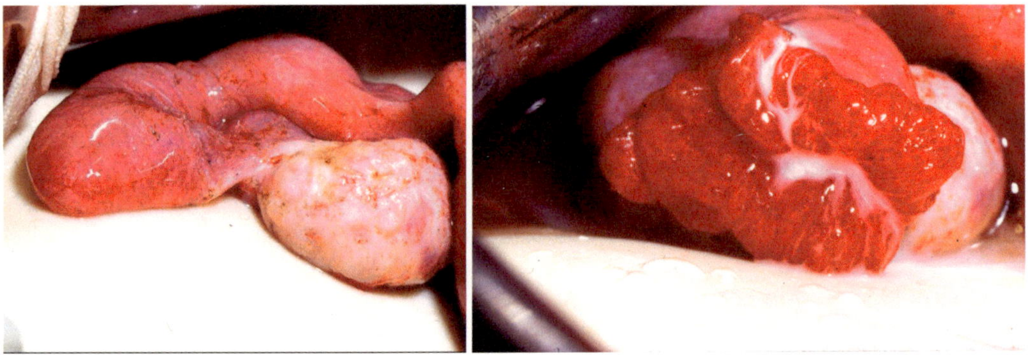

Fig. 4. (a) fimbrial phimosis; (b) fimbrioplasty

2.2.3 Proximal tubal disease: tubo-cornual anastomosis

Case series and cohort studies demonstrated high pregnancy rates following microsurgical tubo-cornual anastomosis (Johnson et al., 2010). A review of eleven case series in women who underwent proximal tubal operations by microsurgery (n = 490) reported a cumulative EP rate of 0% to 12% and a rate of IUP of 22% to 74% concerning to all patients (Posaci et al., 1999). The largest study from 1997 showed an EP rate of 11% and an IUP rate of 74% after a three year follow-up (Dubiusson et al., 1997). Negativ prognostic factors on the pregnancy rate after tubocornual anastomosis are reduced residual length, damaged intramural portion, presence of chronical inflammation and tubal inclusion in the tubal wall, and tubal endometriosis (Posaci et al., 1999).

In our own study with 68 patients, the EP rate was 10.3% (7/68 patients) whereas the IUP rate was 55.9% (38/68 patients) when tubal anastomosis (reversal of sterilization excluded) was performed (Table 2).

3. Conclusion

In cases of tubal infertility, it is today possible to fulfill a couple's desire to have a child either by means of a reconstructive operation of the fallopian tubes or by IVF therapy. The success of treatment - even when attempted multiple times - cannot be guaranteed. In

general, microsurgery and IVF therapy are not competing, but complementary therapeutic options for the treatment of tubal infertility. The definitive decision about which therapy to pursue should always be left to the affected couple after the pertinent information has been competently communicated.
The risk for EP and the chances for an intrauterine ongoing pregnancy following tubal reconstructive surgery, respectively, vary widely depending on the type, location and severity of the tubal disease and the performed surgical procedure.
The ectopic rate for mild aquired tubal disease is reported to be 1%-10% (Boer-Meisel et al., 1986; Winston & Margara, 1991; Nackley& Muasher, 1998) and for reversal of sterilization less than 10% (Practice Committee of American Society for Reproductive Medicine, 2008), but in contrast, EP rates increase up to 40% in the presence of intrinsic tubal damage, salpingitis isthmica nodosa and severe tubal pathology (Taylor et al., 2001; Posaci et al., 1999; Pandian et al., 2008; Marana & Quagliarello, 1988a, 1988b; Akande et al., 2004, Mosgaard et al., 1996). For this reason, patients with dense adhesions like frozen pelvis and a severe tubal pathology are best referred to IVF (Schippert et al., 2010).
In our own patient's collective, the EP rate following reversal of sterilization was 6.7%.
In the presence of acquired tubal disease, mainly because of previous pelvic inflammation and salpingitis, the overall EP rate was 7.9% following microsurgical reconstruction using the techniques of adhesiolysis, salpingostomy, salpinoneostomy, fimbrioplasty and anastomosis.
The risk factors for developing EP after ART still are inconsistent. The incidence is reported to be between 2.1% and up to 11% in tubal infertiltiy. The data of the Geman IVF Registry demonstrate a significantly increased incidence of EP in the presence of tubal pathology (original data from the German IVF Registry). The highest EP rate related to all pregnancies was detected to be 4.5% (95% CI: 3.0-6.0) in women <30 years who firstly had a tubal pathology, who secondly had been treated with IVF, and who thirdly smoked. If these women are non-smokers, the EP rate was 4.2% (95% CI: 3.5 - 5.0).
In summary, the risks for EP after ART and microsurgical tubal reconstruction in women with tubal infertility or tubal co-morbidity are significant and approximately comparable. Surgical tubal reconstruction still remains a significant part in the range of modern infertility treatments, however the success and/or failure of infertility surgery depends on a careful selection of appropiate patients. ART is especially recommended in women with severe tubal pathology and in the case of severe male infertility or ovarial dysfunction.

4. Acknowledgment

The authors wish to thank Professor Dr. Hans Walter Schloesser, a great teacher, character, visionary gynaecologist and microsurgeon.

5. References

Akande, V.A.; Cahill, D.J.; Wardle, P.G.; Rutherford, A.J.; Jenkins, J.M. (2004). The predictive value of the 'Hull & Rutherford' classification for tubal damage. *BJOG*, Vol. 111, pp. 123–141.

Boer-Meisel, M.E.; te Velde, E.R.; Habbena, J.D.F.; Kardaun, J.W.P.F. (1986). Predicting the pregnancy outcome in patients treated for hydrosalpinx; a prospective study. *Fertil Steril*, Vol. 45, pp. 23–29.

Bouyer, J. ; Coste, J. ; Shojaei, T.; Pouly, J.L.; Fernandez, H.; Gerbaud, L. (2003). Risk factors for ectopic pregnancy: a comprehensive analysis based on a large case-control population-based study in France. *Am J Epid,* Vol. 157, pp. 185-194.

Bühler, K.; Bals-Pratsch, M.; Kupka, M.S. and the Board of Trustees (2010). DIR Annual 2009. *J. Reproduktionsmed. Endokrinol,* Vol. 7, No. 6, pp. 470-497.

Clayton, H.B.; Schieve, L.A.; Peterson, H.B.; Jamieson, D.J.; Reynolds, M.A.; Wright, V.C. (2006). Ectopic pregnancy risk with assisted reproductive technology procedures. *Obstet Gynecol,* Vol. 107, No. 3, pp. 595-604.

Donnez, J. & Casanas-Roux, F. (1986). Prognostic factors of fibrial microsurgery. *Fertil Steril,* Vol. 46, pp. 200-204.

Dubuisson, J.B.; Aubriot, F.; Mathieu, L.; Foulot, H.; Mandelbrot, L.; Bouquet de Jolinière, J. (1991). Risk factors for ectopic pregnancy in 556 pregnancies after in vitro fertilization: implications for preventive management. *Fertil Steril,* Vol. 56, pp. 686-690.

Dubuisson, J.B.; Morice, P.; Chapron, C.; De Gayffier, A.; Mouelhi, T. (1996). Salpingectomy - the laparoscopic surgical choice for ectopic pregnancy. *Hum Reprod,* Vol. 11, pp. 1199–1203.

Dubuisson, J.B. ; Chapron, C. ; Ansquer, Y. ; Vacher-Lavenu, M.C. (1997). Proximal tubal occlusion: is there an alternative to microsurgery? *Hum Reprod,* Vol. 12, pp. 692–698.

Feinberg, E.C.; Levens, E.D.; DeCherney, A.H. (2008). Infertility surgery is dead: only the obituary remains? *Fertil Steril,* Vol. 89, No. 1, pp. 232-236.

Lok, F.; Ledger, W.L.; Li, T.C. (2003). Surgical intervention in infertility management. *Hum Fertil (Camb),* Vol. 6, Suppl 1, pp. 52-59.

Gauwerky, J.F.H. Rekonstruktive Tubenchirurgie (Reconstructive Surgery of the Fallopian Tubes). Springer-Verlag, Berlin, Heidelberg, New York, Tokio 1999. ISBN 3-540-62970-X.

Gelbaya, T. (2010). Short and long-term risks for women who conceive through in vitro fertilization. *Hum Fertil (Camb),* Vol. 13, No. 1, pp. 19-27.

Herman, A.; Ron-El, R.; Golan, A.; Weinraub, B.; Bikovsky, I.; Caspi E. (1990). The role of tubal pathology and other parameters in ectopic pregnancies occuring in in- vitro fertilization and embryo transfer. *Fertil Steril,* Vol. 54, pp. 864-868.

Johnson, N.; van Voorst, S.; Sowter, M.C.; Strandell, A.; Mol B.W. (2010). Surgical treatment for tubal disease in women due to undergo in vitro fertilization. *Cochrane Database Syst Rev.* Vol. 20, No 1:CD002125.

Kim, S.H.; Shin, C.J.; Kim, J.G.; Moon, S.Y.; Lee, J.Y.; Chang, Y.S. (1997). Microsurgical reversal of tubal sterilization: a report on 1,118 cases. *Fertil Steril,* Vol. 68, No. 5, pp. 865-870.

Land, J.A. & Evers, J.L. (2002). Chlamydia infection and subfertility. *Best Pract Res Clin Obstet Gynaecol,* Vol. 16, No. 6, pp. 901-912.

Lavy, G.; Diamond, M.P.; DeCherney, A.H. (1987). Ectopic pregnancy: its relationship to tubal reconstructive surgery. *Fertil Steril,* Vol. 47, pp. 543–556.

Lesny, P.; Killick, S.R.; Robinson, J.; Maguiness, S.D. (1999), Transcervical embryo transfer as a risk factor for ectopic pregnancy. *Fertil Steril,* Vol.72, pp. 305-309.

Lundroff, P.; Hahlini, P.; Kallfelt, B.; Thornburn, J.; Lindblom, B. (1991). Adhesion formation after laparoscopic surgery in tubal pregnancy: a randomised trial after laparotomy. *Fertil Steril,* Vol. 55, pp. 911–915.

Marcus, S.F. & Brinsden, P.E. (1995). Analysis of the incidence and risk factors associated with ectopic pregnancy following in-vitro fertilization and embryo transfer. *Hum Reprod,* Vol. 10, pp. 199-203.

Marana, R. & Quagliarello, J. (1988a). Proximal tubal occlusion: microsurgery versus in vitro fertilization-a review. *Int J Fertil,* Vol. 33, pp. 107–115.

Marana, R. & Quagliarello, J. (1988b). Proximal tubal occlusion: microsurgery versus IVF-a review. *Int J Fertil,* Vol. 33, pp. 338–340.

Marana, R.; Catalano, G.F.; Muzii, L. (2003). Salpingoscopy. *Curr Opin Obstet Gynecol,* Vol. 15, No. 4, pp. 333-336.

Marana, R.; Ferrari, S.; Astorri, A.L.; Muzii, L. (2008). Indications to tubal reconstructive surgery in the era of IVF. *Gynecol Surg,* Vol. 5, pp. 85-91.

Mosgaard, B.; Hertz, J.; Steenstrup, B.R.; Soorensen, S.S.; Lindhard, A.; Anderson, A.N. (1996) Surgical management of tubal infertility: A regional study. *Acta Obstet Gynecol Scand,* Vol. 75, No. 5, pp. 469–474.

Nackley, A.C. & Muasher, S.J. (1998). The significance of hydrosalpinx in in-vitro fertilization. *Fertil Steril,* Vol. 69, No. 3, pp. 373-384.

Neuahus, W.; Marx, C.; Hamm, W. (1995). Experiences with definitive contraception - results of a follow-up study of sterilized women. *Geburtshilfe Frauenheilkd,* Vol. 55, pp. 135-139.

Pandian, Z.; Akande, V.A.; Harrild, K.; Bhattacharya, S. (2008). Surgery for tubal infertility. *Cochrane Database Syst Rev,* Vol. 16, No. 3: CD006415.

Posaci, C.; Camus, M.; Osmanagaoglu, K.; Devroey, P. (1999). Tubal surgery in the era of assisted reproductive technology: clinical options. *Hum Reprod,* Vol. 14 Suppl. 1, pp. 120-136.

Practice Committee of American Society for Reproductive Medicine. (2008). The role of tubal reconstructive surgery in the era of assisted reproductive technologies. *Fertil Steril,* Vol. 90, No. 5 Suppl. pp. 250-253.

Schippert, C.; Garcia-Rocha, G.; Kauffels, W.; Schlösser, H.W. (2004). Erneuter Kinderwunsch nach Tubensterilisation - Erfolgsaussichten einer mikrochirurgischen Tubenrekonstruktion im Vergleich zur In-vitro-Fertilisation (IVF). *Geburtshilfe Frauenheilkd,* Vol. 64; pp. 153-159.

Schippert, C.; Hille, U.; Bassler, C.; Soergel, P.; Hollwitz, B.; Garcia-Rocha, G.J. (2010). Organ-preserving and reconstructive microsurgery of the fallopian tubes in tubal infertility: still an alternative to in vitro fertilization (IVF). *J Reconstr Microsurg,* Vol. 26, No. 5, pp. 317-323.

Schlaff, W.E.; Hassiakos, D.; Damewood, M.D.; Rock, J.A. (1990). Neosalpingostomy for distal tubal obstruction: prognostic factors and impact of surgical technique. *Fertil Steril,* Vol. 54, pp. 984–990.

Steptoe, P.C. & Edwards, R.G. (1976). Reimplantation of the human embryo with subsequent tubal pregnancy. *Lancet,* Vol. 24 1 (7965), pp. 880-882.

Strandell, A.; Thorburn, J.; Hamberger, L. (1999). Risk factors for ectopic pregnancy in assisted reproduction. *Fertil Steril,* Vol. 71, pp. 282-286.

Taylor, R.C.; Berkowitz, J.; McComb, P.F. (2001). Role of laparoscopic salpingostomy in the treatment of Hydrosalpinx. *Fertil Steril,* Vol. 75, pp. 594-600.

Thorburn, J.; Berntsson, C.; Philipsson, M.; Lindblom, B. (1986). Background factors for ectopic pregnancy. Frequency distribution in a case-control study. *Eur J Obstet Gynecol Reprod Biol,* Vol. 23, pp. 321-331.

Tuomovaara, L. & Kauppila, A. (1988), Ectopic pregnancy: a case-control study of aetiological risk factors. *Arch Gynecol Obstet,* Vol. 243, pp. 5-11.

Verhulst, G.; Camus, M.; Bollen, N.; Van Steiterghem, A.; Devroey, P. (1993). Analysis of risk factors with regard to the occurrence of ectopic pregnancy after medically assisted reproduction. *Hum Reprod,* Vol. 8, pp. 1284-1287.

Winston, R.M. & Margara, R.A. (1991). Microsurgical salpingostomy is not an obsolete procedure. *BJOG* Vol. 98, pp. 637-642.

Yao, M. & Tulandi, T. (1997). Current status of surgical and non-surgical treatment of ectopic pregnancy. *Fertil Steril,* Vol. 67, pp. 421–433.

6

Persistent Ectopic Pregnancy After Laparoscopic Linear Salpingostomy for Tubal Pregnancy: Prevention and Early Detection

Shigeo Akira, Takashi Abe and Toshiyuki Takeshita
Department of Obstetrics and Gynecology, Nippon Medical School, Tokyo, Japan

1. Introduction

Persistent ectopic pregnancy (PEP) is a condition that occurs due to incomplete removal of trophoblastic tissue during fallopian tube-preservation surgery for tubal pregnancy. According to several studies, the incidence has been reported to be approximately 3%-20%,[1] and the incidence appears to be rising due to the increase in treatment of tubal pregnancies via laparoscopic surgery.[2-4] If treatment for PEP is delayed, tubal rupture and intra-abdominal hemorrhage can occur and may be accompanied by significant morbidity and mortality. Therefore, prevention and early detection of PEP is of great importance.

Methotrexate (MTX), a cytostatic agent with proven anti-trophoblastic activity, has been used for the treatment of ectopic pregnancies, and has also been reported to be useful for treating PEPs.[5-6] Therefore, combined use of MTX following conservative tubal surgery may facilitate prevention of PEP.

Indeed, MTX has thus far been reported to significantly decrease the occurrence of PEP when systemically-administered in a single dose within 24 hours after laparoscopic linear salpingostomy.[7] However, systemic MTX administration has been reported to cause side effects and must be used with caution.[8,9] In contrast, local MTX administration into the tube, either laparoscopically[10,11] or through transvaginal ultrasonography[12,13], has been associated with few side effects, and may be useful as a prophylactic for PEP. Therefore, local MTX administration after linear salpingostomy could prevent PEP without serious side effects.

In this chapter, we examined the efficacy of local MTX administration after linear salpingostomy for tubal pregnancies in preventing PEP, and evaluated the usefulness of postoperative serum human chorionic gonadotropin (hCG) decline (percentage of the preoperative hCG level) for early detection and ruling out of PEP.

2. Subjects and methods

2.1 Patients selection

Patients who underwent linear salpingostomies between January 1996 and December 2010 were enrolled in the study. A linear salpingostomy was indicated according to the following criteria: 1) stable circulatory dynamics; 2) desired future pregnancy; 3) no tubal rupture; 4) absence of marked tubal adhesions; 5) ectopic pregnancy diameter $\leq$ 5 cm; 6) absence of a fetal heart beat; and 7) absence of a recurrent ectopic pregnancy in the ipsilateral fallopian tube. For patient selection, we did not limit the gestational age or pre-operative serum hCG level.

2.2 Surgical procedure

Following confirmation of indication criteria for laparoscopy, 5 IU of vasopressin was injected into the mesosalpinx. After making a linear incision on the distended portion of the fallopian tube with electrocautery, the products of conception were removed *en bloc* using forceps or by hydrodissection. Trophoblasts were macroscopically confirmed in water and sent for pathologic evaluation. The diagnosis of ectopic pregnancy was pathologically-confirmed in all cases. Surgery was performed using an identical technique by several physicians under the guidance of a supervising physician.

2.3 Serum hCG measurement

Preoperative serum hCG levels were obtained ≤ 24 hours before surgery. Serum hCG levels during the first postoperative week were measured at 2-3 day intervals. The intervals between hCG measurements were determined by the attending physician based on clinical symptoms. Serum hCG levels were followed postoperatively until serum hCG levels < 5 IU/ml or until the diagnosis of PEP.

Serum hCG levels were determined by an electrochemiluminescence immunoassay (ECLIA), which is based on a sandwich antibody principle (Elecsys 2010 Systems; Roche Tokyo, Japan). The inter-assay coefficient of variation was 5.8; the intra-assay coefficient of variation was 4.5.

2.4 Prevention of PEP

Patients were divided into two groups (prophylaxis and control groups). In the prophylaxis group, MTX (50 mg) was serially administered into the tubal wall near the lesion immediately after linear salpingostomy. Patients who underwent surgery without MTX administration were assigned to the control group. All patients gave informed consent to the procedures, and this study was approved by the Nippon Medical School Hospital Ethics Committee.

PEP was defined as an increase in the serum hCG level or a decline of < 20% between measurements taken 3 days apart.[14]

The incidence of PEP between groups was analyzed using Fischer's exact test. In addition, statistical analysis for both groups used the Student's t-test or the Mann-Whitney test, as appropriate (STATMATE for Windows). Significance was defined as a $P < 0.05$.

2.5 Early detection of PEP

The 53 patients without prophylactic MTX injection were divided into two groups, as follows: patients with an increase in the serum hCG level or a decline in the serum hCG level < 20% between measurements taken 3 days apart (PEP group); and successfully-treated patients with a marked decrease in hCG (control group). The clinical and laboratory characteristics of both groups were compared with respect to maternal age, parity, gestational age at enrollment, specimen diameter, and pre-operative serum hCG levels.

The postoperative course was divided into 4 periods, as follows: period A, days 1–2; period B, days 3–4; period C, days 5–6; and period D, days 7–8. The serum hCG declines during each period in the PEP and control groups were compared.

A cut-off value for serum hCG to rule out a PEP was established using receiver operating characteristic (ROC) curve analysis. The two groups were compared using the Student's t-test, and when appropriate, Fisher's exact test was used. Significance was defined as a $P < 0.05$.

3. Results

3.1 Prevention of PEP

One hundred two patients were enrolled in the present study. The prophylaxis and control groups consisted of 55 and 47 patients, respectively, with no intergroup differences in age, gestational age, or preoperative hCG levels. PEP were not noted in the prophylaxis group, but occurred in 8 patients (17.0%) in the control group ($p<0.05$; Table 1).

The 8 patients in the control group who developed PEP received a single systemic administration of MTX (50 mg/m^2) between postoperative days 7 and 10, the period during which the diagnosis was made. One patient had a poor decline in serum hCG and required an additional administration of MTX (50 mg/m^2) 7 days later. In addition, another patient developed lower abdominal pain and a hemoperitoneum 4 days after MTX administration, and underwent laparoscopic salpingectomy. The remaining six patients had a steady decline in serum hCG levels. Patients in both groups who did not develop PEP reached undetectable serum hCG levels, and thus completed the recommended follow-up by post-operative day 28. In contrast, patients who developed PEP required a mean follow-up of 51.7±17.2 days ($p<0.05$; Table 2).

No side effects attributable to MTX, such as dermatitis, alopecia, dyspepsia, and hepatic or bone marrow toxicity, were observed in the prophylaxis group.

3.2 Early detection of PEP

In 42 of the 53 patients, no postoperative symptoms of PEP were noted, and the serum hCG levels dropped to pre-pregnancy levels; the PEP was located in 11 patients. Table 3 presents the clinical characteristics of both groups. No statistically significant differences existed between the PEP and control groups with respect to age, parity, gravidity, gestational age, specimen diameter, or preoperative serum hCG levels.

	Prophylaxis Group (n = 55)	Control Group (n = 47)
Age (yr)	30.2 +/- 4.3	29.7 +/- 5.1
Gestational age (wk)	7.2 +/- 1.3	7.0 +/- 1.5
Preoperative hCG (mIU/ml)	3257 +/- 3380 (250 to 13012)	3118 +/- 3051 (198 to 12756)
Persistent ectopic pregnancy	0	8 *

Data are presented as mean +/- standard deviation with ranges in parentheses.
*$P < 0.05$ compared with the prophylaxis group

Table 1. Patient characteristics and frequency of persistent ectopic pregnancy.

	Prophylaxis Group (n = 55)	Control Group (n = 39)	PEP Group (n = 8)
Length of follow up (days)	20.3 +/- 5.7	21.6 +/- 6.4	51.7 +/- 17.2*

Data are presented as mean +/- standard deviation.
*P < 0.05 compared with the prophylaxis group and control group without persistent ectopic pregnancy (PEP).

Table 2. Duration of follow up.

	Total n = 53	Control n = 42	PEP n = 11	p value
Maternal age (y)	29.6 +/- 5.4	30.0 +/- 5.1	28.0 +/- 6.3	0.367
Parity	0.18 +/- 0.44	0.16 +/- 0.37	0.27 +/- 0.64	0.813
Gravidity	0.62 +/- 0.83	0.52 +/- 0.67	1.00 +/- 1.26	0.281
Gestational age at enrollment (w)	6.96 +/- 1.40	6.95 +/- 1.43	7.00 +/- 1.34	0.964
Diameter of tumor (cm)	2.90 +/- 1.55	3.08 +/- 1.61	2.30 +/- 1.30	0.339
hCG at diagnosis (IU/L)	3078.9 +/- 2915.1	3046.9 +/- 3208.9	3201.2 +/- 1396.4	0.160

Data are presented as mean +/- standard deviation or number (%).

Table 3. Clinical characteristics of subjects in the study of postoperative declines in serum human chorionic gonadotropin (hCG) levels and persistent ectopic pregnancy (PEP).

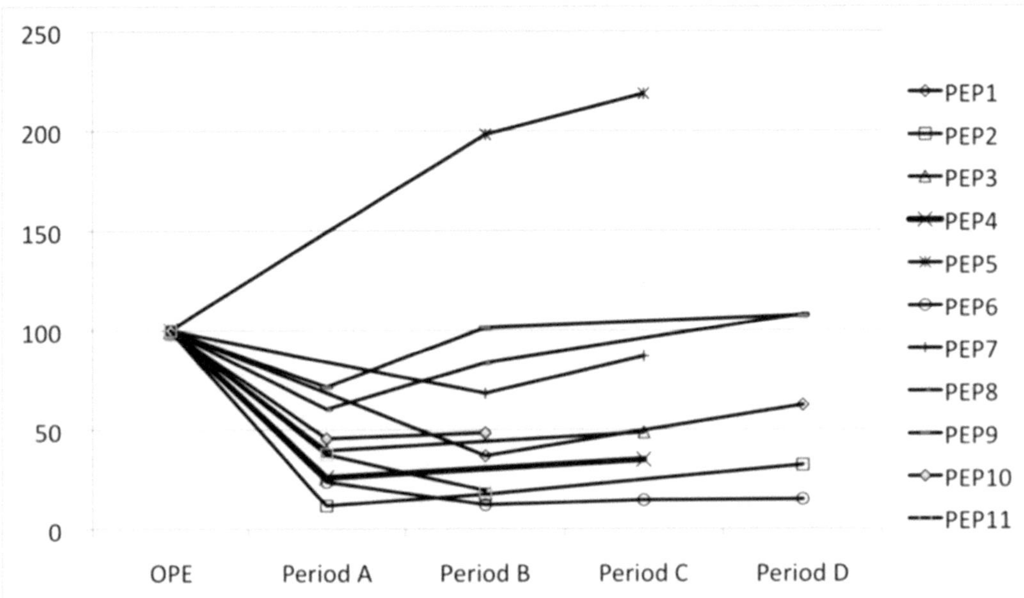

Fig. 1. Postoperative declines in serum human chorionic gonadotropin (hCG) levels (percentages of preoperative hCG levels) during the first week after laparoscopic salpingotomy in the persistent ectopic pregnancy patients.

Figure 1 shows the postoperative hCG declines in the PEP group. In one patient, the post-operative serum hCG levels steadily increased post-operatively, and in the other nine patients, the levels of serum hCG decreased transiently, then increased. After period C, the hCG levels of all patients in the PEP group increased and did not decrease until the second intervention. In these patients, systemic administration of one additional dose of MTX (50 mg/m^2) was given.
Figure 2 compares the variance in the hCG decline for each study period between the control and PEP groups. After period B, the hCG decline was significantly less in the PEP group than the control group.

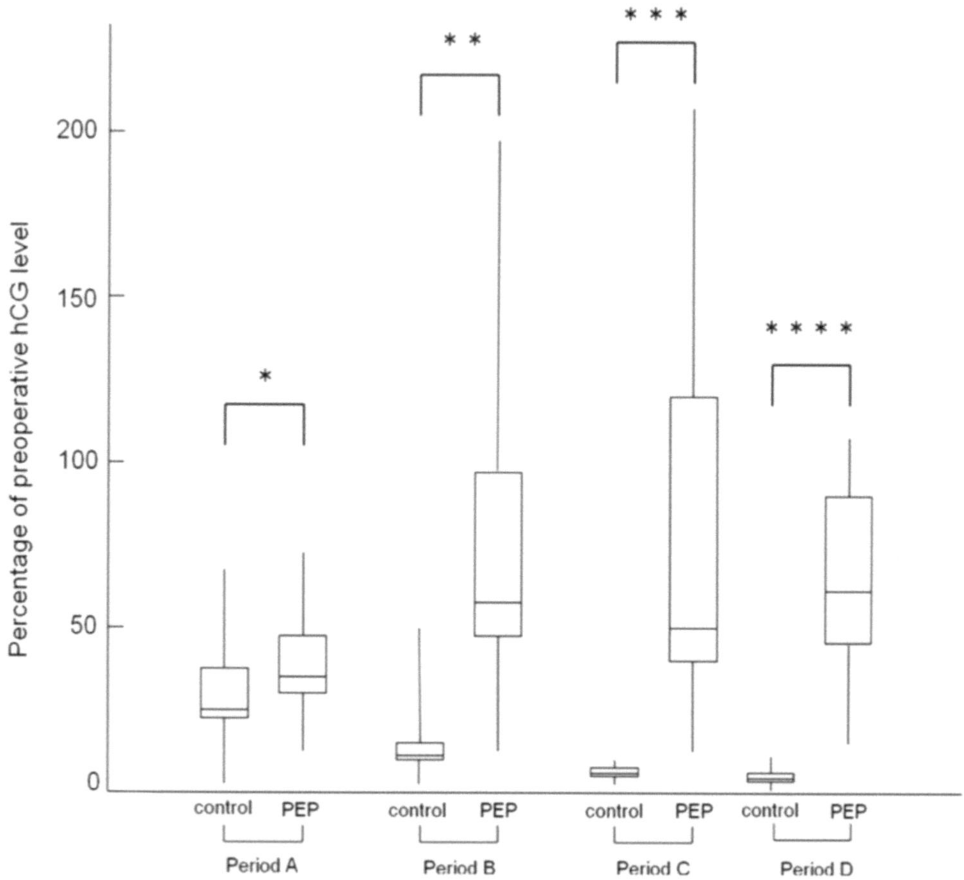

Fig. 2. Comparison of the variance in the serum human chorionic gonadotropin (hCG) decline for each period between the control and persistent ectopic pregnancy (PEP) groups. Data are presented as median value and interquartile ranges (IQR) in each period.

Figure 3 presents the 95% confidence interval (CI) of the hCG decline for 1 week after surgery in the control group, and the postoperative hCG decline in the PEP group. In the PEP group, the hCG decline after period C was outside the 95% CI of the control group.
Analysis by ROC, sensitivity and specificity were calculated with optimal points in each period, and 14% of preoperative hCG valued in period C and D revealed that the specificity and sensitivity of the test were equal to 100% (Figure 4).

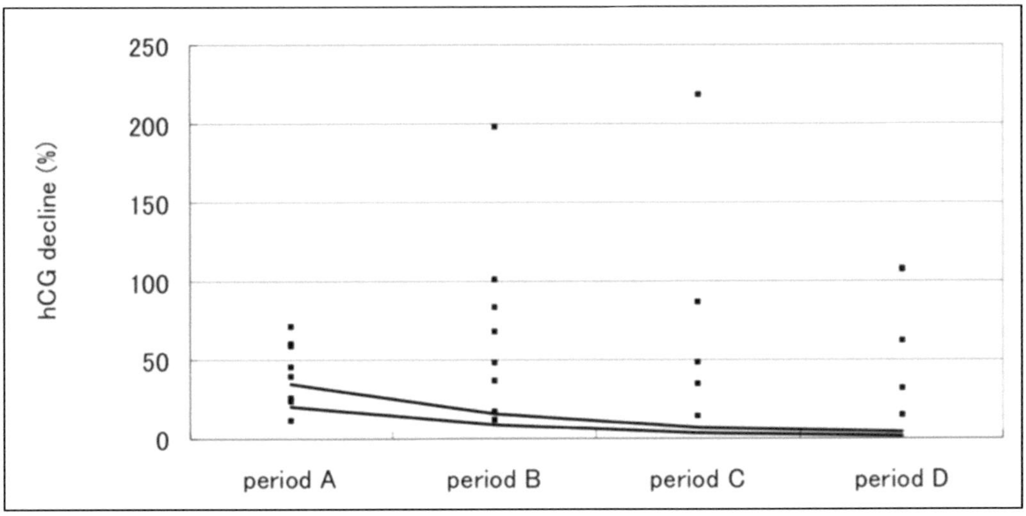

Fig. 3. Postoperative declines in serum human chorionic gonadotropin (hCG) levels during the first week after laparoscopic salpingotomy in the successfully treated patients (control group, black line [95% confidence interval]) an PEP patients (Black boxes [individual hCG declines]). Between the black lines is presented 95% confidential interval of the control group. Black boxes present individual preoperative hCG values.

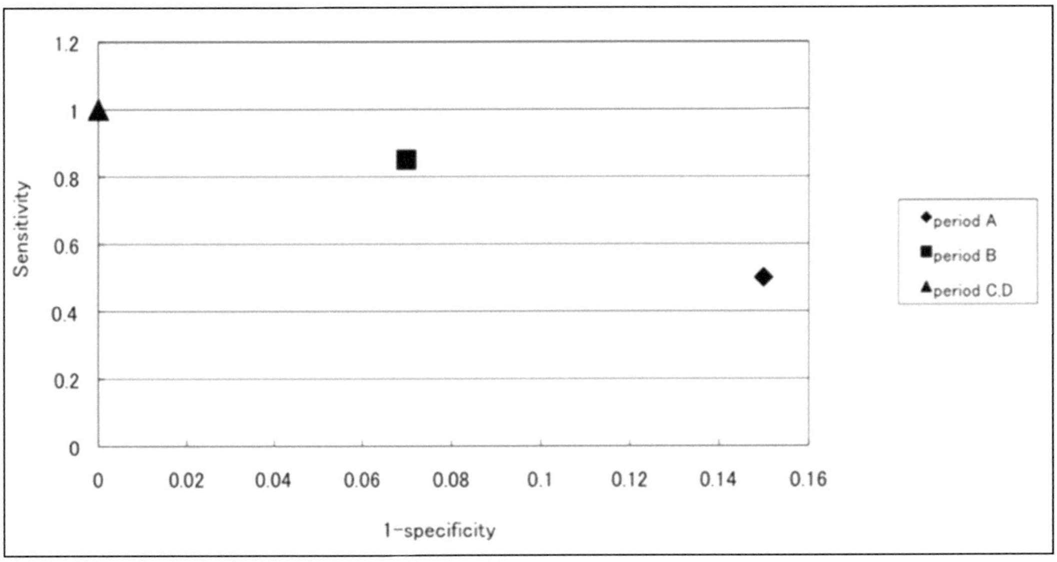

Fig. 4. Analysis by receiver operating characteristic curve correlating sensitivity of the test with the false-positive rate (1-specificity) for each postoperative period for the first week following laparoscopic salpingotomy. Sensitivity and specificity were calculated with optimal points in each period, and the excellent sensitivity and false positive rate (1-specificity) were plotted on this figure. A 14% of preoperative serum human chorionic gonadotropin (hCG) value in period C and D revealed that the specificity and sensitivity of the test were equal to 100%.

4. Discussion

As indicated by the results of the present study, prophylactic local administration of MTX into the tubal wall immediately after linear salpingostomy is extremely effective in preventing post-operative PEP. In addition, even when systemic MTX administration was effective, patients who developed PEP required a significantly longer follow-up of hCG level than patients without PEP.

MTX has been shown to have no adverse effects on future pregnancies as long as pregnancy is avoided for a certain period of time,[15] and may thus be proactively used as prophylaxis following salpingostomy. Graczykowski et al.[7] reported that the incidence of PEP was reduced to 1.9% following a single systemic administration of prophylactic MTX (1 mg/kg) within 24 hours after salpingostomy. However, although generally mild, side effects related to systemic MTX administration have been reported in up to 24% of cases,[8] including some cases of serious side effects.[9] Therefore, the implementation of prophylactic systemic administration of MTX for all patients remains controversial. Importantly, local intratubal administration of MTX has been reported to enhance local anti-trophoblastic activity,[16] in addition to reducing side effects,[17,18] and may thus be a more effective and safer regimen for preventing PEP. This assumption is supported by the fact that no cases of PEP or side effects were observed in the MTX group in the present study, while PEP was observed in 1.9% of cases in a study involving single systemic administration of MTX.[8]

Regarding the toxicity to the tube of local administration of MTX (50 mg), no effects were reported in a histologic study of intratubal injection of MTX (100 mg).[19] Furthermore, subsequent fertility after local MTX injection was satisfactory.[13,20] Therefore, local administration of MTX (50 mg) was thought to have no toxicity in the tube.

Administration of prophylactic MTX to all patients remains a controversial issue. Prophylactic administration of MTX may be appropriate for patients at increased risk for developing PEP, such as patients with a short duration of amenorrhea, a small ectopic pregnancy (< 2 cm in size), and a preoperative hCG level ≥ 2500 IU/ml.[21] Considering that no side effects were reported after local MTX administration in the present study, and in light of the risk of salpingectomy and the need for long follow-up in cases of PEP, it may be appropriate to consider prophylactic local administration for all patients.

This study also showed that age, parity, gravity, gestational age, specimen diameter, and preoperative serum hCG levels are not predictive of a PEP following a laparoscopic salpingostomy. Several attempts have been made to predict a PEP; however, no effective predictive protocols for PEP currently exist.[22] Because our results were comparable and decreasing pattern of serum hCG has been reported to be helpful aid in avoiding further surgery,[23] serum hCG levels must be closely monitored in all patients who have had a salpingostomy before PEP is ruled out.

In the current study, no difference existed in the decline in serum hCG postoperatively between the PEP and control groups during period A; however, after period B, the decline in serum hCG in patients with PEP was significantly less than the control group. This finding indicates that a subsequent increase in the serum hCG level occurs during period B in the PEP group (approximately 3-4 days postoperatively).

Previous studies have used the decline in serum hCG to detect a PEP[24-26]; however, all of the studies have used a single early post-operative hCG measurement. We indicated that the future course of serum hCG cannot be predicted reliably from a single early postoperative measurement. In our study, during period B, the hCG decline in patients with PEP began to be less than the 95% CI of the control group, and from period C, the decline in PEP group was

completely outside the 95% CI of the control group. In addition, the subsequent increase in hCG was observed after period C in all PEP patients. Furthermore, once an increase in the serum hCG levels was observed, the serum hCG levels never decreased until the second intervention. Therefore, the decision to perform a second intervention, including MTX treatment, should be made by confirming a rise in the hCG levels from period A or B to period C.
We also evaluated the appropriate duration of intensive hCG measurement to rule out a PEP. After period C, the hCG decline in all patients with PEP was completely outside the 95% CI of the control group. Furthermore, based on the results of the ROC analysis of the two groups, the specificity and sensitivity were equal to 100% from period C (Figure 4). These results indicate that intensive serum hCG monitoring after laparoscopic salpingostomy must be continued through period C; if the level of the hCG declines to < 14% of the preoperative level, PEP can be ruled out and the serum hCG monitoring interval can be extended.

5. Conclusions

We suggest that prophylactic intratubal injection of MTX after a linear salpingostomy for tubal pregnancy is a safe and effective regimen for preventing PEP, enhances the possibility of tubal preservation, and contributes to improvements in the postoperative QOL of patients.
The decision-making for a second intervention to PEP should be made by confirming an increase of the serum hCG levels from period A or B to period C. Intensive hCG follow-up after laparoscopic salpingostomy for tubal pregnancy must continue through period C; if the serum hCG decline is < 14%, a PEP can be ruled out and the serum hCG monitoring interval can be extended.
In view of these findings, serum hCG follow-up after laparoscopic salpingostomy can be as follows (Figure 5).

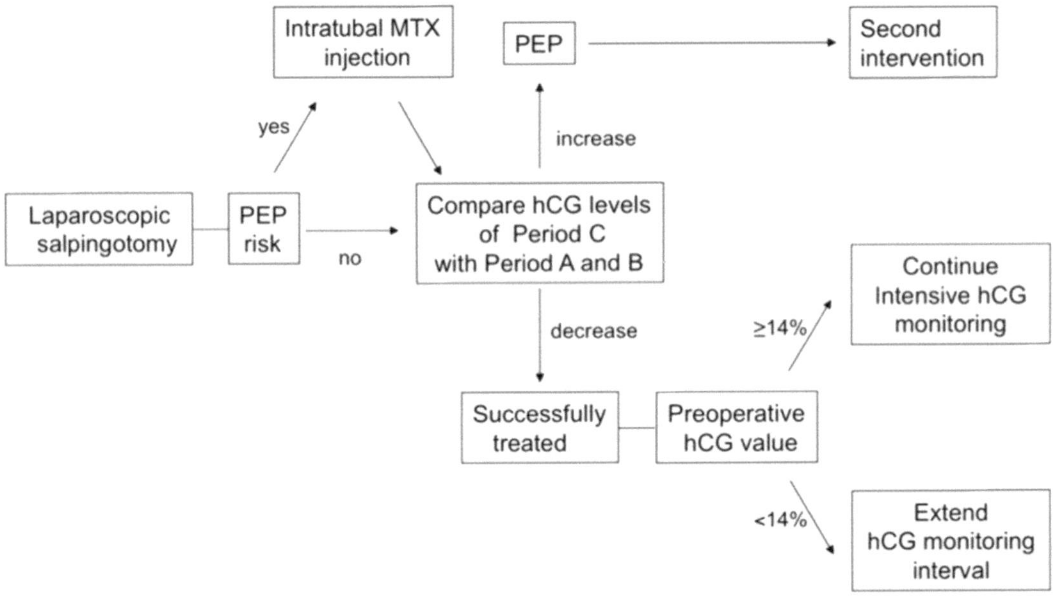

Fig. 5. Strategy for management of ectopic pregnancy after laparoscopic salpingotomy. hCG: human chorionic gonadotropin, MTX: methotrexate, PEP: persistent ectopic pregnancy.

Prophylactic local administration of MTX after laparoscopic salpingostomy may be appropriate for patients at increased risk for PEP[20,27-29], specifically patients with a short duration of amenorrhea and a small ectopic pregnancy site. The hCG decline in periods A and B should be compared with period C and if a rise in serum hCG occurs, MTX should be administered. Conversely, if a continuous decline in serum hCG is confirmed and if the serum hCG decline is < 14% in period C, the measurement interval for serum hCG can be extended to once every 2 weeks until the level becomes undetectable.

6. References

[1] Seifer DB, Diamond MP, Decherny AH: Persistent ectopic pregnancy. Obstet Gynecol Clin North Am 1991;18:153-159.
[2] Vermesh M, Silva PD, Rosen GF, et al.: Management of unruptured ectopic gestation by linear salpingotomy: a prospective, randomized clinical trial of laparoscopy versus laparotomy. Obstet Gynecol 1989;73: 400-404.
[3] Murphy AA, Nager CE, Wujek JJ, et al.: Operative laparoscopy versus laparotomy for the management of ectopic pregnancy: A prospective trial. Fertil Steril 1992;57:1180-1185.
[4] Seifer DB, Gutmann JN, Grant WD, et al.: Comparison of persistent ectopic pregnancy after laparoscopic salpingostomy versus salpingostomy at laparotomy for ectopic pregnanacy. Obstet Gynecol 1993;81:378-382.
[5] Tanaka T, Hayashi H, Kutsuzawa T, et al.: Treatment of interstitial ectopic pregnanacy with methotrexate: report of a successful case. Fertil Steril 1982;37:851-852.
[6] Ory SJ, Villanueva AJ, Sand PK, et al.: Conservative treatment of ectopic pregnancy with methotrexate. Am J Obstet Gynecol 1986;154:1299-1306.
[7] Graczykowski JW, Mishell DR: Methotrexate prophylaxis for persistent ectopic pregnancy after conservative treatment by salpingostomy. Obstet Gynecol 1997;89:118-122
[8] Parker J, Bisits A, Proietto AM: A systematic review of single-dose intramuscular methotrexate for the treatment of ectopic pregnancy. Aust N Z Obstet Gynecol 1998; 38:145-150Z rnecol 1998;38:145-150.
[9] Isaacs JD Jr, McGehee RP, Cowan BD: Life-threating neutropenia following methotrexate treatment of ectopic pregnancy: a report of two case. Obstet Gynecol 1996; 88:694-696.
[10] Pansky M, Bukovsky I, Golan A, et al.: Local methotrexate injection : a nonsurgical treatment of ectopic pregnancy. Am J Obstet Gynecol 1989;161:393-396.
[11] Akira S, Ishihara T, Yamanaka A, et al.: Laparoscopy with ultrasonographic guidance of intraamniotic methotrexate injection for ectopic pregnancy: a report of two cases. J Reprod Med 2000;45:844-846.
[12] Menard A, Crequat J, Mandelbrot L, et al.: Treatment of unruptured tubal pregnancy by local injection of methotrexate under transvaginal sonographic control. Fertil Steril 1990;54:47-50.
[13] Fernandez H, Benifla J-L, Lelaidier C, et al.: Methotrexate treatment of ectopic pregnancy: 100 cases treated by primary tranvaginal injection under sonographic control. Fertil Steril 1993;59:773-777.

[14] Vermesh M, Silva PD, Sauer MV, et al.: Persistent tubal ectopic gestation: Patterns of circulating β-human chorionic gonadotropin and progesterone, and management options. Fertil Steril 1988;50:584-588.
[15] Yao M, Tulandi T: Current status of surgical and nonsurgical management of ectopic pregnancy. Fertil Steril1997;76: 421-433.
[16] Sand PK, Stubblefield PA, Ory JS: Methotrexate inhibition of normal trophoblasts in vitro. Am J Obstet Gynecol 1986;155:324-329.
[17] Haans LCF, vanKessel PH, Kock HCLV: Treatment of ectopic regnancy with methotrexate. Eur J Obstet Gyne4col Reprod Biol 1987;24:63-67.
[18] Stovall TG, Ling FW, Buster JE: Outpatient chemotherapy of unruptured ectopic pregnancy. Fertile Steril 1989;51:435-438.
[19] Kooi S, van Etten FHPM, Kock HCLV: Histopathology of five tubes after treatment with methotrexate for a tubal pregnancy. Fertile Steril 1992;57:341-345.
[20] Stovall TG, Ling FM, Gray LA, et al: Methotrexate treatment of unruptured ectopic pregnancy: A report of 100 cases. Obstet Gynecol 1991; 77: 749-753.
[21] Seifer DB, Gutmann JN, Doyle MB, et al.: Persistent ectopic pregnancy following laparoscopic linear salpingostomy. Am J Obstet Gynecol 1990;76:1121-1125.
[22] Lund CO, Nilas L, Bangsgaard N, et al.: Persistent ectopic pregnancy after linear salpingostomy: a non-predictable complication to conservative surgery for tubal gestation. Acta Obstet Gynecol Scand 2002;81:1053-1059.
[23] Kamrava MM, Taymor ML, Berger MJ, et al.: Disappearance of human chorionic gonadotropin following removal of ectopic pregnancy. Obstet Gynecol 1983;62:486-488.
[24] Mock P, Chardonnens D, Stamm P, et al.: The apparent late half-life of human chorionic gonadotropin (hCG) after surgical treatment for ectopic pregnancy. A new approach to diagnose persistent trophoblastic activity. Eur J Obstet Gynecol Reprod Biol 1998;78:99-102.
[25] Spandorfer SD, Sawin SW, Benjamin I, et al.: Post-operative day 1 serum human chorionic gonadotropin level as a predictor of persistent ectopic pregnancy after conservative surgical management. Fertil Steril 1997;68:430-434.
[26] Poppe W.A.J, Vandenbussche N. Postoperative day 3 serum human chorionic gonadotropin decline: a predictor of persistent ectopic pregnancy after linear salpingotomy. Obstet Gynecol Reprod Biol 2001; 99: 249-252.
[27] Lundorff P, Hahlin M, Sjoblom P, Lindblom B. Persistent trophoblast after conservative treatment of tubal pregnancy: prediction and detection. Obstet Gynecol 1991; 77: 129-133.
[28] Hagstrom HG, Hahlin M, Bennegard-Eden B, Sjoblom P, Thorburn J, Lindblom B. Prediction of persistent ectopic pregnancy after laparoscopic salpingostomy. Obstet Gynecol 1994; 84: 798-802.
[29] Hoppe DE, Bekkar BE, Nager CW, et al.: Single-dose systemic methotrexate for the treatment of persistent ectopic pregnancy after conservative surgery. Obstet Gynecol ;1994: 83: 51-55.

Part 3

Diagnosis of Ectopic Pregnancy

7

Management and Outcome of Ectopic Pregnancy in Developing Countries

Buowari Yvonne Dabota
Medical Women Association Of Nigeria, Rivers State Branch
Nigeria

1. Introduction

Ectopic pregnancy is a common life-threatening emergency in the developing world and its frequency is still high. Ectopic pregnancy is the commonest cause of maternal morbidity and mortality in the first trimester of pregnancy (Airede & Ekele 2005, Grimes 1994, Okunlola et al 2006). Complications of early pregnancy are common clinical conditions that often require emergency care. The patient may or may not be aware that she is pregnant at the time of evaluation at the emergency department (Complications of pregnancy, 2007). Diagnosis is frequently missed and should be considered in any woman in the reproductive age group presenting with abdominal pain or vaginal bleeding especially when combined with an episode of collapse or syncope. Ectopic pregnancy is a complication of pregnancy in which the products of conception develop outside the uterine cavity. With rare exceptions, ectopic pregnancies are not viable. By far the commonest site is the fallopian tube (Hanretty, 2004). It is a tragedy of reproduction and a form of reproductive failure in the index pregnancy of affected women. Such women have a 7-15% chance of recurrence and only 40-60% chance of conceiving after surgery (Aboyeji et al, 2002). Ectopic pregnancy remains a major gynaecological problem in contemporary gynaecological practice. Not only do women die from this disease but also of greater clinical importance is the indirect morbidity of poor fertility prognosis and adverse outcome in subsequent pregnancies (Musa et al, 2009). Ectopic pregnancy may not necessarily be managed by a gynaecologist especially in hospitals in rural settings where there are no specialist doctors or if present are limited in number. In such district hospitals, general practitioners with surgical and gynaecological skills manage them in low-income countries where most patients present late as emergencies.

Gynaecological emergencies form a large proportion of the workload of a gynaecologist. Gynaecological emergencies, diagnosis, and treatment have progressed in the light of evidence-based medicine combined with a good clinical assessment. This allows for appropriate management. Any primary health care doctor should be prepared to encounter and to handle gynaecological emergencies in patients even those in critical ill states. Ectopic pregnancy is a condition that occurs in all races, in all countries and in any socio-economic class of women during the reproductive years. It is a life threatening surgical gynaecological emergency in our environment (Nwagha et al 2007, Adesiyun et al 2001). Whilst there are many conditions that may lead to an emergency presentation, there are four emergencies, which account for the great majority. These are spontaneous abortion, pelvis sepsis including bartholin's abscess, ectopic pregnancy, and accidents to an ovarian cyst. These common conditions should be at the forefront of the doctors' mind when asked to see a patient presenting as a gynaecological emergency whether she is referred by her general practitioner or presents herself to the casualty department. It is only when these diagnosis have been excluded should one consider alternative less common gynaecological emergencies.

Ectopic pregnancy presents a major health problem for women of childbearing age. If not treated vigorously and early enough, it may be fatal. It is of immerse concern to reproductive health and it is associated with significant maternal morbidity and mortality and is fatal to the embryo. The future reproductive potential of the woman after an ectopic pregnancy is compromised. Ectopic pregnancy accounts for 73 % of early pregnancy mortalities. Ectopic pregnancy is derived from the Greek word 'Ekpos' meaning out of place and it refers to implantation of a fertilised egg in a location outside of the uterine cavity. In many parts of the world, there has been a dramatic increase in the incidence over recent decades with studies showing at least a doubling of the rate (Rajkhowa et al, 2000). Ectopic pregnancy is one of the most critical and life threatening emergencies in gynaecological practice (Olarewaju, 1994). It is also known as extra uterine pregnancy.

Sites where an ectopic pregnancy can occur are the fallopian tube which is the commonest site, ovary, cervix, and the abdomen. When it occurs in the fallopian tube, it is known as tubal pregnancy. Implantation can occur at any point along the tube, although the ampulla is the commonest site. The isthmus is the next in frequency and the interstitial portion least common. While interstitial pregnancies represent a small fraction of ectopic gestations, they are especially feared due to their devastating outcomes (Fisch et al, 1998). Ectopic pregnancies that involves implantation in the cervix, the interstitial portion of the fallopian tube, the ovary, the abdomen or a scar from a caesarean section account for less than 10 % of all ectopic pregnancies. These unusual ectopic pregnancies are difficult to diagnose and are associated with high morbidity (Barnhart, 2009). The risk of reoccurrence of ectopic pregnancy is approximately 10% among women with 1 previous ectopic pregnancy and at least 25% among women with 2 or more previous ectopic pregnancies. Women in whom the affected fallopian tube has been removed are at increased risk for ectopic pregnancy in the remaining tube. Case series have suggested that approximately 60% of women who receive a diagnosis of an ectopic pregnancy are subsequently able to have an intrauterine pregnancy (Barnhart, 2009). Ipsilateral ectopic pregnancy occurs rarely and may be difficult to diagnose in low resource settings where there are no diagnostic tools. Few cases have been reported (Faleyimu, 2008). When the ectopic pregnancy is located in the abdomen, it is known as abdominal pregnancy. Patient with ectopic pregnancies are widely reported to be of low parity (Onwuhufua et al, 2001, Abdul, 1999, Baffoe & Nkyekyer, 1991). In a study in Benin city, Nigeria, majority of the patients with ectopic pregnancies were nulliparous and in their mid twenties (Gharoro & Igbafe, 2002). It remains a major challenge to the reproductive performance of women worldwide. The abnormally implanted gestation grows and draws its blood supply from the site of abnormal implantation. As the gestation enlarges, it creates the potential for organ rupture because only the uterine cavity is designed to expand and accommodate foetal development. Ectopic pregnancy can lead to massive haemorrhage, infertility, or death. Of all ectopic pregnancies, 97 % occur in the fallopian tube. Of all tubal pregnancies, 55 % are at the ampulla, 25 % at the isthmus, and 17 % at the fimbria (Complications of pregnancy, 2007). In rare cases of ectopic pregnancy, there may be two fertilized eggs one outside the uterus and the other inside. This is called heterotopic pregnancy. Often the intrauterine pregnancy is discovered later than the ectopic pregnancy mainly because of the painful emergency nature of the ectopic pregnancies. The ectopic pregnancies are normally discovered and removed early in the pregnancy. Naturally occurring heterotopic pregnancy is rare (Odewale & Afolabi, 2008). Heterotopic pregnancy is on the increase because of increasing incidence of ectopic pregnancy. Heterotopic pregnancy is associated with a high maternal morbidity and foetal loss. This is probably due to delayed diagnosis resulting from confusing clinical features especially when diagnostic facilities are not available.

The importance of ectopic pregnancy in our environment is peculiar because rather than join the global trend of early diagnosis and conservative approach in management, we are challenged by late presentations with rupture in more than 80% in most cases (Igbarese et al, 2005). We are also challenged by poor diagnostic tools, limited capacity to handle emergencies and consequent burden of increased maternal morbidity and mortality and consequent reproductive failure (Udigwe et al, 2010).

The ectopic pregnancy may be ruptured or unruptured at the time of diagnosis. The unruptured variety may be intact or the slowly leaking type. The rupture can occur early in the gestation and a delay in diagnosis, potentially limits conservative treatment option (Fylstra, 2002).

Cervical ectopic pregnancy is the implantation of a pregnancy in the endocervical canal (Leeman & Wendland, 2000). Interstitial pregnancies represent a small fraction of ectopic gestations; they are especially feared due to their often devastating outcomes. The standard treatment for interstitial pregnancies have been laparatomy and cornual resection with hysterectomy required in many cases in order to control bleeding (Fisch et al, 1998). Interstitial implantation is rare but very dangerous because it ends in rupture of the uterine muscle.

Ipsilatetral ectopic pregnancy occurs rarely and may be difficult to diagnose in low resource settings where there are no diagnostic tools (Bode-Law et al, 2008). Bode-law et al reported an ipsilateral ectopic pregnancy ectopic pregnancy occurring in the stump of a previous ectopic site.

Heterotopic pregnancy is the simultaneous occurrence of an ectopic pregnancy with an intrauterine pregnancy. Assisted fertilization is a major risk factor for heterotopic pregnancy. Its presentation is similar to ectopic pregnancy with simultaneous evidence of an intrauterine pregnancy. Laparatomy is preformed to selectively remove the ectopic pregnancy. The intrauterine pregnancy survives to delivery in 66% of cases after treatment of the ectopic pregnancy (Wagner & Promes, 2007). Maternal deaths may occur and morbidity rates are high usually resulting from complications such as haemoperitoneum and peritonitis due to rupture of the extra uterine pregnancy site (Abedi et al, 2010). In 2008, Odewale and Afolabi in Nigeria published a report of heterotopic pregnancy, an ectopic pregnancy at the ampullary portion of the right fallopian tube and co-existent intrauterine pregnancy, which spontaneously aborted on the 10th postoperative day. Abasiattai et al reported a case of spontaneous heterotopic pregnancy with tubal rupture and delivery of a live baby at term (Abasiattai et al, 2010).

The implantation of a pregnancy within the scar of a previous caesarean delivery is the rarest form of ectopic pregnancy. Ibekwe in 2004 reported a case of ruptured ectopic pregnancy presenting as uterine rupture at 23 weeks. Mutihir and Nyango in 2010 reported a 34-year-old nullipara managed for ruptured ectopic pregnancy from endometriosis. This work was carried out at a general hospital located in a rural setting in northern Nigeria.

2. Incidence of ectopic pregnancy

There have been different hospital based studies in Nigeria and other developing countries on ectopic pregnancy. The incidence of ectopic pregnancy varies from country to country and within the same country, it varies from one community to another. In Nigeria, there are several private hospitals owned by individuals where patients can seek for medical treatment. Most Nigerian studies on ectopic pregnancies were carried out in the government owned hospitals; hence, this may not give a true picture of the incidence, as those in the private hospitals are not included. Also, some women may have died at home, as many people seek medical care late in Nigeria.

Some of these ectopic pregnancies may be terminated spontaneously before they give rise to notable clinical symptoms. There is currently an increased incidence of ectopic pregnancy globally. This incidence may be related to a higher incidence of tubal disease notably salpingitis. Other reasons for the rising incidence of ectopic pregnancy are adequate treatment for pelvic inflammatory disease, which in the past rendered women sterile. The use of intrauterine contraceptive device, increase in surgical procedures for tubal disease and improved diagnostic technique. The increase in the incidence of ectopic pregnancy is also associated with advances in assisted reproductive technology, tubal surgeries, and sterilizations and earlier diagnosis with more sensitive methods of cases that otherwise could have resolved without causing any symptoms (Arup et al, 2007). There is evidence that the overall incidence of ectopic pregnancy has been rising in many countries depending on the prevalence of risk factors and the methods of diagnosis available while the case fatality have been decreasing (Jurkovic, 2007, Morcau et al, 1995, Thonneau et al, 2002). Ectopic pregnancy is a global problem and has shown a rising incidence during the last three decades the world over (Arup et al, 2007). The incidence of recurrent ectopic pregnancy is approximately 15 % and this rises to 30 % following two previous ectopic pregnancies (Tulandi, 1988). A figure of 1 in 4000 to 7000 pregnancies is currently quoted for heterotopic gestation (Jurkovic, 2007). The incidence of a simple ectopic gestation varies from 1 in 300 pregnancies in Europe to as high as 1 in 20 to 50 pregnancies in Africa and West Indies (Piam & Otubu, 2006). Only a few reports of heterotopic pregnancy are reported (Aliyu et al, 2008, DeVoe & Pratt, 1998). The once extremely rare condition of heterotopic pregnancy is now more common with the advent of in vitro fertilization and embryo transfer. It is 1-3 % of all pregnancies and 10-15% of all ectopic pregnancies following in vitro fertilization and embryo transfer (Aliyu et al, 2008).

Ectopic pregnancy occurs approximately in 1.5 to 2.0 of pregnancies and is potentially life threatening (Barnhart, 2009). Despite the continued increase in the incidence of ectopic pregnancy, the rate of death from ectopic pregnancy has declined in developed countries primarily because of earlier diagnosis before tubal rupture. The incidence of ectopic pregnancy depends on the population studied and ranges from 1 % in rural general practice to 13 % in urban emergency department (Kaplan et al, 1996, Erondu et al, 2010).

The incidence of ectopic pregnancy in western countries has generally shown a rising trend with a decreased mortality mainly because of availability of modern diagnostic methods, which makes early diagnosis before tubal rupture, occurs in over 70 % of cases (Rajkhowa et al, 2000). The incidence of ectopic pregnancy was found to be 2.0 % in France (Coste et al, 1994), 2.8 % in Finland (Markinen, 1993) and 2.2 % in the United States (CDC, 1992). Another study over an 18-year period in America reported a rising incidence from 0.45 % to 1.68 % (Ory, 1992). It was reported to 1.24% in England (Rajkhowa et al, 2000). In most of Europe and North America, the incidence of ectopic pregnancy is estimated at 2 % of livebirths (Moore et al, 2000). A study in Norway found out that the incidence of ectopic pregnancy in that country increased from 1.4% to 2.2% of livebirths between 1976 and 1993 (Bergsjo et al, 1990). In England and Wales, the incidence of ectopic pregnancy increased by five times between 1966 and 1996 from 0.3% to 1.6% of livebirths (Rajkhowa et al, 2000). The incidence also increased from 1.9 % to 2.3 % of livebirths between 1981 and 1991 in the United States (Berg, 1999). In another study conducted in the United States, the annual incidence of ectopic pregnancy increased from 0.37 % of pregnancies in 1948 to 1.97 in 1992 (Lipscomb et al, 2000). At the Royal Commission Medical Centre, Yanbe Industrial city in the Kingdom of Saudi Arabia the incidence between 2005 to 2008 was found to be 1 in 171 deliveries that is 0.58 % (Aziz et al, 2011). In India, the incidence of ectopic pregnancy is 1 in 161 (0.6%) deliveries (Arup et al, 2007).

In recent decades majority of methodological limitations in various African published literature make it impossible to draw formal conclusions concerning the incidence of ectopic pregnancy in Africa (Goyaux et al, 2003). In African developing countries, a majority of hospital-based studies have reported ectopic pregnancy case fatality rates of around 1-3 %, ten times higher than that reported in industrialised countries (Goyaux et al, 2003). Late presentation to a health facility, late diagnosis leading in almost all cases to majority of complications and emergency surgical treatment are the key factors accounting for such high fatality rates in women suffering from ectopic pregnancy in Africa. The incidence of ectopic pregnancy was found to be 0.79% in Yaoundé, Cameroun (Leke et al, 2004). This value may be considered a minimum due to probably underestimation. Nevertheless, this rate is lower than currently observed in industrialised countries. Late diagnosis, low percentage of conservative treatment and subsequent maternal deaths are important findings that should encourage African gynaecologists to promote ectopic pregnancy prevention programs and to improve the care given to women with ectopic prevention. The case fatality rate of ectopic pregnancy in Ghana was found to be 27.9/ 1000 (Baffoe & Nkyekyer, 1999). A study conducted in 1992 and 1993 at the Umtata General Hospital in Transkei, South Africa reported an ectopic incidence of 1.1% (Amoko et al, 1995). Between 1993 to 1995, the hospital based ectopic pregnancy incidence at Nosy Be Hospital, Madagascar was 2.9 % (Ratinahirana et al, 1997). It was 4 % at the gynaecology and obstetrics clinic of the national teaching hospital in Cotonou republic of Benin (Perrin et al, 1997). In Gabon University Medical Centre, Libreville it doubled between 1977 and 1989 from 1 % to 2.3 % (Picaud et al, 1990). At Yaoundé University Teaching Hospital, Cameroon, the incidence of ectopic pregnancy increased from 0.9% to 1.7 % between 1984 and 1992 (Kouam et al, 1996). The incidence of ectopic pregnancy increased in two maternities in Conakry at the Donka and Ignace Dean University Hospital, Guinea from 0.41 % to 1.5 % from 1995-1999 (Thoneau et al, 2002).

In Nigeria, an incidence of 1:287 deliveries or 0.35 %(Egwuatu & Ozumba, 1987) and 1:43 deliveries or 2.31% (Oronsange & Odiase, 1984) were reported from two institutions. These incidences may probably be an underestimation as many cases are managed in private hospitals and are not reported. A study by Oloyede et al in Sagamu, Nigeria over a 12-year review reported an incidence by 3.1% or 1 in 32 of all births (Oloyede et al, 2002). Ectopic pregnancy is an important cause of maternal death in Nigeria and in other developing countries. In Lagos, Nigeria, ectopic pregnancy was found to be responsible for 8.6 % of maternal deaths and had a case fatality rate of 3.7%. An incidence of 23.1 / 1000 deliveries was reported and ectopic pregnancy was found to be responsible for 48.5% of gynaecological emergencies (Anorlu et al, 2005). In another study in the same Lagos, Nigeria, it was responsible for 30 % of emergency gynaecological admissions with a case fatality rate of 3.7 % (Abudu, 1999). It was also found to be responsible for 8.6% of maternal deaths in Lagos, Nigeria (Abudu & Olatunji, 1996). Data obtained from various studies from different parts of Nigeria, showed that the perceived lower prevalence of chronic pelvic inflammation in the northern part of Nigeria might explain the comparatively lower incidence of ruptured tubal pregnancy (Essel et al, 1980). The incidence of ectopic pregnancy in two cities in northern Nigeria is 18.1 / 1000 deliveries in Sokoto (Airede & Ekele, 2005) and 1.14 % in Zaria (Adesiyun et al, 2001). It is 1.7% in Jos (Olarewaju et al, 1994) and 1.68 % in Benin City, Nigeria (Gharoro & Igbafe, 2002). A previous study on ectopic pregnancy done at Benin City, Nigeria revealed an incidence of 3.5 % of the total hospital births. In Markudi, Nigeria, ruptured tubal pregnancy of 0.87 % accounted for foetal births and 94.6 % of all ectopic pregnancies. There is a rising trend in the incidence of ruptured tubal pregnancy from 0.65 % in 2004 to 1.09 % in 2006 (Jogo & Swende, 2008). At the Nnamdi Azikiwe Teaching Hospital in southern Nigeria, ectopic pregnancy was responsible for 6.5 % of gynaecological admissions with an incidence of 1.3 % (Udigwe et al, 2010), 3.30 per 100 deliveries in Calabar (Ekanem et al, 2009). It increased from 0.4 % to 1.7 % between 1977 to 1987 at the Obafemi Awolowo University Teaching Hospital, Ile-Ife (Makinde & Ogunnniyi, 1990). While it decreased at the University of Nigeria Teaching Hospital, Enugu between 1978 to 1981 to 0.53 % to 0.21% of deliveries (Egwuatu & Ozumba, 1987). These observations suggest that the incidence of ectopic pregnancy in developing countries especially on the African continent has probably increased in recent decades (Thoneau et al, 2002).

3. Risk factors

Multiple factors contribute to the relative risk of ectopic pregnancy although some patients may not have any risk factor yet developed ectopic pregnancy. In theory, any thing that hampers or delays the migration of the embryo to the endometrial cavity could predispose women to ectopic pregnancy. Age, marital status, and parity have been found not to be significant risk factors for ectopic pregnancy (Anorlu et al, 2005). The reported aetiological factors for ectopic pregnancy include pelvic inflammatory disease, post abortal sepsis, postpartum sepsis, previous ectopic pregnancy, reversal of previous tubal sterilization, tubal spasm, long defects of the fallopian tubes and psychological and emotional factors (Doyle et al, 1991).

Pelvic inflammatory disease: Pelvic inflammatory disease from inappropriate obstetric care or from unsafe abortion is a risk factor for ectopic pregnancy (Onwuhafua et al, 2001). These infection causes distortion in the genital tract and the fallopian tube in particular. Unsafe abortion leads to post abortal sepsis. Induced abortion and sexually transmitted disease increases the risk four fold and nine-fold respectively (Anorlu et al, 2005). Also, multiple sexual partners predispose the patient to acquiring sexually transmitted disease. Pelvic inflammatory disease is a major risk factor for developing ectopic pregnancy in Nigeria (Olarewaju, 1994, Egwuatu & Ozumba, 1987). Induced abortion as a significant risk factor for ectopic pregnancy was not observed in studies from countries where abortion is legalised (Atrash et al, 1997). This is because qualified medical personnel carry it out under aseptically clean environment with sterile instruments. Biologically the adolescent is particularly at risk of sexually transmitted disease because the columnar epithelium, which is susceptible to *Chlamydia* and *gonococci* organism extends from the endocervical canal to the ectocervix making it fully exposed to pathogens. Adolescents also lack immunity to certain pathogens. Early sexual debut may also lead to adolescent pregnancy which is often unwanted and which usually end up with induced abortion in unsafe places and in the hands of quacks. Late age of sexual debut on the other hand, significantly reduces the risk of ectopic pregnancy (Anorlu et al, 2005). In a study in France by Coste J et al, found that *Chlamydia trachomatis* seropositively appeared to be an important risk factor in the development of ectopic pregnancy. Pelvic inflammatory disease is a risk factor for ectopic pregnancy especially salpingitis. A case control study conducted showed that the risk of ectopic pregnancy was showed that the risk of ectopic pregnancy was increased four fold with induction of ovulation (Fernandez et al, 1991).

Assisted conception: Ectopic pregnancy is one of the recognised complications of in-vitro fertilization and embryo transfer (Okohue et al, 2010). Ectopic pregnancy can present following an in vitro fertilization procedures. A high index of suspicion is necessary even in cases with previous bilateral salpingectomies or easy embryo transfer.

Intrauterine contraceptive device (IUCD): The use of intrauterine contraceptive device increases the risk of developing an ectopic pregnancy almost four fold (Anorlu et al, 2005).

Previous history of ectopic pregnancy: Previous history of an ectopic pregnancy increases the risk for another ectopic pregnancy. The risk of recurrent ectopic pregnancy is 12-18 % (Jurkovic, 2007). Every woman with a previous ectopic pregnancy would be at a high risk of recurrence of another ectopic pregnancy. This should be excluded when a patient with a previous ectopic pregnancy presents in early pregnancy.

Tubal surgery: Scarring following tubal surgery causes anatomical abnormalities of the fallopian tube, which presents abnormal embryo transport increase the risk of ectopic pregnancy (Doyle et al, 1991).

Previous caesarean delivery: There has not been any evidence of increased risk of ectopic pregnancy related to previous caesarean section (Kendrick et al, 1996). However, there are reports of ectopic pregnancies implanting on previous caesarean section scars. Endometrial and myometrial disruptions or scaring can predispose to abdominal pregnancy implantation (Fylstra, 2002).

4. Research methodology

4.1 Study design

This is a prospective study carried out at General Hospital Aliero, Kebbi State, Nigeria from February 2006 to January 2007. General Hospital Aliero is a general hospital and a secondary health facility that was upgraded from a primary health centre. At the time of the study, the three doctors at the hospital were general practitioners with no specialist training in obstetrics and gynaecology. The hospital manages patients with various illnesses and cases requiring specialist care are referred to the nearest tertiary health facility. The hospital does not have a gynaecological ward therefore patients with gynaecological problems are admitted into the female medical ward and those who had surgeries are admitted into the female surgical ward. The hospital is a general hospital, which does not have an active gynaecological unit as the patients are being managed by general practitioners posted to the hospital.

4.2 Study area

General hospital Aliero is located in Kebbi State of Nigeria. The capital of Kebbi State is Birnin Kebbi. The state was formed from part of the former Sokoto State in 1991. Kebbi State is bordered by Sokoto State, Niger State, Dosso region in the Republic of Niger and the Nation of Benin. Kebbi state is traditionally considered to belong to the Banza Bakwai States of Hausa land. Kebbi State has the slogan 'Land of Equity'. At the time of the study, General Hospital Aliero is located in Aliero, which is the capital of Aliero Local Government Area. The study was conducted during the author's National Youth Service Corps at Kebbi State, Nigeria. National Youth Service Corps is a one-year compulsory posting of Nigerian graduates outside the area of there abode within the country to serve their fatherland for one year.

4.3 Study population

All patients managed for ectopic pregnancy during the study period were included in this study. The patients were admitted through the casualty department as they all presented as emergencies. Once a patient is diagnosed with ectopic pregnancy, blood sample was sent to the laboratory for haemoglobin estimation and whole blood is grouped and cross-matched against the patients' serum as blood products are not available at the centre. The patient is counselled for surgery and informed consent obtained. At presentation, a brief history was obtained and physical examination carried out for pallor, jaundice, cyanosis and any form of bleeding and pain. History of any previous ectopic pregnancy and tubal and pelvic infections are obtained. Including any previous treatment for pelvic inflammatory disease. Urinalysis is done and venous intravenous access established.

5. Results

During the period of study, 13 patients were managed for ectopic pregnancy making 8.23 % of gynaecological emergencies at the hospital. One hundred and fifty eight patients were managed for various gynaecological emergencies during the study period. The other gynaecological emergencies are spontaneous abortion, ovarian cyst, hydantidiform mole, and uterine fibroid. All the patients had a history of collapse at home before presenting in hospital. The age of patients ranged from 20 to 42 years with a mean of 25.12 years. All the patients were married and were accompanied by there spouses and family members to the hospital. Ten of the patients were nullipara, one primipara, and two Para three. All patients in the study have never been treated for pelvic inflammatory disease and none of them have used any form of contraception. Most of the women in the community prefer to have their babies at home with the assistance of a traditional birth attendant also known as traditional midwife. Some of these traditional birth attendants and traditional midwives have received some form of training. Therefore, it is difficult to calculate the incidence as per the number of deliveries.
Twelve patients presented with ruptured ectopic pregnancy. Only one patient had an unruptured ectopic pregnancy. All the patients had emergency exploratory laparatomy, as laparoscopic services are not available at the centre at the time of the study. Also, methotrexate was not available at the centre at the time of the study. The patients had an uneventful postoperative period and were discharged home with an advise to complete there course of antibiotics, analgesics, and haematinics. The twelve patients that presented with ruptured ectopic pregnancy received whole blood intra-operatively as blood products are not available at the centre. Findings at laparatomy were right fallopian tube ectopic pregnancy in eleven patients and two patients had left ampullary ectopic pregnancy. Salpingectomy was done for all the patients. There was no history of previous ectopic pregnancy in the patients. The patients' were followed up until after discharge from hospital.

6. Clinical manifestations

There is no pelvic condition that gives rise to more diagnostic errors than ectopic pregnancy. There are no specific signs and symptoms that are pathnognomonic but a condition of findings may be suggestive of an ectopic pregnancy. Therefore, there should be high index of suspicion all the time when symptoms of early pregnancy are followed by irregular vaginal bleeding, lower abdominal pain, tenderness, fainting attack, shoulder tip pain, signs and symptoms of massive blood loss and diarrhoea and vomiting. The signs and symptoms depend on the amount and pattern of bleeding. In slowly leaking ectopic pregnancy, the bleeding occurs slowly. A delayed period is followed by spotting to continuous bleeding and unilateral pelvic pain with an adnexal mass. Rupture is signalled by hypotension, marked tenderness and severe pain radiating to the shoulder. A ruptured ectopic pregnancy typically presents with abdominal pain and can be in hypovolaemic shock. Some patients may have a paradoxical bradycardia despite a large amount of blood loss. Syncope or collapse is also common. An unruptured ectopic pregnancy presents with abdominal pain with or without vagina bleeding (Wagner & Promes, 2007).

The clinical presentation of ectopic pregnancy depends on whether it has ruptured or not. Ruptured ectopic pregnancy presents usually from 6 to 12 weeks of pregnancy. Ruptured ectopic pregnancy can lead to massive haemorrhage and death. The presentation is variable. The combination of pain, vagina bleeding, and shock is the classical presentation of ruptured ectopic pregnancy. Some patients may have syncope attacks while others may just have a sudden excruciating abdominal pain. This may be associated with severe cardiovascular compromise.

Patients usually present with the ruptured variety with attendant peritoneal flooding and its clinical consequence unlike the situation in the developed countries where up to 75 % are unruptured (Kouam et al, 1996, Morcau et al, 1995). This is because they present early to a health facility. Ectopic pregnancy has a protean manifestation (Ilesanmi & Shobowale, 1992). The delayed diagnosis of ruptured ectopic pregnancy is an important cause of death in women (Fowler, 2006). A dilemma may arise when there is a properly and reliable diagnosis of ectopic pregnancy with a live foetus. Nevertheless, the magnitude of complications of ruptured ectopic gestation is enormous. Delaying the patient of an a reliable diagnosis of ectopic pregnancy to a time of rupture or imminent rupture in other to justify not tampering with life may be considered unethical and illegal (Dickens at al, 2003).

Abdominal pain: Patients with ectopic pregnancy may have abdominal pain. This may be sharp or sudden tearing pain in the patient with ruptured ectopic pregnancy. It may start in any of the flanks or iliac fossa depending on the affected fallopian tube if the ectopic pregnancy is implanted in the fallopian tube. This gradually moves towards the umbilical region and becoming generalised. When it is an unruptured ectopic pregnancy, or slowly leaking, the abdominal pain is dull and continuous. Depending on the intensity of the pain, some patients may seek medical attention now. Ectopic pregnancy can lead to massive haemorrhage or death. It mimics virtually every condition that causes acute abdomen in women of the reproductive age group (Kigbu et al, 2006). Abdominal pain is the commonest symptom of ectopic pregnancy. The pain may be present even prior to rupture. When there is a rupture, the pain becomes sudden with each bleeding continuous and extensive intraperitoneal bleeding, the pain becomes generalized because of irritation of the diaphragm by the haemoperitoneum can cause shoulder tip pain. The abdominal pain is caused by distension of the gravid tube, by its efforts to contract and expel the ovum and by irritation of the peritoneum by leakage of blood.

Shoulder tip pain: Some patients present with shoulder tip pain. There is extensive intraperitoneal bleeding with irritation of the diaphragm by the haemoperitoneum causing irritation of the phrenic nerve.
Vagina bleeding: There may be vagina bleeding with passage of decidua cast.
Amenorrhea: This is evidence that the woman is pregnant
Dizziness and weakness: This is due to the ongoing peritoneal haemorrhage.
Nausea and vomiting: This is not specific to ectopic pregnancy. It is due to irritation of the bowel causing negative peristalsis.
Fever: It is not common and is due to irritation of the peritoneum by blood. There may be other concurrent infections and infestations such as malaria in malaria endemic areas.
The classic triad of amenorrhea, irregular vaginal bleeding and abdominal pain is not always present and occurs usually at more advanced gestational age and in patients in whom ectopic pregnancy has ruptured. In unruptured or slowly leaking ectopic pregnancy, the patient may be haemodynamically stable. A stable patient may have ill-defined abdominal pain and amenorrhea. A stable patient with ectopic may suddenly rupture and decompensate. It is because as the gestation enlarges, it creates the potential for organ rupture because only the uterine cavity is designed to expand and accommodate foetal development. The clinical manifestations in slowly leaking ectopic pregnancy are on and off lower abdominal pain, amenorrhea, irregular scanty vaginal bleeding, and with or without spells of dizziness. In unruptered ectopic pregnancy, the clinical manifestations are stable haemodynamic state, lower abdominal pain, amenorrhoea, may be symptomless and diagnosis aided by ancillary diagnostic tests.

7. Clinical findings

Evidence of blood loss: There will be evidence of blood loss. Rapid pulse rate, pallor, and reduced blood level. In severe haemorrhage, there is be hypotension.
Shock / syncope: This is a clinical manifestation of ruptured ectopic pregnancy. Any female in the reproductive age group with a history of collapse without any trauma should be considered to have ectopic pregnancy until proven otherwise. The collapse is due to massive haemorrhage from the rupture with massive haemoperitoneum. The fainting attack is due to blood loss and weakness. The syncope can sometimes coincide with the rupture. The shock is due to hypovolaemic shock due to heamoperitoneum. It is due to circulating failure from reduction in effective circulating blood volume. There will be clinical features of shock such as tachycardia, hypotension, oliguria and occasionally bradycardia, pallor, sweating, confusion, cold, and clammy peripheries. There is inadequate left ventricular preload, significant fall in cardiac output, low central venous pressure and decreased urine output. Further haemorrhage results in decreased cardiac out, sympathetic over activity, further reduction in tissue perfusion, worsening hypoxia, cellular damage, and release of inflammatory cytokines. Decrease in the intravascular blood volume leads to decrease in cardiac output and tissue perfusion. Also, the decrease in intravascular blood volume causes diversion of blood from the skin to maintain organ perfusion giving rise to pale cool skin, hypotension, and tachycardia. Blood is diverted preferentially to the heart and brain. Therefore, thirst, oliguria, tachycardia, and labile blood pressure occurs. Reduced blood flow to the brain and heart results in restlessness, agitated, confusion, hypotension, tachycardia, and tachypnea.

Pelvic examination: It may be difficult to define the uterus because of pain. There is severe cervical tenderness in the presence of pelvic inflammatory disease. The pouch of Douglas is full. There may be identification of a pelvic mass separate from the uterus.
Haematosalpinx: This is due to accumulation of blood in the fallopian tube.
Haematocele: This is due to progressive bleeding with haematoma formation in the pouch of Douglas (Coutrin et al, 2007).
Haematoperitoneum: Bloody perfusion into the peritoneal cavity secondary to rupture of the fallopian tube and its blood vessels (Coutrin et al, 2007). This is the clinical picture seen most commonly in rural areas.

8. Management of ectopic pregnancy

In managing ectopic pregnancy, there is the need for a high index of suspicion (Ibekwe, 2004). Investigations must not delay resuscitation. The initial management of the acute patient involves correction of shock with rapid fluid replacement, cross matching of blood, check on the haemoglobin and immediate recourse to laparatomy to stern the source of the haemorrhage (Pitkin et al, 2003).

8.1 Investigations

Haemoglobin estimation: There is a drop in the haemoglobin level. Also, there is a gradual drop if serial haemoglobin estimation is done in ruptured or slowly leaking ectopic pregnancy. The haemoglobin level in an unruptured ectopic pregnancy may not give a clue to the condition.
Pregnancy test: This measures the human chorionic gonadotrophin level. A negative test does not exclude an ectopic pregnancy. Ectopic pregnancy does not produce as much human chorionic gonadotropihn as much as intrauterine pregnancy. A pregnancy test is only valuable if it is positive (Coutin et al, 2007).
Ultrasonography: Diagnostic ultrasound also referred to as sonography is the method of imaging structures inside the body by using high frequency sound waves with no ionizing radiation involved. Ultrasound is safe and non-invasive. In ectopic pregnancy, pelvic ultrasound shows an empty uterus and an ectopic gestation sac with a living embryo if the ectopic pregnancy has not ruptured. There is fluid in the cul-de-sac of the perineum. Real time ultrasound shows foetal heart motion. Real time ultrasonography is of great help in establishing the diagnosis of unruptured ectopic pregnancy. Its primary role lies in documenting a normal intrauterine pregnancy about five to six weeks of gestation. Such a finding essentially excludes the possibility of ectopic pregnancy because the incidence of coexisting ectopic pregnancy and intrauterine pregnancy is about 1 in 30,000 pregnancies. Ultrasound examination may be of secondary importance in supporting a diagnosis of possible ectopic pregnancy by showing an adnexa mass or fluid within the cul-de-sac or both. The ability to identify an adnexa mass as an ectopic pregnancy rather than a large ovarian cyst, hydrosalpinx, tubo-ovarian abscess or other causes of adnexa enlargement varies from centre to centre. Ultrasonography has been found to be promising in the confirmatory diagnosis of ectopic pregnancy (Ikpeze, 1991). Use of ultrasonographic imaging should never preclude adequate resuscitation or definitive surgical therapy in a patient who is haemodynamically unstable and in whom ectopic pregnancy is a highly suspected. The goal of bedside ultrasonography is to diagnose an intrauterine pregnancy as heterotopic pregnancy although rarely still occurs. Bedside ultrasonography should not be

performed if it delays resuscitation or definitive surgical care in an unstable patient. Transvaginal sonography facilities diagnose the location of the gestational sac, age, size, and viability of an ectopic pregnancy even within a uterine scar (Herman et al, 1995). Bedside ultrasonography is the test of choice in unstable patients. Ectopic pregnancy within a previous caesarean section scar is best diagnosed by transvaginal ultrasound. However, a delay in either diagnosis or treatment can lead to uterine rupture, hysterectomy, and significant maternal mortality. As soon as the diagnosis is confined, proper surgical treatment by laparatomy should be arranged. Ultrasound evaluation especially transvaginal scan is invaluable but where there result is equivocal, ancillary tests should be done (Tenore, 2000). The ultrasonographic findings of a ruptured ectopic pregnancy are absence of an intrauterine gestational sac, fluid particularly haemorrhagic in the pelvis or perineum, adnexal masses or haematosalpinx. Transvaginal ultrasound provides improved resolution allowing descriptions of early embryonic development characteristics. Improvement in the identification of the sonographic landmark of normal embryonic development and awareness of the sonographic risk factors of pregnancy failure may lead to more successful management strategies. Diagnosis of suspected ectopic pregnancy often involves an assessment of both hormonal markers and sonographic features (Lucie et al, 2005). Ultrasound that demonstrates an intrauterine pregnancy is reassuring because heterotopic pregnancy occurs in only 1: 7000 to 1: 30,000 of spontaneously conceived pregnancies (DeVoe & Pratt, 1948). The sonographic appearance of an ectopic pregnancy is varied. There may be simple adnexal cyst, complex adnexal mass, tubal ring, free fluid in the adnexal cul-de-sac, a live extra uterine foetus or an empty uterus with no other sonographic findings (Lucie et al, 2005). A live extra uterine embryo is diagnostic of an ectopic pregnancy. Isolated free fluid in the pelvis is rarely the only sonographic findings. Presence of an adnexal mass and / or free pelvic fluid is strong predictor of an ectopic pregnancy (diagnostic imaging). Where ultrasound is not available and there is still some doubt, two other diagnostic procedures can be used. They are culdocentesis, which is puncture of the pouch of Douglas and abdominis parencentesis.

Culdocentesis: This involves aspiration of fluid from the pouch of Douglas through the posterior fornix of the vagina.

Parencentesis abdominis: This involves aspiration of non-clotting blood from the abdomen. It is not diagnostic because the needle used for aspiration can go into the inferior vena cava, or rectum. It is technically difficult in the obese patient. The pouch of Douglas may be full. There can be adhesions therefore the needle may not get to the abdomen.

8.2 Resuscitation

Volume replacement is done with plasma expanders and preparations for the definitive therapy. In developing countries and low resource settings, colloids are not readily available. In severe anaemia, blood transfusion is commenced before surgery. In ruptured ectopic pregnancy, intravenous access is established with a wide bore cannula and rapid infusion of a plasma expander done if the patient is in shock or in the presence of hypotension. If there is evidence of haemoperitoneum with clinical shock following rupture, there is little room for delay. Blood sample is collected for haemoglobin estimation, grouping, and crossmatching of at least two units of blood. Occasionally a delay in red blood cell transfusion poses a substantial risk to the patient. In these circumstances, transfusion with non-crossmatched type O rhesus negative blood may be necessary. The disadvantages of using non-cross matched blood include possible transfusion of incompatible blood owing to clinically significant antibodies to blood groups other than ABO.

8.3 Treatment

Ectopic pregnancy can be treated surgically or non-surgically depending if it is ruptured or not and the equipments available at the centre. Due to advances in the diagnostic techniques, it has become possible to identify and manage ectopic pregnancy before they cause clinical symptoms in many developed countries. (Amok & Buga, 1995). This is not so in most developing countries. Subsequent fertility is substantially improved when conservative surgery is utilised instead of salpingectomy. Subsequent intrauterine pregnancy rates have been found to be 76% when conservative surgery is performed and 44% when salpingectomy is performed (Sherman et al, 1982). In patients with adhesive disease in the contra-lateral adnexa and a history of infertility, conservative management of ectopic pregnancy has produced good results with restoration of tubal potency in over 80 % in some cases if the ectopic pregnancy has not ruptured (Rajkhowa et al, 2000, Ekele, 2001, Lipscomb et al, 2000). The management of ectopic pregnancy has been improved upon by the use of ultrasound, laparoscopy, and monitoring of the beta subunit of the Human Chorionic Gonadotrophin (Gracia & Barnhan, 2001). Early diagnosis before tubal rupture is important in reducing mortality as well as preserving the potential for future fertility through conservative management (Gazvani, 1996). If not treated vigorously and early enough, ectopic pregnancy may be fatal. Women with ectopic pregnancy continue to present late precluding early diagnosis and use of conservative modalities of management. Morbidity remains high but mortality has declined. Blood bank services and availability of antibiotics are necessary in the management of most gynaecological emergencies. This is a problem in some developing countries and sometimes absent in some hospitals in rural areas. Transportation to an appropriate health facility can be a cause of late presentation.

8.3.1 Surgical therapy

Surgical treatment of ectopic pregnancy can be by laparatomy or minimally invasive surgery that is laparoscopy. Laparatomy involves removing the affected fallopian tube (salpingectomy) or dissecting the ectopic pregnancy with conservation of the fallopian known as salpingostomy. Laparatomy is reserved for patients with extensive intraperitoneal bleeding, intravascular collapse, or poor visualisation of the pelvis at the time of laparoscopy. The decision to perform a salpingostomy or salpingectomy is often made intra-operatively based on the extent of damage to the affected and contra-lateral tubes but it is also dependent on the patient's history of previous ectopic pregnancy and wish for future fertility, availability of assisted reproductive technology and the skill of the surgeon (Barnhart, 2009). Most gynaecological emergencies that are managed by laparatomy can be treated by laparoscopy and benefit both patient and the health facility (Baumann et al, 1989). Not all cases of ectopic pregnancy can be treated with laparoscopy especially ruptured ectopic pregnancy. The treatment of ectopic pregnancy is influenced by the clinical state of the patient, the site of the ectopic gestation, the reproductive wish of the patient and available facilities and technology. Surgical treatment for ectopic pregnancy is still the norm and gold standard. The surgical procedure may also be radical (salpingectomy) or conservative (linear salpingostomy). In the surgical management of ectopic pregnancy, the benefits of salpingectomy over salpingostomy are uncertain (Farquhar, 2005). In developed countries, most ectopic pregnancies are diagnosed before rupture and there is room for conservative surgical procedures (Ibekwe, 2004). The emphasis in the management of ectopic pregnancy is on early diagnosis before rupture and conservative surgery. However, in most developing countries especially Nigeria where patients still present late after rupture, salpingectomy remains the operative procedure (Ibekwe, 2004). Salpingectomy is the commonest surgical management for tubal pregnancy in Nigeria because most of the women present late (Egwuatu & Ozumba, 1987, Gharoro & Igbafe, 2002). Salpingectomy, which leads to tubal loss and reduced reproductive potentials is the commonest management option in low resource settings (Eze, 2008). Intrauterine pregnancy rate after salpingectomy is about 45 % with a 9 % repeat ectopic pregnancy (Eze, 2008). In salpingostomy, tissue handling is minimized to reduce tissue trauma and prevent tubal occlusion or peritubal adhesions. The success of reconstructive tubal surgery for ectopic pregnancy can be only measured in terms of subsequent live births the individual achieves. During the surgical treatment of ectopic pregnancy by both laparatomy and laparoscopy, the state of the contra-lateral tube is noted. The condition of the contra-lateral tube has been reported to play a crucial role in subsequent fertility of patients with ectopic pregnancy (Kjellberg & Lalos, 2000, Tuomivaara & Kauppila, 1988). An ectopic pregnancy with a ruptured or severely damaged tube renders little choice but salpingectomy (Nannie et al, 2003). Salpingostomy is where the ectopic conceptus is removed from the affected tube through a linear incision of the tube overlying the ectopic pregnancy. This incision is not surgically closed and is allowed to heal through secondary intention. This surgical treatment conserves the affected tube (Varma & Gupta, 2008).

8.3.1.1 Ectopic pregnancy in caesarean section scar

Although the expedient and medical management have been reported, termination of a caesarean section scar pregnancy by laparatomy and hysterectomy with repair of the accompanying uterine scar dehiscence may be the best option (Fylstra, 2002).

8.3.2 Laparoscopy

This service is not readily available in developing countries especially those in low resource areas and in underequipped hospitals. Elsewhere in the developed world, minimal access laparoscopic surgery has become the preferred technique unless the woman is haemodynamically unstable (Tulandi & Saleh, 1997). Laparoscopic surgery has brought a lot of revolution in the field of medicine. Its evolution and spread was rapid in developed countries. In the industrialized countries, it is often the first choice intervention when surgery is needed. However, there is still a major gap in the implementation of laparoscopic surgery in under resourced settings often due to restricted availability to access to the equipment and lack of training. Laparoscopic surgery compared to open surgery may offer advantages such as less infections, complications, minimal tissue trauma, faster recovery, and shorter stay in hospital. Its implementation is associated with some constraints such as the surgeons' skills, the cost of acquisition and maintenance of the laparoscope, need for a trained anaesthetist, the availability of electricity and medical carbon dioxide.

Diagnostic and therapeutic laparoscopy has increased over the last decade without increase in maternal and foetal complications. Laparoscopic approach is useful for haemodynamically stable patients. The choice of laparoscopic surgery versus laparatomy depends on the clinical experience of the surgeon, equipment availability, and patients' physical status (Ling & Stovall, 1994). In women desiring fertility, conservative tube sparing surgery has been recommended, as it does not increase the subsequent recurrence of ectopic pregnancy (Arora et al, 2005). Salpingectomy is the procedure of choice if the woman has no desire for future pregnancy. Laparoscopic management of ectopic pregnancy has been demonstrated to be safe and an effective alternative to conventional management by laparatomy. Laparoscopic procedures are associated with less intra-operative blood loss, lower analgesic requirements, shorter hospital stay and a quicker return to normal activities (Qureshi et al, 2006). Experienced operators may be able to manage laparoscopically women with even large haemoperitoneum safely but the surgical procedure, which prevents further loss quickly should be used (Guideline: 2004). In most centres, this will be by laparatomy. A pregnancy ectopically implanted into the fallopian tube, ovary or other distant sites may also be associated with the accumulation of fluid in the uterine lumen at five weeks gestation. This absence of a chorionic sac however leads to the appearance of only a single ring or pseudo sac in the uterus, in contrast to the double ring of an intrauterine pregnancy. The identification of a cystic mass with complex shadows in the adnexa may give a further clue to the presence of an ectopic pregnancy although it is often impossible to determine the exact site of origin of such a mass on ultrasound. Finally, bleeding associated with ectopic pregnancy may manifest itself as free fluid in the pouch of Douglas (Loughney & Stirges, 2004). Ectopic pregnancy can occur in the absence of either a single uterine ring, an adnexa mass or free peritoneal fluid.

8.3.3 Medical treatment

Medical therapy has an established place in the treatment of ectopic pregnancy and in carefully selected patients; it appears to be effective as surgery (Sowter & Farquhar, 2004). For medical therapy of ectopic pregnancy, systemic methotraxate is usually employed. However, ultrasonographic or laparoscopic guide injection into the gestational sac can lead to resolution in asymptomatic patients. There are numerous reports describing successful treatment of all varieties of ectopic pregnancies using a number of methotrexate (MTX) regimens. It is clear that many women with an ectopic pregnancy are not suitable for medical therapy. Active intra-abdominal haemorrhage is a contraindication. The size of the mass is important. Medical therapy for ectopic pregnancy involves also monitoring the patients' quantitative beta human chorionic gonadotropihn concentrations and this is not available in low resource areas. Single dose methotrexate is associated with a higher risk of rupture than multiple doses (Buster & Barnhart, 2004). Medical management is indicated with no viable intrauterine pregnancy, absence of rupture, adnexal mass of 4 cm or less and beta Human Chorionic Gonadotrophin levels are below 10,000 iu/ml (Buster & Barnhart, 2004). Some of the side effects of methotrexate are abdominal discomfort, chills and fever, dizziness, immunosuppression, leucopoenia, malaise, nausea, ulcerative stomatitis, photosensitivity and undue fatigue. Breastfeeding is an absolute contraindication to methotrexate therapy. Relative contraindications to methotrexate therapy are abnormal liver function test, blood dyscrasias, ongoing radiotherapy, excessive alcohol consumption, HIV / AIDS, psoriasis, rheumatoid arthritis and significant pulmonary disease. There is no role for medical management in the treatment of ruptured tubal pregnancy or suspected tubal pregnancy when a patient shows signs of hypovolaemic shock (Guideline, 2004).

8.4 Postoperative management

The patient may still require blood transfusion if anaemia is still present. Intravenous fluids are administered until bowel sounds return and the patient is able to take orally. Antibiotics and analgesics are administered. Haematinics is commenced once the patient has commenced oral feeding. The patient is encouraged to ambulate especially if obese. On discharge, the patient is counselled for family planning and follow-up. Follow-up visit is necessary. Broad-spectrum antibiotics are administered.

8.5 Blood transfusion

Blood transfusion involves the infusion of whole blood or blood component from one individual to another. In an emergency with massive blood loss that threatens life, it is permissible to transfuse group O negative packed cells but blood sample must be taken for grouping and crossmatching prior to transfusions (Simmons, 2008). Blood transfusion is associated with significant risk hence it calls for great caution. Transfusion safety lies on the avoidance of transfusion reaction. Blood transfusion services are necessary in the management of ectopic pregnancy because of the intraperitoneal haemorrhage. Some patients may present in haemorrhagic shock. Blood transfusion could be life saving in cases of ruptured ectopic pregnancy. Blood products are scarce resources in developing countries especially in low resource centres although blood transfusion carries its own risks. Transfusion of safe blood when life-threatening conditions cannot be prevented or managed by other means. Blood transfusion is just a part of clinical management. Blood loss can be massive requiring blood transfusion. Autologous blood transfusion is done in most rural centres. Blood from the intraperitoneal haemorrhage is scooped out and filtered through five to eight layers of sterile gauze to remove large blood clots. This filtered blood is introduced into a blood bag, which contains an anticoagulant to prevent clotting of the filtered blood, and transfused to the patient via blood giving set.

8.6 Patients who refuse blood transfusion

Even after extensive counselling regarding the risks and benefits of blood transfusion, some patients still refuse blood transfusion even under life threatening conditions. These are due to religious and traditional beliefs. Written informed consent concerning this issue should be obtained in the presence of a witness because if death of the patient occurs, the patient will no longer be there to attest herself. Initial management with intravenous fluids sufficient to maintain perfusion and haemodynamic stability should be commenced.

9. Discussion

Ectopic pregnancy is a cause of maternal morbidity and mortality and is reduced where there are emergency surgical facilities and blood transfusion services. All the patients in this study had laparatomy as in most studies conducted in Nigeria. This is because laparoscopic services are not available at the centre. Laparatomy for now remains the most common surgical intervention method at our disposal for the management of ectopic pregnancy. This is due in part to non-availability of operating laparoscopes, which have been shown to be very useful (Barnhart et al, 1980). Moreover, significant haemoperitoneum from ruptured tubal pregnancy makes laparoscopic surgery less than ideal. The doctors at the study centre do not have specialist training in obstetrics and gynaecology hence salpingectomy is done in all patients diagnosed with ectopic pregnancy. Referral of a patient with ectopic pregnancy to a centre with laparoscopic service may lead to death during transportation and transfer because there is continuous intraperitoneal bleeding which can lead to exsanguination. Blood transfusion services are necessary in the management of ectopic pregnancy. Mortality and morbidity are low when diagnosis is made before rupture occurs. The most common cause of these deaths is massive bleeding after rupture of the ectopic pregnancy. Absence of cross-matched blood should not be a deferment to exploratory laparatomy because intraperitoneal haemorrhage is on going. In developed countries, diagnosis is made before rupture occurs however most cases in our environment still present late with severe intraperitoneal haemorrhage (Nwagha et al, 2007).

Early presentation, high index of suspicion and use of modern diagnostic techniques will improve overall clinical outcome in patients. Promotion of family planning, early treatment of pelvic inflammatory disease and good quality obstetric care could be important preventive intervention.

Abdominal pain and tenderness are the most frequent sign and symptom of ectopic pregnancy (Airede & Ekele, 2005). Diagnosis was usually based on clinical findings augmented by procedures such as parencentesis abdominis, abdominal and pelvic examination, and urine pregnancy test. Blood products are not available at the centre hence all the patients received transfusion of whole blood.

10. Case series

10.1 Case 1

A 24-year-old nullipara presented with complaints of abdominal pain and vaginal bleeding of one-week duration. The pain was cramp-like and sharp at the umbilicus. She had amenorrhea for six weeks. Physical examination revealed a young woman in painful distress that was very pale. Pulse rate was 120 beats per minute and blood pressure 90/60 mmhg. The abdomen was distended and tender. It was difficult to palpate abdominal organs because of guarding. Pelvic examination showed an uneffaced cervix, which was firm, tender, and central. Cervical Os was closed. The uterus was empty with free adnexa, full, tender, and cystic pouch of Douglas on pelvic examination. There was cervical excitation tenderness and the examining gloved finger was stained with altered blood. The packed cell volume was 22%. A diagnosis of ruptured ectopic pregnancy was made. Abdominal ultrasound showed a bulky uterus, which was anteverted. The endometrial cavity was empty and intact. There was significant decidual reaction suggestive of ruptured ectopic gestation. The entire pelvic organs was floating on fluid suggestive to be internal haemorrhage. Differential diagnosis of massive peritoneum, ascitis, very bulky uterus with decidual reaction and ruptured ectopic pregnancy was made. At laparatomy, there was seropurulent peritoneal fluid with a gangrenous 80 cm of the terminal ileum, gangrene of 10 cm of the sigmoid colon trapped in a sigmoid volvolus. The gangrenous segment of bowel was excised and resected with an ileo-ileal and colo-colic anastomosis done.

10.2 Case 2

A 30-year-old woman presented with complaints of six hours severe abdominal pain and eight weeks of amenorrhoea. Clinical findings showed tender right iliac fossa and lumber region. She was in painful distress and pale. Cervical excitation tenderness was tender on pelvic examination and tenderness of the right adnexa. Abdominal ultrasound suggested right ovarian cyst torsion. Laparatomy findings was a right ruptured ectopic pregnancy.

10.3 Case 3

32-year-old nullipara presented with complaints of bleeding altered blood per vaginum of four weeks duration with associated offensive discharge, abdominal pain of three weeks duration, generalized body weakness, abdominal swelling, two episodes of fainting attacks and vomiting of one-week duration. She never used any form of contraceptives and has had two terminations of pregnancies. On examination, she was pale with an unrecordable blood pressure at presentation. She was resuscitated with intravenous normal saline and the blood pressure became 100/ 60 mmhg. Abdomen was distended with guarding. The abdominal organs were difficult to palpate due to tenderness with the presence of ascitis evidenced by positive shifting dullness, the cervix was firm and uneffaced. Uterus was bulky and the left adnexa were bulky and tender on pelvic examination. The packed cell volume was 10 % with a positive pregnancy test. At laparatomy, there was haemoperitoneum of 3L with a right ruptured ampullary gestation with normal right ovary. Right partial salpingectomy was performed.

10.4 Case 4

A 26-year-old nulliparous undergraduate presented with six weeks of amenorrhea, fainting attacks, and severe abdominal pain. On examination, she was in shock with a fast and thready pulse and unrecordable blood pressure. She was resuscitated with 1.5 L of normal saline. Packed cell volume was 20%. Pelvic examination showed a bulky uterus with cervical excitation tenderness and full pouch of Douglas. A diagnosis of ruptured ectopic gestation was made. She was immediately planned for laparatomy. At laparatomy, there was haemoperitoneum of 3L with a ruptured left ovarian ectopic pregnancy. Left partial salpingecyomy with left oophprecytomy was performed. She received two units of blood intra-operatively and one unit of whole blood postoperatively.

10.5 Case 5

A 35-year-old Para two woman with one previous caesarean section was diagnosed to have slowly leaking ectopic pregnancy. She refused surgical intervention. After surfing the internet, she found out that ectopic pregnancy could be treated medically. Without finding out the criteria for medical therapy of ectopic pregnancy, she was able to obtain methotraxate on her own. One week later, she collapsed while at work and was rushed to a nearby hospital where emergency laparatomy and right salpingectomy for ruptured ectopic pregnancy was performed.

11. Prognosis

Ectopic pregnancy results in significant morbidity for the mother and inevitable loss of the pregnancy. Apart from foetal wastage, maternal morbidity and mortality occurs, ectopic pregnancy is also associated with repeat ectopic gestation and impairment of subsequent fertility (Abdul, 1999). The survival rate of ectopic pregnancy has improved with great improvements in anaesthesia, antibiotics, and blood transfusion. Maternal morbidity and mortality can be reduced with an early diagnosis of ectopic pregnancy. Early diagnosis before tubal rupture is important in reducing mortality as well as preserving the potential for future fertility through conservative management (Gazvani, 1996). In many cases, early diagnosis allows a conservative approach resulting in a normal macroscopic appearance and thereby preserving tubal potency and function.

12. Conclusion

Ectopic means out of place. The egg settles in the fallopian tube in more than 95% of cases. This is why it is commonly called tubal pregnancy. The egg can also implant in the ovary, abdomen, or cervix. None of these areas has as much space for nurturing tissue as a uterus for a pregnancy to develop. As the foetus grows, it will eventually burst the organ that containing it causing severe bleeding and endanger the mothers' life.

Ectopic pregnancy remains the leading cause of maternal morbidity and mortality in the first trimester of pregnancy and is a significant cause of reproductive failure in Nigeria (Igberase et al, 2005). It remains a major public health challenge among women of the reproductive age group in this region. Community based comprehensive health education programme focusing on contraception, sex education, prevention and treatment of post abortal sepsis, pelvic inflammatory disease and puerperal sepsis are urgently needed. It continues to be an important contributor to maternal morbidity and mortality and early wastages in the first trimester of pregnancy in our environment mainly because of the late diagnosis because of seeking for medical help late with attendant risk of tubal rupture and haemorrhage (Igberase, 2005, Kora et al, 1996). A high prevalence of sexually transmitted infections and unsafe abortions results in a high incidence of ectopic pregnancy. Poverty, ignorance, late presentation, non-availability of modern diagnostic tools is the basis of significant improvement in the detection and prompt treatment of ectopic pregnancy in developing nations. Emphasis should be placed on prevention and early detection as to give patients the opportunities for tubal conservative treatment. The incidence of ruptured ectopic pregnancy is decreased in westernised and developed countries because of increased awareness of the disease condition, early referral and better techniques and diagnostic instruments such as quantitative beta human chorionic gonadotrophin and vagina ultrasound probe.

The importance of ectopic pregnancy in our environment is peculiar because rather than join the global trend of early diagnosis and conservative approach in management we are challenged by late presentations with rupture in more than eight percent in most of the cases (Gharoro & Igbafe, 2002).

Promotion of family planning, early and prompt treatment of pelvic inflammatory disease and good quality obstetric care could be important in preventive intervention measures (Adesiyun & Adze, 2001). The high incidence of ectopic pregnancy may be related to a higher incidences of tubal disease notably salpingitis. Technological advances have led to earlier diagnosis of ectopic pregnancy with a decline in morbidity and mortality in developed countries. Early presentation, high index of suspicion and use of modern diagnostic techniques will improve overall clinical outcome of patients. Considerable progresses have been accompanied in the diagnosis and treatment of ectopic pregnancy (Ayoubi & Fanchin, 2003). The combination of abdominal pain, vaginal bleeding, and shock is the classical presentation of ruptured ectopic pregnancy though the presentation can be varied. Although advances in earlier diagnosis have led to reduced case fatality rates and conservative laparoscopic treatments have enabled improved outcomes (Doyle et al, 1990). Ectopic pregnancy accounts for a sizable proportion of infertility and ectopic reoccurrence (Dolye et al, 1990). Health education of women in the reproductive age on safe sex and eradication of unsafe abortion and early treatment of pelvic infections and good quality obstetric care will prove useful as preventive measures.

A high index of suspicion and up to date diagnostic methods, proper sex education, prevention of unwanted pregnancy, prevention and proper treatment of sexually transmitted infections will reduce the incidence of ectopic pregnancy. Ectopic pregnancy presents a major health problem for women of childbearing age. It is the result of a flaw in the human reproductive physiology that allows the conceptus to implant and mature outside the endometrial cavity, which ultimately ends in death of the foetus. Without timely diagnosis and treatment, ectopic pregnancy can become a life-threatening situation. In addition to the immediate morbidity caused by ectopic pregnancy, the woman's future ability to reproduce may be adversely affected as well.

Ectopic pregnancy should be considered a relevant public health indicator in developing countries. An overall picture of the capacity of a health system to deal with the diagnosis and treatment of emergencies especially in the field of obstetrics and gynaecology (Goyaux et al, 2003). Ectopic pregnancy remains a major cause of maternal mortality and morbidity as well as early foetal wastage in Nigeria and other developing countries (Okunlola et al, 2006, Makinde et al, 1990, Baffoe & Nkyekyer, 1991, Abdul, 1999, Elhelw, 2003). A classical ectopic pregnancy does not develop into livebirth. Ectopic pregnancy can be difficult to diagnose because symptoms often mimic those of a normal early pregnancy. The first warning signs of an ectopic pregnancy are often pain or vaginal bleeding. Ectopic pregnancies continue to be a significant cause of maternal morbidity, mortality, and reproductive failure in Nigeria (Faleyimu et al, 2008). Ipsilateral ectopic pregnancy occurs rarely and may be difficult to diagnose in low resource settings where there are no diagnostic tools especially vaginal ultrasound probe. When vaginal ultrasound probe is available, there are no trained medical personnel to operate such sophisticated equipments. There are few reported cases of ectopic pregnancy on a previous ectopic pregnancy stump. Ectopic pregnancy may pose a diagnostic dilemma where facilities are not available. In developed nations, treatment options have shifted from laparatomy to conservative surgical and non-surgical techniques. The availability of high-resolution ultrasonography with vaginal transducers in combination with the discriminatory zone of the beta subunit of human chorionic gonadotrophin has increased early diagnosis of the ectopic pregnancy in centres, which have such facilities (Ory, 1992). As the ability to diagnose ectopic pregnancy improves, physicians will be able to intervene sooner, preventing life threatening sequalae and extensive tubal damage, which could preserve future fertility. Already with improving technology, physicians are treating ectopic pregnancies with minimally invasive surgery or no surgery at all. Physicians have been able to reduce the mortality rate secondary to ectopic pregnancy despite its growing incidence.

Efforts to improve early diagnosis prior to tubal rupture however remain a great challenge in the developing countries and under equipped hospitals. The future fertility outcome is improved if the contra-lateral tube is normal. However, it is subjective to assess the normalcy of the tube by gross assessment since the pathology that usually predisposes to the ectopic pregnancy is intraluminal and may be present in the contra-lateral tube. Nevertheless, the practice of examination and documentation of the status of the contra-lateral tube during laparatomy for ectopic pregnancy is important. Late diagnosis leading to almost all cases of major complications and emergency surgical treatments are key elements accounting for such high fatality rates in women suffering from ectopic pregnancy in Africa. Transportation to an appropriate health facility can be a cause of late presentation. Ectopic pregnancy should be considered a relevant public health indicator in developing countries providing an overall picture of the capacity of a health system to deal with the diagnosis.

13. Acknowledgement

Dr Emmanuel Etriem and Dr Aliyu Abdullahi both medical officers at General hospital Aliero Kebbi State, Nigeria at the time of the study are both acknowledged.

14. References

Abasiattai AM, Utuk MN, Ugege W. (2010). Spontaneous Heterotropic Pregnancy with Tubal Rupture and Delivery of a Live Baby at Term: A Case Report. *Nigerian Journal of Medicine*. Vol 19. No 2. (April-June 2010). Pp 236-238. ISSN 1115 - 2613

Abdul IF. (1999). Ectopic Pregnancy in Ilorin, Nigeria. *International Journal of gynecology and obstetrics* Vol 66. Pp 179-80. ISSN 0020-7292

Abedi HO, Okonta PI, Igberase GO. (2010). Heterotropic Gestation: Successful Vaginal Term Delivery after Laparatomy in the First Trimester. *Nigerian Journal of General Practice*. Vol 8. No 5. Pp 8-10. ISSN 1118-4647

Aboyeji AP, Fawole AA, Ijaiya MA. (2002). Trends in Ectopic Pregnancy in Ilorin, Nigeria. *Nigerian Journal of Surgical Research*. Vol 4. No 1-2. (March-June 2002). Pp 6-10. ISSN: 1595-1103

Abudu OO, Egwatu JI, Imosemi OO, Ola ER. (1999). Ectopic Pregnancy: Lagos University Teaching Hospital Experience over a Five-Year Period. *Nigerian Quarterly Journal of Hospital Medicine*. Vol 9. Pp: 100-3. ISSN 0189-2657

Abudu OO, Olatunji AD. (1996). A Review of Maternal Mortality in Lagos University Teaching Hospital. *Nigerian Medical Practitioner*. Vol 31. Pp: 12-6. ISSN 0189-0964

Adesiyun GA, Adze J, Onwuhafua A, Onwuhafua PI. (2001). Ectopic pregnancies at Ahmadu Bello University Teaching Hospital, Kaduna, Northern Nigeria. *Tropical Journal of Obstetrics and Gynaecology*. Vol 18. No 2. Pp: 82-86. ISSN 0189-5178

Airede LR, Ekele BA. (2005). Ectopic Pregnancy in Sokoto, Northern Nigeria. *Malawi Medical Journal*. Vol 17. No 1. Pp: 14-16. ISSN 1995-7262, online 1995-7270

Aliyu JA, Eigbefoh JO, Mabayoje PS. (2008). Heterotropic Pregnancy: A Report of Two Cases. *Nigerian Journal of Clinical* Practice. (March 2008). Vol 11. No 1. Pp: 85-87. ISSN 1119-3077

Amoko DH, Buga GA. (1995). Clinical Presentation of Ectopic Pregnancy in Transkei, South Africa. *East African Medical Journal*. Vol 72. No 12. (December 1995). Pp: 770-3. ISSN 0012-835X

Anorlu RI, Oluwole A, Abudu OO, Adebajo S. (2005). Risk Factors for Ectopic Pregnancy in Lagos, Nigeria. *Acta Obstetricia et Gynecologica Scandinavica*. Vol 84. No 2. (February 2005). Pp: 184-8. ISSN 1600-0412

Arora D, Bhattacharyya TK, Kathpalia SK, Kochar SPS. (2005). Acute abdomen in Gynaecologic Practice. *Medical Journal Armed Forces India*. Vol 61. Pp 66-70. ISSN 0377-1237

Arup KM, Niloptal R, Kakali SK, Pradip KB. (2007). Ectopic Pregnancy: An Analysis of 180 Cases. *Journal of the Indian Medical Association*. Vol 105. Pp 308-314. ISSN 0019-5847

Atrash HK, Strauss LT, Kendrick JS, Skjeldestad FE, Ahn YW. (1997). The Relationship between Induced Abortion and Ectopic Pregnancy. *Obstetrics and Gynaecology*. Vol 89. Pp 512-8. ISSN 0029-7844

Ayoubi J, Fanchin R. (2003). Ectopic Pregnancy: Which Side to Operate? *The Lancet*. Vol 362. No 9391. (October 11, 2003). Pp 1183. ISSN 0140-6736 retrieved from <www.thelancet.com>

Aziz S, Al-Wafi B, Swadi HA. (2011). Frequency of Ectopic Pregnancy in A Medical Centre, Kingdom of Saudi Arabia. *Journal of Pakistan Medical Association*. Vol 61. No 3. (March 2011). Pp 221-224. ISSN 0030-9982

Baffoe S, Nkyekyer K. (1999). Ectopic Pregnancy in Korle Bu Teaching Hospital, Ghana: A Three-Year Review. *Tropical Doctor*. Vol 29. No 1. (January1999). Pp: 18-22. ISSN 0049-4755

Barnhart KT. (2009). Ectopic Pregnancy. *New England Journal of Medicine*. Vol 361. No 4. (July 23, 2009). Pp 379-387. ISSN 0028-4793 retrieved from <www.nejm.com>

Baumann R, Magos Al, Turnbull AC. (1989). Managing Gynaecological Emergencies with Laparoscopy. *Maternal Mortality Journal*. Vol 299. Pp 371-4

Berg CI, Shulman H, Green GA, Atrash HK et al.(1999). Estimates of the Annual Number of Clinically Recognised Pregnancies in the United States 1981-91. *American Journal of Epidemiology*. Vol 149. Pp: 1025-9. ISSN 0002-9262

Bergsjo P, Storeide O, Veholmen M, Eide M, Sandvei R. (1997). The Incidence of Ectopic Pregnancy in Holland Country, Norway 1976-1993. *Acta Obstetetricia ET Gynecologica Scandinavica*. 1997. Vol 76. Pp: 345-9. ISSN 1600-0412

Bode-Law F, Igberase GO, Momoh MO. (2008). Ipsilateral Ectopic Pregnancy Occurring In the Stump of a Previous Ectopic Site: A Case Report. *Cases Journal*. No 1. Vol 343. November 21, ISSN 1757-1626 retrieved from www.casesjournal.com

Bruhat MA, Menhes H, Mage G, Pouly Pl. (1980). Treatment of Ectopic Pregnancy By Means Of Laparoscope. *Fertility and Sterility*. Vol 33. Pp 411-14. ISSN 0015-0282

Buster JE, Barnhart K. (2004). Ectopic Pregnancy: A Five-Step Plan for Medical Management. *OBG Management*. November 2004, Pp 74-85 retrieved from <www.obgmanagement.com>

CDC (1992) (Centers for Disease Control and Prevention) Ectopic Pregnancy in the United States of America 1978-1989. CDC Surveillance Summaries. *Morbidity and Mortality Weekly Report*. Vol 41. Pp 591-594. ISSN 0149-2195

Complications of Pregnancy Part 1. (2007). Early Pregnancy. Vol 9 No 6 retrieved from <www.ebmedicine.net>

Condous G. (2006). Ectopic Pregnancy: Risk Factors and Diagnosis. *Australian Family Physician*. Vol 35. No 11. November 2006. Pp 854-857. ISSN 0300-8495

Coste J, Job-Spira N, Aublet- Cuvellier B Et Al. (2003). Incidence of Ectopic Pregnancy: First Results of a Population Based Register in France. *American Journal of Epidemiology.* (February 2003). Vol 157. No 3. Pp 185-94. ISSN 0002-9262 retrieved from <http://aje.oxfordjournals.org>

Coutin A, Grouzard V, Henkens M, Marquard TT. (2007). *Obstetrics in Remote Settings Practical Guide For Non-Specialised Health Care Professionals.* Médècins sans Frontiers, Paris. Pp 29-32. ISBN 2-906498-67X retrieved from <www.msf.org>

DeVoe RW, Pratt JH. (1948). Simultaneous Intrauterine and Extrauterine Pregnancy. *American Journal of Obstetrics and Gynaecology.* Vol 56. Pp 1119-21. ISSN 0002-9378

Diagnostic Imaging Pathways retrieved from <www.imagingpathways.health.wa.gov.au>

Dickens BM, Feweders A, Cook RJ. (2003). Ectopic Pregnancy and Emergency Care: Ethical and Legal Issues. *International Journal of Gynecology and Obstetrics.* Vol 82. No 1. Pp 121-6. ISSN 0020-7292

Doyle MB, Decherney AH, Diamond MP. (1991). Epidemiology and Aetiology of Ectopic Pregnancy. *Obstetrics and Gynaecology Clinics of North America.* Vol 18. No 4. (March 1991) Pp 1-17. ISSN 0889-8545

Egwuatu VE, Ozumba BC. (1987). Unexpected Low Ratio And Falling Incidence Rate Of Ectopic Pregnancy In Enugu, Nigeria 1978-1981. *International journal of Fertility.* Vol 32. Pp 113-121. ISSN 0020-725X

Elhelw B. (2003). Ectopic Pregnancy. *Middle East Fertility Society Journal.* Vol 8. No 2. Pp 103-116. ISSN 1110-5690

Ekanem EI, Ekott M, Udoma E, Udofia O, Udo A, Iklaki C. (2009). Incidence Of Ectopic Pregnancy In Calabar, Nigeria: Two Halves Of The Last Decade Compared. *Global Journal of Community Medicine.* Vol 2. No 1 & 2. ISSN: 1597-9857. retrieved from <www.ajol.info>

Ekele BA. (2001). Medical Treatment Of Ectopic Pregnancy Using Parenteral Methotrexate. *West African Journal of Medicine.* Vol 20. Pp 181-183. ISSN 0189-160X

Erondu FO, Okoro CR, Aniemeka JI, Ugwu AC, Ohuegbe CI. (2010). Atypical Clinical Sonographic Presentation of Ectopic Pregnancy: A Case Report. *Journal of Medicine and Medical Sciences.* Vol 1. No 4. (May 2010). Pp 087-090. ISSN 1119-3999 retrieved from <www.intersjournals.org/JMMS>

Essel EK, Ezem BU, Otubu JA. (1980) Ruptured Tubal Pregnancy In The Northern Part Of Nigeria. *East African Medical Journal.* 1980. Vol 57. Pp: 574-584. ISSN 0012-835X

Eze JN. (2008). Successful Intrauterine Pregnancy Following Salpingostomy: Case Report. *Nigerian Journal of Medicine.* Vol 17. No 3. (July-August 2008). Pp 360-362. ISSN 1115-2613

Faleyimu BL, Igbarase GO, Momoh MO. (2008). Ipsilateral Ectopic Pregnancy Occurring In the Stump of a Previous Ectopic Site: A Case Report. *Cases Journal.* Vol 1 No 1. (November 2008). Pp 343. ISSN 1757-1626 retrieved from <www.ncbi.nlm.nih.gov>

Farquhar CM. (2005). Ectopic Pregnancy. *The Lancet.* Vol 366. Pp 583-591. ISSN 0140-6736 retrieved from <www.thelancet.com>

Fernandez H, Coste J, Job-Spira N. (1991). Controlled Ovarian Hyperstimulation As A Risk Factor For Ectopic Pregnancy. *Obstetrics and Gynaecology*. Vol 78. Pp 656. ISSN 0029-7844

Fisch JD, Ortiz BH, Tazuke SI, Chitkara U, Giudice LC. (1998). Medical Management of Interstitial Ectopic Pregnancy: A Case Report and Literature Review. *Human Reproduction*. Vol 13. No 7. July 1998. Pp 1981-1986. ISSN 1355-4786

Fowler PBS. (2006). Ectopic Pregnancy. *The Lancet*. Vol 367. Pp 27. ISBN 0140-6736 retrieved from <www.thelancet.com>

Fylstra Dl. (2002). Ectopic Pregnancy within a Caesarean Section Scar: A Review. *Obstetric and Gynaecologic Survey*. Vol 57. Pp 537-43. ISSN 0029-7828

Fylstra Dl, Pond-Chang T, Miller MG, Cooper A, Miller KM. (2002). Ectopic Pregnancy within a Caesarean Section Delivery Scar: A Case Report. *American Journal of Obstetrics and Gynaecology*. Vol 187. Pp 302-4. ISSN 0002-9378

Gazvani MR. (1996). Modern Management of Ectopic Pregnancy. *British Journal of Hospital Medicine*. Vol 56. Pp 597-599. ISSN 0007-1064

Gharoro EP, Igbafe AA. (2002). Ectopic Pregnancy Revisited In Benin City, Nigeria: Analysis of 152 Cases. *Acta Obstetricia* et *Gynecologica Scandinavica*. Vol 81. No 12. (December 2002). Pp: 1139-1143. ISSN 1600-0412

Goyaux N, Leke R, Keita N, Thonneau P. (2003). Ectopic Pregnancy in African Developing Countries. *Acta Obstetetricia et Gynecologica Scandinavica*. Vol 82. No 4. April 2003. Pp: 305-12. ISSN 1600-0412

Gracia CR, Barnhan KT. (2001). Diagnosing Ectopic Pregnancy: Decision Analysis Comparing Six Strategies. *Obstetrics and Gynaecology*. Vol 97. Pp 469-70. ISSN 0029-7844

Grimes DA. (1994). The Morbidity and Mortality of Pregnancy: Still Risky Business. *American Journal of Obstetrics and Gynaecology*. Vol 170. Pp 1489-1494. ISSN 0002-9378

Hanretty KP. (2003). *Obstetrics Illustrated*. Churchill Livingstone. Sixth Edition. ISBN 044-307268-X. London. Pp 161-69.

Herman A, Weinraub Z, Avrech O, Maymon R, Ron-El R, Bukovsky Y. (1995). Follow Up and Outcome of Isthmic Pregnancy Located In A Previous Caesarean Section Scar. *British Journal of Obstetrics and Gynaecology*. Vol 102. Pp 839-41. ISSN 0368-2315

Ibekwe PC. (2004). Ruptured Advanced Tubal Pregnancy Simulating Uterine Rupture: A Case Report. *Nigerian Journal of Medicine*. Vol 13. No 2. (April-June 2004). Pp 196-198. ISSN 1115-2613

Igbarase GO, Ebeigbe PN, Igbekoyi OF, Ajufoh BI. (2005). Ectopic Pregnancy, an 11 Year Review in A Tertiary Centre in the Niger Delta. *Tropical Doctor*. Vol 35. No 3. Pp 175-177. ISSN 0049-4755

Ikpeze OC. (1991). A Critical Assessment of the Usefulness of Abdominal Ultrasound in the Diagnosis of Ectopic Pregnancy. *Nigerian Journal of Surgical Sciences*. Vol 1. Pp 25-27. ISSN 1116-5898

Ilesanmi OA, Shobowale OA. (1992). Ectopic Pregnancy in Ibadan, Nigeria. *Nigerian Medical Journal*. Vol 23. No 1. Pp 11-14. ISSN 0300-1652

Jogo AA, Swende TZ. (2008). Ruptured Tubal Pregnancy in Makurdi, North Central Nigeria. *Nigerian Journal of Medicine*. Vol 17. No 1. (January-March 2008). Pp: 75-77. ISSN 1115-2613

Jurkovic D. (2007) Ectopic Pregnancy. In Edmonds DE (Ed) *Dewhurst's Textbook of Obstetrics and Gynaecology for Postgraduates*. (Seventh Edition), Blackwell Science Limited, Pp 106-116. ISBN 978-1-405-3355-5. London

Kaplan BC, Dart RG, Moskos M, Kharwadkar E, Chun B, Hamid MA (1996) Ectopic Pregnancy: Prospective Study With Improved Diagnostic Accuracy. *Annals of Emergency Medicine*. Vol 28. Pp 10-17. ISSN 1097-6760 Retrieved from <www.annemermed.com>

Kendrick JS, Tiemey EF, Lawson HW, Strauss LT, Klein L, Atrash HK. (1996). Previous Caesarean Delivery and the Risk of Ectopic Pregnancy. *Obstetrics and Gynaecology*. Vol 87. No 2. February 1996. Pp 297-301. ISSN 0029-7844

Kigbu JH, Pam IC, Ekwempu CC, Swen PD. (2006). Splenic Rupture Masquerading Ruptured Ectopic Pregnancy. *Highland Medical Research Journal*. Vol 4. No 1. Pp 119-122. (2006). ISSN 1596-2407

Kjellberg L, Lalos O. Lalos A. (2000). Reproductive Outcome after Surgical Treatment of Ectopic Pregnancy. *Gynaecologic and Obstetric Investigation*. Vol 49. Pp 227-230. ISSN 1423-002X

Kouam L, Kamdom-Moyo J, Ngassa P. Doh AS. (1996). Treatment of Ectopic Pregnancy by Laparatomy in Under-Equipped Countries: A Series of 144 Cases at the Yaoundé University Hospital Centre, Cameroun. *Journal de Gynécologie et Obstétrique Biologie de Reproduction (Paris)*. Vol 25. Pp 804-808. ISSN 0368-2315

Leeman LM, Wendland CL. (2000). Cervical Ectopic Pregnancy, Diagnosis with Endovaginal Ultrasound Examination and Successful Treatment with Methotrexate. Ach Family Medicine. Vol 9. (January 2000). Pp 72-77 retrieved from <www.archfammed.com>

Leke RJ, Goyaux N, Matsuda T, Thonneau PF. (2004) Ectopic Pregnancy In Africa: A Population Based Study. *Obstetrics and Gynaecology*. Vol 103. No 4. April 2004. Pp 692-7. ISSN 0029-7844

Lucie M, Montreal QC, Michael C, Halifax NS. (2005). Ultrasound Evaluation of First Trimester Pregnancy Complications. *Journal of Obstetrics and Gynecology of Canada*. Vol 161. (June 2005). Pp 581-585. ISSN 1701-2163

Ling FW, Stovall TG. (1994). Update On the Management of Ectopic Pregnancy. *Advanced Obstetrics and Gynaecology*. Vol 1. Pp 57. ISSN 0029-7844

Lipscomb GH, Stovall TG, Ling FW. (2000). Nonsurgical Treatment of Ectopic Pregnancy. *New England Journal of Medicine*. Vol 343. No 18. November 2. Pp 1325-1329. ISSN 0028-4793 retrieved from <www.nejm.com>

Loughney A, Stirgess S. (2004). Obstetric and Gynaecological Emergencies in Brooks A, Connolly J, Chan O (Eds). *Ultrasound in Emergency Care*. BMJ Books. Blackwell Publishing. Massachusetts. Pp 79. ISBN 0-7279-1731-5

Makinde OO, Ogunniyi SO. (1990). Ectopic Pregnancy in a Defined Nigerian Population. *International Journal of Gynecology and Obstetrics*. Vol 33. Pp 239-41. ISSN 1471-0528

Makinem J. (1993). Is The Epidemic Of Ectopic Pregnancy Over? In: Proceedings of the 10th Meeting of the International Society for Sexually Transmitted Disease Research. Helsinki, Finland. 29th August/ September 1993: Pp 71-79

Moore J, Tay JI, Walker J. (2000). Ectopic Pregnancy. *British Medical Journal*. Vol 320. Pp: 916-9. ISSN 0959-8138

Morcau JC, Rupari L, Dionne P et al. (1995). Epidemiological and Anatomo-Clinical Features Of ExtraUterine Pregnancy at the Dakar University Hospital Centre. *Dakar Medicine*. Vol 40. Pp 175-179. ISSN 0049-1101

Musa J, Daru PH, Mutihir JT, Ujah IAO. (2009). Ectopic Pregnancy in Jos Northern Nigeria: Prevalence and Impact on Subsequent Fertility. *Nigerian Journal of Medicine*. Vol 18. No 1. (January-March 2009). Pp 35-38. ISSN 1115-2613

Mutihir JT, Nyango DD. (2010). Massive Haemoperitoneum from Endometriosis Masquerading As Ruptured Ectopic Pregnancy: Case Report. *Nigerian Journal of Clinical Practice*. Vol 13. No 4. (October-December 2010). Pp 477-479. ISSN 1119-3077

Nannie B, Claus OL, Bent O, Nilas L. (2003). Improved Fertility Following Conservative Surgical Treatment Of Ectopic Pregnancy. *British Journal of Obstetrics and Gynaecology*. Vol 110. August 2003. Pp 765-770. ISSN 0306-5456

Nwagha UI, Iyioke C, Nwagha TU. (2007). Current Trends in the Management of Ectopic Pregnancy: A Review. *Journal of the College of Medicine*. Vol 12. No 2. Pp 67-75. ISSN 188-2601

Odewale MA, Afolabi MO. (2008). Heterotopic Pregnancy: A Clinical Case Report from Rural Nigeria. *Rural and Remote Health*. Vol 8: 979 online (September 2008) ISSN 1445-6554 retrieved from <http://rrh.org.au>

Okohue JE, Ikimalo JI, Omoregie OB. (2010). Ectopic Pregnancy Following In vitro Fertilization and Embryo Transfer. *West African Journal of Medicine*. Vol 29. No 5. (September-October 2010). Pp 349-351. ISSN 0189-160X

Okunlola MA, Adesina OA, Adekunle AO. (2006). Repeat Ipsilateral Ectopic Gestation: A Series of Three Cases. *African Journal of Medicine and Medical Science*. Vol 35. Pp 173-5. ISSN 1116-4077

Olarewaju RS. (1994). Trends of Ectopic Pregnancy at Jos University Teaching Hospital. *Nigerian Medical Journal*. Vol 26. No 2. Pp: 57-59. ISSN 0300-1652

Oloyede OAO, Lamina MA, Odusoya OL et Al. (2002). Ectopic Pregnancy in Sagamu: A 12-Year Review. *Tropical Journal of Obstetrics and Gynaecology*. Vol 19. Supplementary 2. Pp: 34-35 ISSN 0189-5178

Oronsanye AU, Odiase GI. (1981). The Prevalence of Ectopic Pregnancy in Benin City, Nigeria. *Tropical Doctor*. Vol 11. No 4 (October 1981). Pp 160-3. ISSN 0049-4755

Ory SJ. (1992). New Options for Diagnosis and Treatment of Ectopic Pregnancy. *Journal of American Medical Association*. Vol 267. Pp: 534-537. ISSN 0098-7484 Retrieved from <www.jama.com>

Otubu JAM, Piam IC. Ectopic Pregnancy In: *Textbook of Obstetrics and Gynaecology for Medical Students*, Agboola A (ED). Pp 101-105. Second Edition. Heinemann Educational Books (Nigeria) Plc. 2006. ISBN 978-193-024-1. Ibadan

Perrin R, Boco V, Bilongo B, Akpovi B, Alihonou E. (1997). Management of Ectopic Pregnancies at the University Clinic of Obstetrics and Gynaecology in Cotonou, Benin. *Santé*. 1997. Vol 7. Pp: 201-3. ISSN 1192-4829

Picaud A, Nlome-Nze AR, Ogowet-Igumu N. (1990). Diagnostic Echography of Extrauterine Pregnancy (EUP) Apropos Of 228 Extrauterine Pregnancies Confirmed By Laparatomy. *Journal De Gynécologie, Obstétrique et Biologie de la Reproduction*. Vol 19. Pp 817-21. ISSN 0368-2315

Pitkin J, Peattie AB, Magowan BA. (2003). *Obstetrics and Gynaecology: An Illustrated Colour Text*. Churchill Livingstone. London. Pp 98-99. ISBN 044305035X

Qureshi NS, Wiener JO, Weerakkody ANA. (2006). Laparoscopic Management of Tubal Pregnancy: Availability of Training. *The Obstetrician and Gynaecologist*. Vol 8. Pp 251-255 retrieved from <www.rcog.org.uk>

Rajkhowa M, Rutherford AJ, Sharma V, Glass MR, Balen AH, Cuckle HS. (2000). Trends in the Incidence of Ectopic Pregnancy in England and Wales from 1966 to 1996. *British Journal of* Obstetrics *and Gynaecology*. Vol 107. Pp 369-374. ISSN 0306-5456

Ratinahirana S, Razanamparany PV, Radaniarison H, Ratsimanohatra E, Rakotozafy G.(1997). Current Aspects of Extrauterine Pregnancy in Nosy Be (Madagascar) From November 1993 to February 1995. *Santé*.. Vol 7. Pp: 19-23. ISSN 1192-4829

Royal College of Obstetricians and Gynaecologists. (2004) The Management of Tubal Pregnancy. Guideline. No 21. London. RCOG Press. May 2004. Retrieved from <www.rcog.org.uk>

Safdarian L, Mossayebi E, Badehnoosh B. (2008). Medical Management of Ectopic Pregnancy with High HCG Levels: A Case Series. *Middle East Fertility Society Journal*. Vol 13. No 1. (2008). Pp 57-58. ISSN 1110-5690

Sherman D, Langer R, Sadovsky G, Bukovsky I, Caspi E. (1982). Improved Fertility Following Ectopic Pregnancy. *Fertility and Sterility*. Vol 38. Pp 427-430. ISSN 0015-0282

Simmons ED. (2008). Transfusion Therapy. In Bongard FS, Sue DY, Vintch JRS. (EDS). *Current Diagnosis and Treatment Critical Care*. Third Edition. New York. McGraw-Hill Medical. Pp 71-87. ISBN 0-07-143657-X

Sowter MC, Farquhar CM (2004). Ectopic Pregnancy: An Update. *Current Opinion in Obstetrics and Gynaecology*. Vol 16. No 4. Pp 289-293. ISSN 1473-656X

Tenore JL. (2000). Ectopic Pregnancy. *American Family Physician*. Vol 61. Pp 1080-8. ISSN 0002-838X

Thonneau P, Hijazi Y, Goyaux N, Calvez T, Keita N. (2002). Ectopic Pregnancy in Conakry, Guinea. *Bulletin of the World Health Organization*. Vol 80. No 5. Pp 365-370 Retrieved from <www.who.int>

Tulandi T. (1998). Reproductive Performance of Women after Two Tubal Ectopic Pregnancies. *Fertility and Sterilization*. Vol 50 Pp 164. ISSN 0015-0282

Tulandi T, Saleh A. (1997). Surgical Management of Ectopic Pregnancy. *Clinical Obstetrics and Gynaecology*. Vol 42. (1997). Pp 31-35. ISSN 1532-5520

Tuomivaara L, Kauppila A. (1988). Radical or Conservative Surgery for Ectopic Pregnancy. A Follow-Up Study of Fertility of 323 Patients. *Fertility and Sterility*. Vol 50. (1988). Pp 580. ISSN 0015-0282

Udigwe GO, Umeonunihu OS, Mbachu II. (2010) Ectopic Pregnancy: A Five Year Review Of Cases At Nnamdi Azikiwe University Teaching Hospital (NAUTH), Nnewi, Nigeria. *Nigerian Journal of Medicine.* Vol 51. No 4. (October-December 2010). Pp 160-165. ISSN 1115 - 2613

Varma R, Gupta J. (2009). Tubal Ectopic Pregnancy. *Clinical Evidence.* Vol 04. Pp 1406. ISSN 1462-3846

Wagner MJ, Promes SB. (2007). *Last Minute Emergency Medicine.* McGraw Companies Limited. New York. Pp 310-311. ISSN 0-07-150975-5

8

Clinical Application of One-Step Diagnosis for Ectopic Pregnancy by HCG Ratio: Hemoperitoneum Versus Venous Serum

Yu-dong Wang, Wei-wei Cheng and Xiao-ping Wan
International Peace Maternal and Child Health hospital, Shanghai Jiaotong University
China

1. Introduction

Suspected ectopic pregnancy (SEP) means a woman whose hemoperitoneum and pregnancy test are positive but the gestational sac is uncertain, which is finally diagnosed as an ectopic pregnancy (EP) or a hemoperitoneum with intrauterine pregnancy (hIUP). For emergency physicians, it is mostly important to differentiate EPs rapidly from hIUPs of which the vast majority can be managed without surgery. The combination of transvaginal ultrasound and serum HCG determination seem to be reliable for the early diagnosis of EP (Kaplan et al., 1996; Mol et al., 1998.). However, in most of the emergency rooms (especially on the night shift) in the general hospital, transvaginal ultrasound is often unavailable or instead of transabdominal ultrasound operated by a nonprofessional gynecologist in developing countries, which limits the prompt and accurate diagnosis of EP. Besides, the serial transvaignal ultrasound and HCG quantity result in a lot of workload for the gynecologist and additional medical costs for the patients (Condous et al., 2005.).

A serum: cerebrospinal fluid (CSF) HCG ratio less than 40 is an accurate indication of the presence of brain metastases of gestational trophoblastic tumor, and may have considerable predictive value. However, false-negative serum: CSF HCG ratio (greater than 40) frequently occur in patients with proven brain deposits, and the cerebrospinal fluid puncture or lumbar puncture is difficult to perform for the gynecologist (Bakri et al., 2000.). Magnetic resonance imaging head scan, hence, is now preferred as the most sensitive and safe technology available for brain metastases of gestational trophoblastic tumor.

Culdocentesis is the transvaginal passage of a needle into the posterior cul-de-sac in order to determine whether free blood is present in the abdomen. It is a simple procedure to determine whether there is intraperitoneal hemorrhage. It has been used less frequently in recent years because many gynecologists think it useless for the diagnosis of EP. In the light of the idea that serum: CSF HCG ratio is indication of the presence of brain metastases, making use of the simple operation of culdocentesis, we have proved that HCG ratio of hemoperitoneum versus venous serum (Rp/v-HCG) of EPs is apparently different from that of hIUPs (Wang, et al., 2010.). Hence, in order to provide a single-visit method for predicting EP from SEP, we want to prospectively further assess the diagnostic value of the Rp/v-HCG for early EP. Furthermore, we want to discuss the availability of Rp/v-HCG for rare EP such as abdominal pregnancy et cetera.

2. Materials, methods and results

From March 2005 to Apr 2008, 103 SEPs were retrospectively analyzed for the cut-off value (Rp/v-HCG = 1.0) between EPs and hIUPs (Wang, et al., 2010.). From May 2008 to Nov 2010, we performed this prospective study to prove the diagnostic value of Rp/v-HCG for EPs. All of the 299 patients with stable vital signs were enrolled and evaluated at the out-patient department, in-patient department or emergency center of the Hospital affiliated to JiaoTong University, Shanghai, China.

The hemoperitoneum was collected by culdocentesis (n=255) before surgery or by aspiration during surgery (n=44, thirteen patients among of them rejected the culdocentesis before surgery). Once the hemoperitoneum was obtained, the venous serum was prepared within 1h. The HCG levels of venous serum and hemoperitoneum were quantified by chemiluminescence at the same batch with the same set and HCG kit (Strada per Crescentino, snc, 13040 Saluggia-Ital). Those SEPs with a Rp/v-HCG of ≥ 1.0 were presumed as EPs, those SEPs with a Rp/v-HCG of < 1.0, however, were classified as hIUPs. The SEPs were finally performed by laparotomy (n=50), laparoscopy (n=141), D&C (n=59) or serial transvaginal ultrasound (n=49).

The final diagnoses of hIUPs were confirmed by sonography during follow up with the presence of a intrauterine fetal heartbeat, by D& C in the presence of chorionic villi or falling serum HCG levels (<5 U/L) after D& C. A final diagnosis of EP was confirmed by surgical histological pathology, or by exclusion of an hIUP.

The following parameters were recorded in the medical history: gestational age, the existence of vaginal bleeding, venous and peritoneal serum HCG concentration (U/L), ectopic position of sac, with or without active bleeding, the times and the complications of the culdocentesis. A quantitative estimate of the hemoperitoneum was carried out during surgery by calculating the volume of aspirated and irrigated fluid.

As the routine method in the present medical treatments, both the culdocentesis （18 G long needle, 5 ml syringe and a disposable speculum are enough）and quantitative HCG used in the study were carried out simply and safely (no complications were recorded in this study) for the diagnosis of EP by the gynecological resident and laboratory technicians.

The study was performed in accordance with the 1975 Helsinki Declaration on Human Experimentation and approved by Institutional Review Board (IRB). The patient consent forms for culdocentesis, surgery and collecting private medical information were obtained.

2.1 Inclusive criteria

All the suspected ectopic pregnancy (SEP) patients whose peritoneal blood and urine HCG test are positive were enrolled.

2.2 Excluded criteria

All those whose vital sign is unstable or whose hemoperitoneum is absent were excluded.

2.3 Study design

This was a retrospective development of a protocol, followed by a prospective trial.

2.4 Statistical analysis

Analyses were carried out using a statistical package for social sciences (SPSS, Ver 13.0). Unless otherwise stated, values were expressed as means ± SD or percentage. The

independent sample wilcoxon test or chi-squared test was used to compare variables between the two groups.
The diagnostic performance of Rp/v-HCG for active tubal hemorrhage was expressed using a scatter diagram. The one-step diagnostic value of the Rp/v-HCG for EP was evaluated in terms of the sensitivity, specificity, positive predictive value (PPV) and negative predictive value (NPV) with 95% confidence intervals (CI). The simple kappa coefficient of Rp/v-HCG test was also given for the 2×2 table to assess how the prediction of Rp/v-HCG agreed with the final diagnosis of the EPs.
Significance was defined as p-values less than 0.05 for all the tests and two sided P-values were reported.

2.5 Results

A total of 299 SEPs (average age, 33.1 years; range, 19-42 years) were enrolled and followed to the final diagnosis, which were finally divided into EP group (248 cases, 82.9 percent of SEPs) and hIUP group (51 cases, 17.1 percent of SEPs).
Table 1 shows a statistically significant difference ($P < 0.001$) between the EP group and the hIUP group in terms of the Rp/v-HCG (18.1 ± 40.75 and 0.72 ± 0.29, respectively) and the conservative treatment (23.0 % and 90.2 %, respectively). The culdocentesis before surgery was performed successfully for 255 SEPs except thirteen patients who rejected the culdocentesis, the success rate of the culdocentesis was 89.2 % (255/ 286), the success rate of the "first-time-right" was 76.9 % (220/ 286), even though the peritoneal fluid depth by ultrasound was only 8-12 mm (Figure 1). No complications of culdocentesis were recorded in this study. Of all the hIUPs, 90.2 percent of patients (46/ 51) were cured relying on the hemostatic therapy (Reptilase) instead of the surgical intervention (laparoscopy). 77.8 percent of patients (14/ 18) who desire to fertility succeeded to continue pregnancy with miscarriage treatment (progesterone).

Group	EP (n=248)	hIUP (n=51)	*P value*
Rp/v-HCG	18.1±40.75	0.72±0.29	$P < 0.001$
Successful culdocentesis	89.2 % (215/241)	88.9 % (40/45)	$P > 0.05$
PFD (mm)	39±24	41±22	$P > 0.05$
Non-surgical treatment	23.0 % (57/248)	90.2 % (46/51)	$P < 0.001$

*P<0.001 vs hIUP
EP: ectopic pregnancy; hIUP: hemoperitoneum or hematocolpos with intrauterine pregnancy; Rp/v-HCG: HCG ratio of peritoneal serum versus venous serum; PFD: peritoneal fluid depth by ultrasound.

Table 1. Comparison of managements between hIUP guoup and EP group.

We further confirmed the same cut-off value of the Rp/v-HCG (Rp/v-HCG = 1.0) as the previous results. At this point, the sensitivity and specificity was 98.5% and 100%, respectively (Figure 2).
The SEPs were predicted as EP group and hIUP group according to the Rp/v-HCG cut-off value. The final diagnosis versus the "predicted" diagnosis for suspected EPs were represented in Table 2. When the protocol was tested prospectively on the 299 SEPs, The overall sensitivity of Rp/v-HCG in the diagnosis of ectopic pregnancy was 98.4 % with a specificity of 100 %, a PPV of 100 % and an NPV of 93 %, whilst the likelihood ratio of a

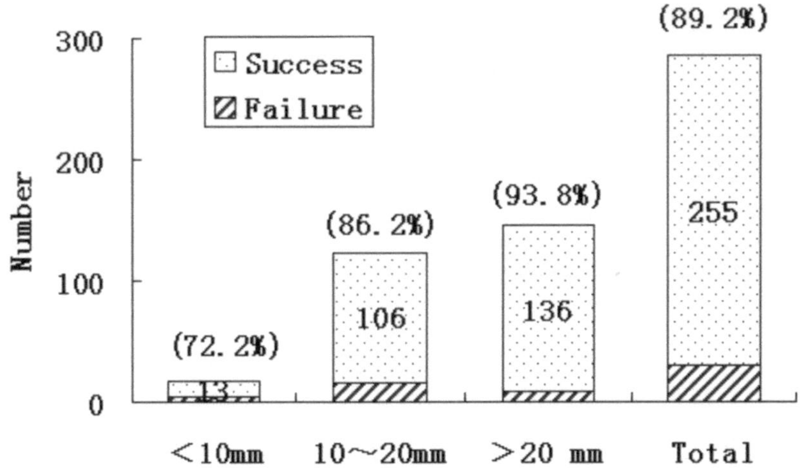

Fig. 1. The success rate of the culdocentesis. The culdocentesis was performed successfully for 255 SEPs in all of the 286 patients, the total success rate of the culdocentesis was 89.2 % (255/ 286). 84.4% (119 /141) percent of SEPs were successfully performed even when the peritoneal fluid depth by ultrasound was of < 20 mm.

negative test (LR-) decreased to 1.5 percent on the test set. The small kappa coefficient of 0.956 (P = 0.022) for the prospective test demonstrated that the predicted diagnosis according to the Rp/v-HCG agreed extremely with the final true diagnosis.

For active bleeding of EP, Figure 3 sees no suggested Rp/v-HCG cut-off value for predicting the active tubal hemorrhage.

Four cases of EPs whose Rp/v-HCG was of <1.0 were performed by laparoscopy, which saw no active bleeding but swollen fallopian, or pink peritoneal fluid from the ruptured ovarian luteinized cyst (surgery sees a tension-free cyst). Most of all the other hemoperitoneum of EPs were dark red fluid.

Two cases of abdominal pregnancy (one is splenic pregnancy) with hemoperitoneum were confirmed during surgery according to intact adnexa uteri (the absence of ectopic gestational sac or chorionic villi) and a Rp/v-HCG of > 1.0.

2.5.1 Retrospective analysis: cut-off value of Rp/v-HCG=1.0 between hIUP and EP

SEPs comprise of EPs (or heterotopic pregnancy, HP) and hIUPs (including hemorrhagic corpus luteum combined with pregnancy and hemorrhagic salpingitis, etc.). HP (coexistence of intrauterine and ectopic pregnancy) is a rare entity, the incidence of which has increased with the widespread use of artificial reproductive technology (ART) (Hsieh, et al., 2004.). While the frequency of spontaneous HP varies from 1 : 10,000 to 1 : 50,000 in normal population, the widespread use of ART may play a role in the increased incidence (according to some series nearly 1%) including ampullary and isthmic tubal EP as well as interstitial ectopic ones (Chang, et al., 2003.). Despite increased medical knowledge and use of improved reproductive technologies, an HP or EP still remains a diagnostic and therapeutic challenge to practitioners. Although signs and symptoms such as abdominal pain, adnexal mass, peritoneal irritation, and enlarged uterus have been reported to be predictive of an HP, they are nonspecific and may be confused with other normal or abnormal pregnancy manifestations.

An HP or EP is difficult to ascertain as pain and bleeding might be attributed to a hIUP, such as threatened abortion, hemorrhagic corpus luteum combined with pregnancy (HCLP) or hemorrhagic salpingitis with pregnancy (Barrenetxea, et al., 2007; Cheng, et al., 2004.). Although hemorrhagic corpus luteum cysts are frequently seen during sonography of the female pelvis, their diagnosis is often challenging as a result of variations in size, thickness of the cyst wall, and internal echo pattern depending on the formation and lysis of the clot (Swire, et al., 2004.). It is necessary for gynecological doctor to set up a new method for distinguishing hIUP from EPs.

In tubal EP, the gestational sac is implanted typically in the wall of the tube, in the connective tissue beneath the serosa, where may be little or no decidual reaction and minimal defense against the permeating trophoblast. The trophoblast invades blood vessels so as to cause local hemoperitoneum. A hematoma in the subserosal space enlarges as pregnancy progresses. Distention of the tube then predisposes to rupture or abortion from isthmus or ampullary. For EP, local hCG level of hemoperitonium is much higher than that of venous serum. The reasons of this finding can be: 1) Blood filling the posterior pouch of Douglas or Morisson's space is from the implantation site of gestational sac, into where the hCG secreted by syntotrophablasts directly flows (hCG secreted into venous serum is relatively low). 2) The metabolism of hCG in the hemoperitoneum is slower than that in venous serum. In HCLP, blood in posterior pouch is from ovarian vessels in which the hCG level is near to that of venous serum (Wang, et al., 2010.). The hCG level of venous serum, however, gradually increases as the IUP proceeds. Then, the last Rp/v-HCG is less than or near to 1.0. Therefore, Rp/v-HCG may promptly distinguish EP from hIUP: as the Rp/v-HCG of EP is always greater than 1.0 while the Rp/v-HCG of hIUP is always less than or near to 1.0.

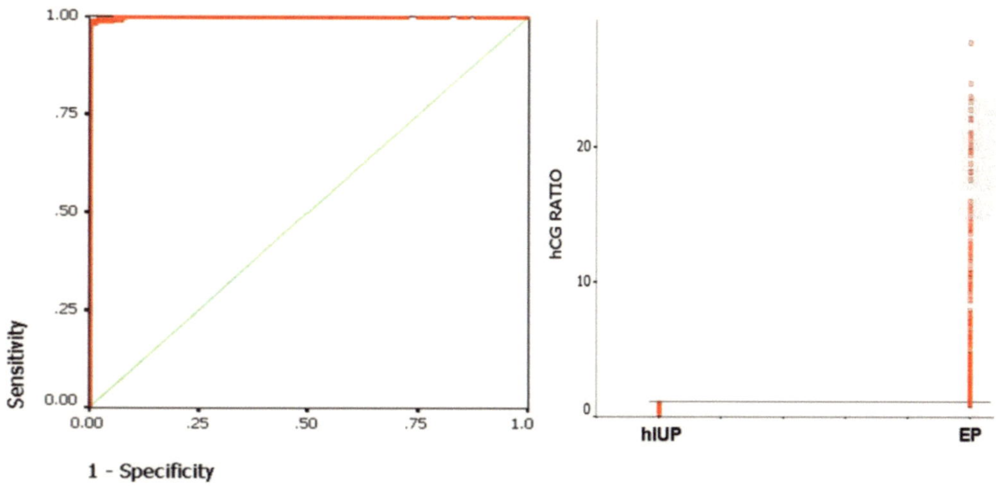

Fig. 2. Cut-off value of the Rp/v-HCG for discriminating EPs from SEPs. ROC analysis showed that the Rp/v-HCG could be used for the differential diagnosis of EP from hIUP, with the area under the curve being 1.0 ($P < 0.001$). The threshold for the diagnosis of EP was 1.0 (at this point sensitivity was 98.5%, and specificity was 100%). Scatter plots of the Rp/v-HCG levels for EPs and hIUPs showed that the Rp/v-HCG levels of EPs mostly located above the value of 1.0. However, the level of hIUPs was absolutely under the suggested cut-off value of 1.0.

In conclusion, in suspected ectopic pregnancy patients, the Rp/v-HCG = 1.0 could be a helpful and practical index for the early differential diagnosis of SEPs. If hemoperitoneum and culdocentesis are positive, the Rp/v-HCG could help discriminate EPs (or HP) from hIUP, and accordingly avoid the unnecessary surgical interventions.

2.5.2 Prospective analysis: Rapid diagnostic value of Rp/v-HCG≥1.0 for EPs before surgery

EP can not be diagnosed solely on the basis of clinical symptoms, such as lower abdominal pain and vaginal bleeding. The ultrasound visualization of heart activity in either intrauterine or extrauterine gestations is important for diagnosis, but rare to accomplish (Oliveira, et al., 2001.). Moreover, during an ultrasound examination, an EP or HP is easily misdiagnosed as a luteal cyst, especially if the concurrent intrauterine pregnancy is reassuring (Habana, et al., 2000.). It is not accurate and rapid enough to meet the need of a clinical gynecologist though a total of 87~93.2% of ectopic pregnancies can be diagnosed using serial transvaginal sound alone (Shalev, et al., 1998; Rosello, et al., 2003.).

Though a single serum hCG value neither identifies an intrauterine or ectopic pregnancy nor predicts ruptured ectopic, it can be used to determine the level of "discriminatory hCG value" at which the sensitivity of ultrasonography for the detection of intrauterine pregnancy approaches 75% and at which the absence of an intrauterine pregnancy suggests abnormal or ectopic gestation. This reported "discriminatory hCG value", however, ranges from 1500 to 3000 mIU per milliliter. The use of a value at the lower end of the range increases the sensitivity for the diagnosis of an ectopic pregnancy, but it also increases the false positive rate, with the attendant risk of interrupting a normal gestation by surgical or medical intervention. In one study, when the hCG value was below 1500 mIU per milliliter, the positive predictive value of ultrasonographic testing for the diagnosis of intrauterine pregnancy was only 80% and the positive predictive value for the diagnosis of ectopic pregnancy was 60% (Barnhart KT, et al., 1999; Romero R, et al., 1985).

When using an HCG ratio (HCG at 48 h/ HCG at 0 h) cut-off of 0.87, the sensitivity and specificity for the prediction of failing Pregnancy of unknown locations were 92.7 and 96.7%, respectively (Condous., 2006.). A rate of decline in serum HCG 21% could define spontaneous resolution of the pregnancy of unknown locations (Barnhart et al., 2004.). Serial quantitative HCG, however, could not meet the rapid diagnosis of EPs.

Laparoscopy is currently considered as the golden standard for the diagnosis of ectopic pregnancy (Ankum et al., 1993.). However, the application of diagnostic laparoscopy is limited to the expensive charge and apparent trauma.

Dilatation and curettage is recommended as a diagnostic method for use in conjunction with low progesterone or β-HCG concentrations and in women in whom transvaginal ultrasound suggests a non-viable intrauterine pregnancy. (McCord et al., 1996; Stovall et al., 1992.) The absence of chorionic villi is associated with an ectopic pregnancy in 40% of women with an empty uterus on ultrasound. An ectopic pregnancy is suggested in women whose β-HCG concentrations do not fall by at least 15 % in the 12 h after dilatation and curettage, or in whom the histological findings do not include chorionic villi. However, use of dilatation and curettage in the diagnostic workup of SEPs has not been widely adopted, in part because some women are reluctant to give up the desiration of fertility, and in part because many women who miscarry can be managed without the need for curettage (Mol, et al., 2002; Wieringa-de, et al., 2002; Dart, et al., 1999.).

Predicted Diagnosis	True diagnosis		Total	
	EP	hIUP		
Rp/v-HCG≥1.0:**EP**	244	0	244	Kappa=0.956
Rp/v-HCG<1.0:**hIUP**	4	51	55	(P<0.001)
Total	248	51	299	
Sensitivity=98.4 %; Specificity=100 %; NPV =93.0 %; PPV =100%; LR(-)=1.5%; п=98.7 %; Youden index=98.4 %				

EP: ectopic pregnancy; hIUP: hemoperitoneum or hematocolpos with intrauterine pregnancy; Rp/v-HCG: HCG ratio of peritoneal serum versus venous serum

Table 2. Evaluation of Rp/v-HCG: final diagnosis versus predicted diagnosis.

It is noted that four cases of SEPs with pink fluid and Rp/v-HCG of < 1.0 were all proved to be EPs, whose hemoperitoneum (pink or bloody-like fluid) were not from fallopian tube rupture or abortion but from the hemorrhagic corpus luteal cyst (3 cases) and hemorrhagic salpingitis (1 case). Therefore, the Rp/v-HCG of < 1.0 could not completely exclude the diagnosis of EP, especially when hemoperitoneum is pink or bloody-like fluid (Qiu, et al., 2010.). That is to say, for SEPs whose Rp/v-HCG of < 1.0, serial transvaginal sound may be followed to prove the intra-uterine pregnancy.

Table 2 shows that the success rate of the culdocentesis is 89.2 % (255 /286) without any complications. 90.2 percent of the hIUPs (46/51) are successfully managed with conservative treatment instead of the surgical intervention (P<0.001). The overall sensitivity of Rp/v-HCG> 1.0 in the diagnosis of ectopic pregnancy is 98.4 % (95% CI: 95.9–99.6) with a specificity of 100 % (95% CI: 93.0–100), a PPV of 100 % (95% CI: 98.5–100) and an NPV of 92.7 % (95% CI: 82.4–98.0). The kappa value of Rp/v-HCG test comparing to the final diagnosis is 0.956 (P < 0.0001). Hence, the Rp/v-HCG≥1.0 is practical and rapid for the diagnosis of EPs.

2.5.3 Rp/v-HCG for predicting the active tubal hemorrhage of EPs

No apparent Rp/v-HCG cut-off value for predicting the active tubal hemorrhage is shown when the HCG level of venous serum is more than 1500U/L. When the HCG level of venous serum is less than 1500U/L, however, few patients have the active tubal hemorrhage. It seems that the Rp/v-HCG is higher; the incidence rate of active tubal hemorrhage is lower. It is very important for gynecological emergency doctor to predict the presence of tubal hemorrhage in EPs. No ideal marker for tubal hemorrhage of EPs, however, has been founded in the present medical procedure till to now.

2.5.4 Rp/v-HCG> 1.0 for diagnosing the abdominal prengancy during surgery

Abdominal pregnancy is an extremely rare form of ectopic pregnancy (EP) with potentially life-threatening complications both to mother and the fetus, which is historically defined as an implantation in the peritoneal cavity, exclusive of tubal, ovarian or intraligamentary pregnancy.

Due to infrequency of abdominal pregnancy, it is often unsuspected and remains a diagnostic challenge despite improvements in imaging techniques (Dassah, et al., 2009.). A retrospective analysis show there were 20 cases of abdominal pregnancy out of 58, 000

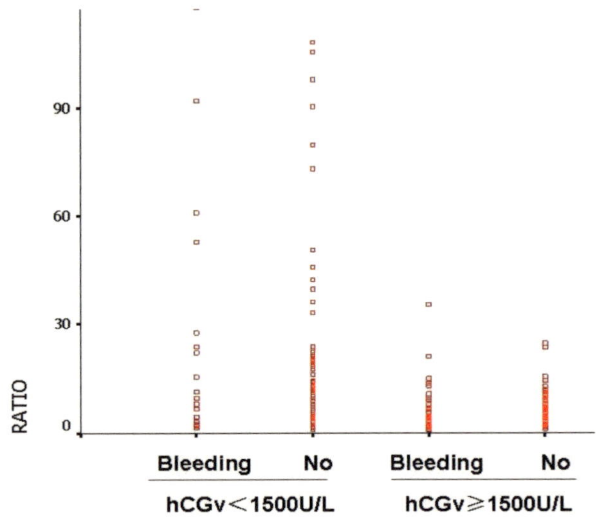

Fig. 3. Scatter diagram of the Rp/v-HCG levels for active bleeding group and without active bleeding (No) group when HCG of venous serum was more than 1500U/L or less than 1500U/L. No suggested Rp/v-HCG cut-off value for the distribution of the active tubal hemorrhage was shown when HCG of venous serum was more than 1500U/L.

deliveries, giving an incidence of 0.34 per 1, 000 deliveries. The diagnoses were missed in 10 cases and there was one maternal death. The rate of 50% missed diagnosis in this analysis highlights the need for a high index of suspicion in the diagnosis of abdominal pregnancies as the clinical features are varied. The maternal and fetal outcomes relate to early diagnosis and skilled management, which calls for vigilance on the part of the obstetrician (Sunday-Adeoye, et al., 2011.).

In this study, two SEPs whose Rp/v-HCG was of > 1.0 showed normal fallopian tube and ovary but hemoperitoneum during the laparotomy. They were both diagnosed as abdominal pregnancy (one was splenic pregnancy) finally after thorough pelvic and abdominal exploration. One of the splenic pregnancy suffered second exploration and splenectomy because it is mistaken as hemorrhagic corpus luteum combined with pregnancy by the gynecologist who ignored of Rp/v-HCG was of > 1.0. Hence, the criteria of diagnosis for abdominal pregnancy may be considered: 1) No evidence of gestational sac or chorionic villi in the adnexa is seen during the surgery, 2) Rp/v-HCG, however, is of > 1.0.

Transvaginal ultrasound and serial β-hCG level are of little use for the differential diagnosis between hemoperitoneum with intrauterine pregnancy and ectopic pregnancy including abdominal pregnancy, however, the overall specificity of Rp/v-HCG> 1.0 in the diagnosis of ectopic pregnancy is 100 % (95% CI: 93.0–100), a PPV of 100 % (95% CI: 98.5–100). Therefore, we may consider the definitive diagnosis of ectopic pregnancy when preoperative Rp/v-HCG is of > 1.0 and consider the diagnosis of abdominal pregnancy when preoperative or intraoperative Rp/v-HCG is of > 1.0, however, the adnexa sees no evidence of gestational sac. It is useful for gynecologists to reduce omission diagnostic rate of abdominal pregnancy, especially during the emergency surgery without enough preoperative preparation. Due to the rare case, further study with more data of abdominal pregnancy is needed.

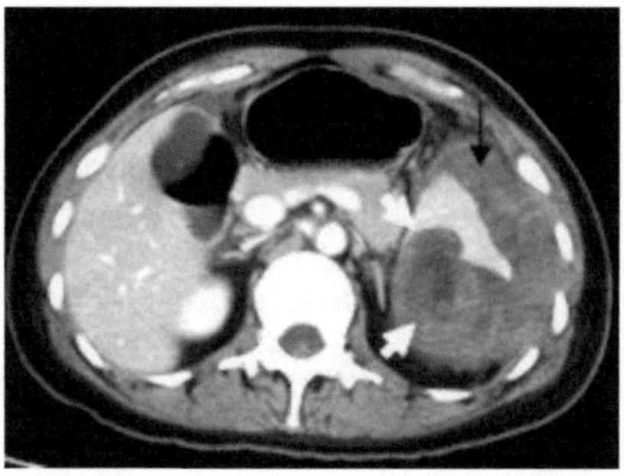

Fig. 4. Contrast enhancement scan of computerized tomography (CT) for splenic pregnancy. One SEP whose Rp/v-HCG = 2.2 (22286 IU/L /9974.9 IU/L) showed intact fallopian and ovary during laparoscopy and then was performed by D &C. Twelve days after operation, CT showed the embryo sac (white arrow) and hematoma under splenic capsule (black arrow).

3. Conclusion

Early diagnosis of ectopic pregnancy is the key to optimal treatment, especially is essential in order to minimize the morbidity and to assess the need for urgent surgical intervention. Intervention prior to rupture prevents hemorrhage, potentially enhances fertility, and allows for nonsurgical methods (Segal, et al., 2010.). Observational studies indicate that among women treated with salpingostomy as compared with those treated with salpingectomy, rates of subsequent intrauterine pregnancy are higher (73% vs. 57%) though the rates of subsequent ectopic pregnancy are also higher (15% vs. 10%) (Seeber, et al., 2006; Mol, et al., 2008.).

Though the advent of β-HCG measurements and improved transvaginal ultrasound techniques has made laparoscopic diagnosis of ectopic pregnancy almost redundant and allowed for both expectant and medical management options, combing transvaginal ultrasonography with gonadotropin quantification could not give the most satisfactory results since it takes an average of 36 h to diagnose EP, not including the resources devoted to collecting blood samples (Garcia, et al., 2001.). Hence, additional new tests or diagnostic methods are necessary to be established for a rapid and accurate diagnosis of EP prior to initiation of either medical or surgical intervention.

Besides laparoscopy and transvaginal sound, serum biomarkers (including HCG) may be helpful for the early diagnosis of EPs. Over 20 serum biomarkers have been identified to date in an attempt to permit earlier diagnosis of ectopic pregnancy, the instigation of earlier management and reduce healthcare costs (Cartwright, et al., 2009; Pedersen, et al., 1991.). The ideal marker for the diagnosis of ectopic pregnancy would be specific for tubal damage or present only after endometrial implantation. Various markers have been assessed, including creatinine kinase (Lavie, et al., 1993.) and fetal fibronectin (Ness, et al., 1998.), but none is sufficiently sensitive or specific for the diagnosis of ectopic pregnancy.

Certain serum biomarkers have been shown initially to be of discriminatory value but then subsequent studies have found them to be of limited use (such as placental protein 14) (Daponte, et al., 2008; Mantzavinos, et al., 1991.). A number of biomarkers (such as estradiol, pregnancy associated plasma protein A, cancer antigen 125) can distinguish a tubal ectopic from a viable intrauterine pregnancy but are unable to distinguish the former from a non-viable intrauterine pregnancy (miscarriage) (Mueller, et al., 2004; Katsikis, et al., 2006).

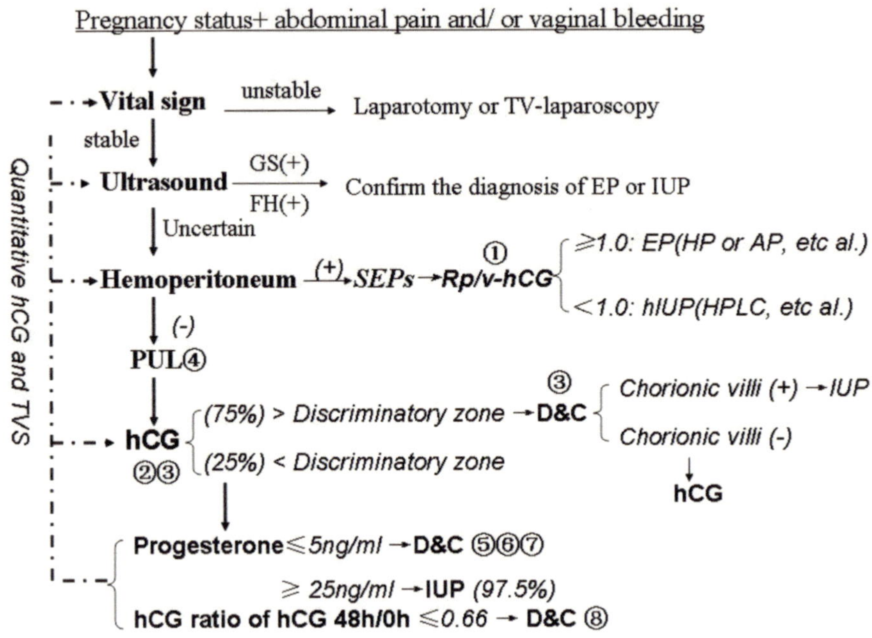

Note: IUP: intrauterine pregnancy; PUL: pregnancies of unknown location; SEP: suspected ectopic pregnancy; GS: gestational sac; FH: fetal heart; Rp/v-hCG: hCG ration of peritoneum versus venous serum. Discriminatory zone or discriminatory concentration is depent on the standard utilized in any given labortory, in general, 6500 IU/L for abdominal ultrasound and 1500 IU/L (or 2400U/L) for transvaginal ultrasound. Uterine curettage may be useful following endocrine documentation that suggests a nonviable pregnancy regardless of it's location.

①Wang et al., 2010; ②Barnhart et al., 1994; ③Barnhart et al., 2002; ④Kirk et al., 2007; ⑤Stovall et al., 1992; ⑥Anonymous., 1992; ⑦Dart et al., 2002; ⑧Kadar et al., 1988.

Fig. 5. Diagnostic flow chart of EP

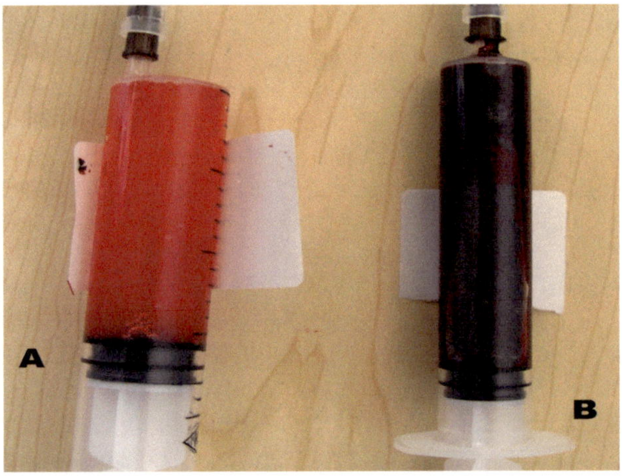

Fig. 6. Pink fluid from not ruptured fallopian tube but hemorrhagic salpingitis of an EP (A); dark red fluid from fallopian tube abortion of an EP (B)

Other markers (such as vascular endothelial growth factor, creatinine kinase and progesterone) have been studied extensively in relation to ectopic pregnancy but the results have been so conflicting that none have been put into clinical use (Develioglu, et al., 2002.). The clinical utility of these biomarkers is limited because of variable results due, for the most part, to limitations in study design. In many studies, the cohort examined was very small and the prevalence of ectopic pregnancy within the study population was not constant. In some studies, patients were not accurately matched for gestation. This reflects the difficulty in determining the gestational age of an ectopic pregnancy. Some of the serum biomarkers also limited their own use, as they did not follow a steady pattern (increase or decrease) with a normal gestation. Moreover, changes in the serum assays and the reagents used to detect the biomarkers over the decades have led to conflicting results between studies.

It was once concluded that culdocentesis is not a useful tool in the diagnosis of suspected ectopic pregnancies because the false negative rate for culdocentesis was 14.8% or so. What is more important, it does not distinguish an ectopic pregnancy from hIUP (Elliot, et al., 1990; Glezerman, et al., 1992.). According to our data, culdocentesis could be routinely, safely and simply performed during clinical practice without any complications. The success rate of the culdocentesis was 89.2 %, even though the peritoneal fluid depth by ultrasound was only 8-12 mm. Moreover, positive culdocentesis could contribute to a quick and accurate differential diagnostic algorithm for SEPs. In this study, we proved that a patient whose Rp/v-HCG is more than 1.0 may be diagnosed and treated instantly as an EP to avoid tubal rupture. The overall sensitivity of Rp/v-HCG $\geq$ 1.0 in the diagnosis of ectopic pregnancy is 98.5 % with a specificity of 100 %, whilst the small kappa coefficient of 0.956 for the prospective test demonstrates that the predicted outcome according to the Rp/v-HCG agreed extremely with the final true diagnosis. At least, Rp/v-HCG involving the culdocentesis provides a new method for rapid diagnosis of EP, which is helpful for fullfilling the diagnostic flow chart of EPs (see Fig 2), though the patients should be managed according to Garcia et al if culdocentesis is negative (Garcia, et al., 2001.).

The culdocentesis will reveal nonclotting blood if intra-abdominal bleeding has occurred. Although nonclotting blood is assumed to be from a ruptured ectopic, similar results can also be obtained under other circumstances (eg, a hemorrhagic corpus luteum), and thus a positive results is not diagnostic of a ruptured ectopic pregnancy. In other words, not all the positive hemoperitoneum on ultrasound examination or by culdocentesis be an absolute contraindication to conservative management of tubal ectopic pregnancy (Bignardi, et al., 2009.). Therefore, whether Rp/v-HCG could predict the existence of active bleeding is important for the prognosis of EPs. Though there was a statistically significant difference between the Rp/v-HCG of the patients with or without active bleeding when the venous hCG (hCGv) of EP was >1500 U/L (Wang, et al., 2010.), no diagnostic value was seen in this study, that is, it is of no use for predicting the prognosis of fallopian tube or EP patient.

In order to expand the application of the new one-step protocol for not only the SEPs whose hemoperitoneum and culdocentesis are positive but also those whose hematocolpos is positive, it is necessary to determine whether the HCG ratio of hematocolpos versus venous serum (RC/V-HCG) alone also could provide a rapid diagnosis of EP.

4. Acknowledgment

We gratefully acknowledge all the postgraduates of JiaoTong University engaged in the study for their detailed record.

Funding

This study was supported by the Foundation of the Sixth People's Hospital, grant no. 0875 (to Y.D.W.), research grants No.044Y06 (to Y.D.W.) from the youth foundation of Shanghai hygiene bureau, and No.30801230 (to Y.D.W.) from the National Natural Science Foundation of China.

5. References

Ankum WM, et al. (1993). Transvaginal sonography and human chorionic gonadotrophin measurements in suspected ectopic pregnancy: a detailed analysis of a diagnostic approach. Hum Reprod 1993;8:1307–1311.

Anonymous. (1992). Serum progesterone in the diagnosis of ectopic pregnancy (editorial). Lancet 1992; 340:583.

Bakri Y, et al. (2000). CSF/serum β-hCG ratio in patients with brain metastases of gestational trophoblastic tumor. Journal of reproductive medicine 2000; 45(2): 94–96.

Barnhart K, et al. (2004). Decline of serum human chorionic gonadotropin and spontaneous complete abortion: defining the normal curve. Obstet Gynecol 2004;104(5 Pt 1):975–981.

Barnhart KT, et al. (1999). Diagnostic accuracy of ultrasound above and below the beta-hCG discriminatory zone. Obstet Gynecol 1999;94:583-7.

Barrenetxea G, et al. (2007). Heterotopic pregnancy: two cases and a comparative review. Fertil Steril 2007; 87(2):417.

Bignardi T, et al. (2009).Does tubal ectopic pregnancy with hemoperitoneum always require surgery? Ultrasound Obstet Gynecol 2009;33(6):711–715.

Cartwright J, et al. (2009). Serum biomarkers of tubal ectopic pregnancy: current candidates and future possibilities. Reproduction 2009;138:9–22. [PubMed: 19321656

Chang Y, et al. (2003). An unexpected quadruplet heterotopic pregnancy after bilateral salpinguectomy and replacement of three embryos. Fertil Steril 2003; 80: 218-22.

Cheng PJ, et al. (2004). Heterotopic pregnancy in a natural conception cycle presenting as hematometra. Obstet Gynecol 2004; 104: 1195-1198.

Condous G, et al. (2005). A prospective evaluation of a single-visit strategy to manage pregnancies of unknown location. Hum Reprod 2005;20:1398–1403.

Condous G. (2006). Ectopic pregnancy--risk factors and diagnosis. Aust Fam Physician 2006;35(11):854–857.

Daponte A, et al. (2008). The value of a single combined measurement of VEGF, glycodelin, progesterone, PAPP-A, HPL and LIF for differentiating between ectopic and abnormal intra- uterine pregnancy. Hum Reprod 2008;20(11): 3163–6. [PubMed: 16055453]

Dart R, et al. (1999). The utility of a dilatation and evacuation procedure in patients with symptoms suggestive of ectopic pregnancy and indeterminate transvaginal ultrasonography. Acad Emerg Med 1999; 6: 1024–1029.

Dassah, et al. (2009). Advanced twin abdominal pregnancy: diagnostic and therapeutic challenges.Acta Obstet Gynecol Scand. 2009;88(11):1291-3.

Develioglu OH, et al. (2002). Evaluation of serum creatine kinase in ectopic pregnancy with reference to tubal status and histopathology. Br J Obstet Gynaecol 2002;109:121–8.

Elliot M, et al. (1990). Serous culdocentesis in ectopic pregnancy: a report of two cases caused by coexistent corpus luteum cysts. Ann Emerg Med. 1990;19(4):407-10.

Garcia CR, et al. (2001). Diagnosing ectopic pregnancy: Decision analysis comparing six strategies. Obstet Gynecol 2001; 97: 464-470.

Glezerman M, et al. (1992). Culdocentesis is an obsolete diagnostic tool in suspected ectopic pregnancy. Arch Gynecol Obstet. 1992;252(1):5-9.

Habana A, et al. (2000). Cornual heterotopic pregnancy:contemporary management options. Am J Obstet Gynecol 2000;182:1264–1270.

Hsieh BC, et al. (2004). Heterotopic caesarean scar pregnancy combined with intrauterine pregnancy successfully treated with embryo aspiration for selective embryo reduction Case report. Hum Reprod 2004; 19: 285-7.

Kaplan, BC. (1996). Ectopic pregnancy: prospective study with improved diagnostic accuracy. *Ann Emerg Med,* Vol.28, No.1, (July 1996), pp. 10-17, PubMed PMID: 8669724.

Katsikis I, et al. (2006). Receiver operator char- acteristics and diagnostic value of progesterone and CA-125 in the prediction of ectopic and abortive intrauterine gesta- tions. Eur J Obstet Gynecol Reprod Biol 2006;125:226–32. [PubMed:16303230]

Kaye SB, et al. (1979). Brain metastases in malignant teratoma: a review of four years' experience and an assessment of the role of tumour markers. Br J Cancer. 1979 Mar;39(3):217-23. PubMed PMID: 88952; PubMed Central PMCID: PMC2009884.

Lavie O, et al. (1993). Maternal serum creatinine kinase: a possible predictor of tubal pregnancy. Am J Obstet Gynecol 1993; 169: 1149–1150.

Mantzavinos T, et al. (1991). Serum levels of steroid and placental protein hormones in ectopic pregnancy. Eur J Obstet Gynecol Reprod Biol 1991;39:117–22. [PubMed: 2050251]

McCord ML, et al. (1996). Single serum progesterone as a screen for ectopic pregnancy: exchanging specificity and sensitivity to obtain optimal test performance. Fertil Steril 1996; 66: 513–516.

Mol B, et al. (2002). Symptom-free women at increased risk of ectopic pregnancy: should we screen? Acta Obstet Gynecol Scand 2002; 81: 661–672.

Mol BW, et al. (1998). Serum human chorionic gonadotropin measurement in the diagnosis of ectopic pregnancy when transvaginal sonography is inconclusive. Fertil Steril 1998; 70(5):972–981.

Mol F, et al. (2008). Current evidence on surgery, systemic methotrexate and expectant management in the treatment of tubal ectopic pregnancy: a systematic review and meta-analysis. Hum Reprod Update 2008;14:309-19.

Mueller MD,et al. (2004). Novel placental and nonplacental serummarkers in ectopic versus normal intrauterine pregnancy. Fertil Steril 2004;81:1106–11. [PubMed: 15066471

Ness R, et al. (1998). Fetal fibronectin as a marker to discriminate between ectopic and intrauterine pregnancies. Am J Obstet Gynecol 1998; 179:697–702.

Oliveira FG, et al. (2001). Rare association of ovarian implantation site for patients with heterotpic and with primary ectopic pregnancies after ICSI and blastocyst transfer. Hum Reprod 2001; 16:2227–2229.

Pedersen JF,et al. (1991). Serum level of secretory endometrial protein PP-14 in intact ectopic pregnancy. Br J Obstet Gynaecol 1991;98:414. [PubMed: 2031903]

Price JM, et al. (2010). Screening for central nervous system disease in metastatic gestational trophoblastic neoplasia. J Reprod Med. 2010 Jul-Aug;55(7-8):301-4. PubMed PMID: 20795342.

Qiu YJ, et al. (2010). Diagnosis of hemorrhagic corpus luteum combined with pregnancy by the hCG ratio of peritoneal serum versus venous serum.Chinese Journal of Obstetrics and Gynecology. 2010;45(8)：639.

Romero R, et al. (1985). Diagnosis of ectopic pregnancy: value of the discriminatory human chorionic gonadotropin zone. Obstet Gynecol 1985;66:357-60.

Rosello N, et al. (2003). Does transvaginal ultrasonography accurately diagnose ectopic pregnancy? Hum Reprod 2003;18 (Suppl 1):160.

Seeber BE, et al. (2006). Suspected ectopic pregnancy. Obstet Gynecol 2006;107:399-43.

Segal S, et al. (2010). Ectopic pregnancy early diagnosis markers.Minerva Ginecol. 2010; 62(1): 49-62.

Shalev E, et al. (1998). Transvaginal sonography as the ultimate diagnostic tool for the management of ectopic pregnancy: experience with 840 cases. Fertil Steril 1998; 69:62–65.

Sunday-Adeoye I, et al. (2011). A 30-year review of advanced abdominal pregnancy at the Mater Misericordiae Hospital, Afikpo, southeastern Nigeria (1976-2006). Arch Gynecol Obstet. 2011 Jan;283(1):19-24. Epub 2009 Oct 30.

Stovall TG, et al. (1992). Serum progesterone and uterine curettage in differential diagnosis of ectopic pregnancy. Fertil Steril 1992; 57: 456–457.

Swire MN, et al. (2004). Various sonographic appearances of the hemorrhagic corpus luteum cyst. Ultrasound Q 2004; 20(2):45-58.

Wang Y, et al. (2010). Human chorionic gonadotropin ratio of hemoperitoneum versus venous serum improves early diagnosis of ectopic pregnancy. Fertil Steril 2010; 93(3): 702–705.

Wieringa-de, et al. (2002). Management of miscarriage: a randomized controlled trial of expectant management versus surgical evacuation. Hum Reprod 2002; 17: 2445–2450.

9

Inhibins and Activins as Possible Marker of Ectopic Pregnancy

Blazej Meczekalski and Agnieszka Podfigurna-Stopa
Department of Gynecological Endocrinology,
Poznan University of Medical Sciences, Poznan
Poland

1. Introduction

The regulation of reproduction is performed by complex hormonal system: hypothalamus - pituitary - ovary. There are a lot of ovarian peptides, playing an essential role in the regulation of this hormonal system. However, the mechanisms of their action are not exactly elucidated. Within ovarian peptides, inhibins are seemed to be consider as very important. The term "inhibin" was indicated by McCullagh in 1932. He described inhibin as a hydrophilic substance and an extract from male gonads, which inhibits the pituitary gland. However, only 53 years later, the isolation of inhibin from follicular fluid in cows for the first has been performed. Inhibin was characterized as a glycoprotein, consisting of two subunits linked by disulfide bond (Yamaguchi et al, 1991).

Inhibins belong to the superfamily of transforming growth factor β (TGF-β). This family contains about 30 peptides, including activin, Anti-Müllerian Hormone (AMH), epithelial growth factor (epidermal growth factor - EGF) and the subfamily of transforming growth factor-β (TGF-β) (de Kretser et al., 2002).Inhibins (inhibin A, B, total inhibin) play a very important role in the regulation of female reproduction.

Inhibins are glycoprotein substances produced mainly in the ovaries and they take part in the regulation of menstrual cycle. They consist of a glycosylated subunit α combined with disulfide bond with one of two different subunits β (betaA or betaB). The resulting inhibin are properly labeled as inhibin A (alpha betaA) and inhibin B (alpha betaB) (Burger & Igarashi, 1988).

Inhibins play an important role in reproductive functions by regulating pituitary follicle-stimulating hormone (FSH) secretion during the menstrual cycle. This regulation is processed by a feedback mechanism. FSH stimulates the maturation of ovarian follicles, where granulosa cells produce inhibins. Increased levels of inhibins in the peripheral blood subsequently inhibit the secretion of FSH (Muttukrishna et al., 2000).

There are studies about possible use of inhibins in reproductive medicine.

Inhibin A is secreted mainly by the dominant follicles and corpus luteum of the ovary. In addition, the sources of this peptide are also adrenal, pituitary, spleen, bone marrow, placenta and fetal membranes (Petraglia et al., 1999). Recent data indicates the evaluation of inhibin A concentration mainly in the obstetric diagnosis (Florio et al., 2004).

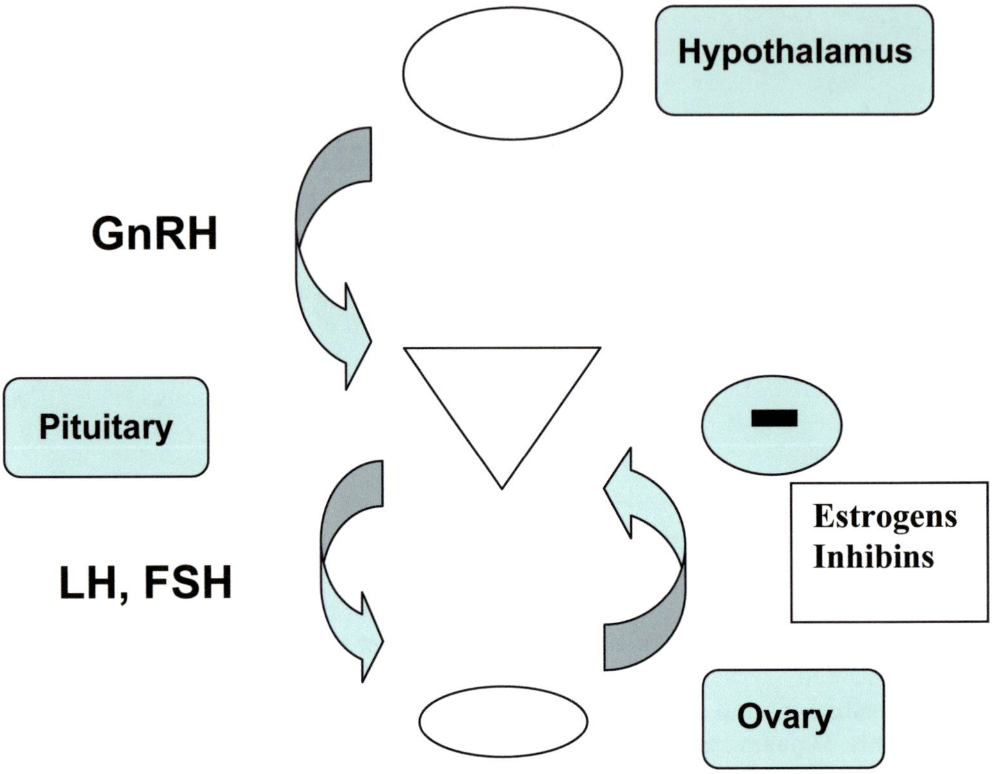

Fig. 1. Role of inhibins in hypothalamic - pituitary – ovarian axis.

According to current knowledge inhibin A can be used in the diagnosis of ectopic pregnancy, mola hydatidosa, threatened abortion, pre-eclampsia and pregnancy associated with Down's syndrome (Meczekalski & Podfigurna-Stopa, 2009).

The concentration of inhibin A in blood serum in the early follicular phase is low. It begins to rise during the late follicular phase, reaching its peak in the middle of the secretion of luteal phase. Throughout the follicular phase of the menstrual cycle inhibin B concentration is higher than the levels of inhibin A in blood serum. Their levels correlate with the concentrations of FSH, luteinizing hormone (LH) and estradiol in the blood serum (Klein et al., 1996).

Inhibin A may be a particular marker of early pregnancy loss (Mattukrishna et al., 2002). Both, single and serial measurements were used to predict subsequent pregnancy loss in women with recurrent miscarriage. There are low serum concentrations of inhibin A at early gestational age in pregnancies destined to miscarry. Its measurement at the time of the first pregnancy test might be able to predict pregnancy outcome (Al-Azemi et al., 2003). Inhibin B is secreted mainly in ovaries and its function is focused on gynecology. Inhibin B is produced by the granulosa cells of early follicles in ovary. The differences in the secretion of inhibin A and B may suggest their different physiological role. Inhibin B seems to play a major role as a marker of follicular growth and could be a potential tool to assess the response to ovulation induction by the action of FSH. It may also play an important role as a prognostic factor in premature ovarian failure and the hypothalamic disturbances (Welt et al., 1997).

In men, only inhibin B is secreted. It is produced by Sertoli cells in the testis, accordingly to the circadian rhythm with a minimum at 10.00 p.m. and the peak from 7.00 to 9.00 a.m. Production

of inhibin B correlates positively with the function of Sertoli cells and the amount of semen. Instead, negative correlation between inhibin B and FSH is recorded (Yamaguchi et al., 1991).
Inhibin B is mainly secreted during the follicular phase of the menstrual cycle. The concentration of inhibin B in serum appears to be growing in the early follicular phase, with a prominent peak occurring after the increase of FSH secretion and gradually decreases in the late follicular phase. Another peak of inhibin B secretion is observed two days after the LH peak, and then its rapid decline, which leads to low levels of inhibin B in the luteal phase (Groome et al., 1996).
Secretion of inhibins changes due to age. In regularly menstruating premenopausal women, in spite of normal levels of estradiol and LH, elevated levels of FSH during the follicular phase of the menstrual cycle was found. This higher concentration of FSH appears for a few years before the onset of menopause, and is accompanied by decreased ovarian reserve and reduced fertility factor. This increased levels of FSH is due to significantly reduced production of inhibin B by a reduced pool of ovarian follicles in the follicular phase. Concentrations of inhibin A, also are reduced in women who are premenopausal. In these patients initially lower the levels of inhibin B in the follicular phase are stated, and only secondly it comes to lower levels of inhibin A. The concentrations of both inhibin A and inhibin B in women during menopause are almost undetectable (Danforth et al., 1998).

	SECRETION
INHIBIN A	dominant follicles and corpus luteum of the ovary Adrenals Pituitary Spleen bone marrow Placenta fetal membranes
INHIBIN B	granulosa cells of early antral follicles

Table 1. Sources of inhibin A and inhibin B secretion in womens' organism.

The measurement of inhibin B can provide useful information about ovarian reserve, and plays an important role in assisted reproductive techniques. Inhibin B can be also regarded as potential marker of diagnosis of premature ovarian failure (POF) and ovarian recovery in hypothalamic disturbances (Meczekalski & Podfigurna-Stopa, 2009).
Both inhibin A and inhibin B can play helpful role in the assessment of ovarian function in patient with Turner syndrome.

	Diagnostic role
INHIBIN A	ectopic pregnancy mola hydatidosa threatened abortion pre-eclampsia pregnancy associated with Down's syndrome
TOTAL INHIBIN	ovarian tumors PCOS

Table 2. Role of inhibin A and total inhibin in obstetrics and gynecology.

Total inhibin is the sum of precursors, subunits of inhibins and molecules. Estimation of total inhibin may play a role in polycystic ovary syndrome (PCOS) and may serve as a potential marker for ovarian cancer (Tsigkou et al., 2007, 2008).

There are requirements of further studies to clarify the use of inhibins in clinical practice of reproductive endocrinology.

Inhibins act indirectly through the antagonistic action to activins, which are dimers with protein molecular weight of about 24,000 Da.

Activins are members of the TGF-β family and they are secreted by the tubal epithelial cells. They are homodimers of inhibin β subunits (β A and β B) and there are distinguished three different glycoproteins: activin A (β A- β A), activin B (β B- β B) and activin AB (β A- β B).

Activins are produced as larger precursor proteins that are subsequently unlinked to excrete the mature C-terminal protein.

Activins regulate their action by binding to a complex of transmembrane serine and threonine kinase receptors. These activin receptors are categorized into two groups: type I receptor group, comprising the activin receptor-like kinase, and type II receptor group comprising the activin type IIA and type IIB receptors (ActRIIA and ActRIIB).

Activin function is regulated by follistatin, which is the binding protein (Refaat et al., 2004). Binding of activin to follistatin is almost irreversible and this harmonized synthesis of follistatin with activin is the main regulator of the local bioactivity of activin.

The activin follistatin complex is most often composed of one activin dimer and two follistatin molecules.

Circulating activin is generally revealed as linked with the long-form follistatin (follistatin-315). The short form of follistatin (follistatin-288) demonstrates high affinity for association with cell membrane proteoglycans. It is said that the affinity of binding activin A, activin B and activin AB to follistatin seems to be similar.

Activins stimulate pituitary FSH secretion and play an important role mainly in the regulation of reproductive, but also in the immunological function.

2. Ectopic pregnancy and serum biomarkers for diagnosis of ectopic pregnancy

Ectopic pregnancy is a situation when fertilized egg has implanted outside the uterus (Walker, 2007). Ectopic means "out of place". The most common site of implantation is fallopian tube (98% of cases), mainly in the ampullary region. Other types of ectopic pregnancy include interstitial, corneal, ovarian, cervical, scar, intraabdominal and heterotopic pregnancy (Condous, 2009).

The incidence of ectopic pregnancy has been increasing in the last decades. The incidence of ectopic pregnancy has increased from 0,37 % of pregnancies in 1948 to approximately 2% of pregnancies in 1992 (Centers for Disease Control). According to the literature from 2002 one in every 80 pregnancy is extrauterines. More than 100 000 cases are reported in each year in United States (Zane et al., 2002). In the developing world the incidence is much higher than in developed countries.

Despite the fact that mortality decreased by almost 90% from 1979 to 1992, ectopic pregnancy remains the leading cause of death during the first trimester of pregnancy with a 9% to 14% mortality rate (Lozeau & Potter, 2005).

Ectopic pregnancy is an increasing health risk for women throughout the world and continues to be the leading cause of maternal death in the first trimester of pregnancy. The cause of this high mortality is very often because of improper examination delayed diagnosis. The early diagnosis of ectopic pregnancy should be based on the transvaginal sonography. However, in some of women with suspected early ectopic pregnancy, the assessment with the transvaginal sonography is inefficient. In these women, biochemical assessment is used to establish the correct diagnosis.

Measurement of biochemical parameters describing ectopic pregnancy is mainly based on the estimation of serum human chorionic gonadotropin (β-hCG) and progesterone concentrations. None of these markers are efficient in the diagnosis of ectopic pregnancy, that is why new screening methods and algorithms are needed.

Short- and long-term consequences on health related quality of life and psychological issues are important but are rarely quantified.

The most important risk factors include a history of ectopic pregnancy, tubal surgery and pelvic inflammatory disease.

Early diagnosis of ectopic pregnancy is critical for conservation of fallopian tubal integrity and prevent potentially life-threatening abdominal bleeding (Lipscomb, 2010).

Ectopic pregnancy can be difficult to diagnose because symptoms often mirror those of normal early pregnancy. The initial evaluation of patients suspected for to have an ectopic pregnancy contain a quantitative measurements of serum human chorionic gonadotropin test (hCG)and transvaginal ultrasonography (US) (Lipscomb, 2010). The use of above-mentioned traditional tool sometimes cannot be fully helpful (Practice Committee of the American Society for Reproductive Medicine, 2006).

Fewer than 50% of tubal ectopic pregnancies are diagnosed at the patient's initial presentation (Munro et al., 2008). Despite clinical advances in imaging ultrasound is non-conclusive in up to 18% of women whom measurement of serial hCG concentration is necessary guide management. Further difficulties are encountered because serial hCG determination cannot separate arrested intrauterine from tubal ectopic pregnancies (Horne et al., 2010). Decelerated increase in hCG concentration cannot be used to discriminate between a miscarriage and an ectopic pregnancy. If hCG levels are found high, the probability of having ectopic pregnancy is about 30%.

A probability of having ectopic pregnancy in women with unknown pregnancy location and progesterone concentrations higher than 5.01 ng/ml is as high as 30% , whereas with progesterone values below the cutoff the probability of having an ectopic pregnancy is about 3.49%.

Multiple visits and tests currently necessary are a real expense for health service. As an example data from Edinburgh indicates that health services in Scotland are spending up to 1,5 million of British Pounds per year diagnosis and excluding ectopic pregnancy (an estimated 9 million of British Pounds in direct costs alone to health services per year throughout the United Kingdom alone) (Florio et al., 2007).

The aim is to find fast and accurate test to diagnose ectopic pregnancy. It would reduce the number of visit of patients during diagnosis process and it would help to avoid unnecessary laparoscopy.

At present, more than 20 biomarkers have been identified to improve earlier diagnosis of ectopic pregnancy. Some of the biomarkers such as placental protein 14 at first was identified as good marker of ectopic pregnancy but further studies revealed its weak discriminatory value. Some of the biomarkers such as cancer antigen 125, pregnancy associated plasma protein A, estradiol are able to discriminate a tubal ectopic pregnancy from a viable intrauterine pregnancy. Unfortunately, they appeared to be unable to distinguish the former from a non-viable intrauterine pregnancy (miscarriage) (Katsikis et al., 2006). The problem is also that other biomarkers such us progesterone, creatinine kinase, vascular endothelial growth factor (VEGF) could not be used in clinical practice because the results of study have been conflicting. (Develioglu et al., 2002).

The best serum biomarker should be easy available, cheap, reliable and based on one measurement. It is important particularly for developing countries that it should be a single marker. These countries have the highest morbidity and mortality problems related to ectopic pregnancy. Therefore essential progress can be observed in the work on new candidate biomarkers for ectopic pregnancy diagnosis. New biomarkers can be based on genomic technology. The attention should be paid on recent discovery the inhibin/activin beta B under-expression in the decidualized endometrium of women with tubal ectopic pregnancies. This kind of discovery can indicate that some secreted proteins associated with uterine decidualization can be useful in the diagnostic process of ectopic pregnancy.

Little is known of the mechanism by which the process of embryo transport is coordinated within the tube. Both cilial activity and tubal peristalsis are believed to be necessary for successful transport of the embryo along the tube and to ensure delivery of the embryo at the endometrial cavity at the optimum time for adhesion and implantation. This is critical for the successful establishment of pregnancy and avoidance of ectopic pregnancy. Therefore, we investigated whether epithelium from Fallopian tubes bearing an ectopic pregnancy differs from a normal tube in expression of TGF-β family and related proteins and their receptors.

3. Inhibins in ectopic pregnancy

3.1 Inhibin A in ectopic pregnancy

There are only few reports on the possible role of inhibin A in ectopic pregnancy.

First report about possible role of inhibin levels in ectopic pregnancy comes from 1996.

It was case-control study and included 19 women who had ectopic pregnancy confirmed at surgery and by pathology (Seifer et al., 1996). Control group was composed of 24 women of similar chronological and gestational age with sonographic evidence of an intrauterine pregnancies that are conceived spontaneously. Serum total and dimeric inhibin concentrations in women with ectopic pregnancy were < 60% of the concentrations for women with single intrauterine pregnancies. Total inhibin, but not dimeric inhibin-A, was elevated in maternal serum before week 8 of gestation relative to normal menstrual cycle levels. Serum inhibin concentrations are lower in ectopic pregnancy as compared with intrauterine pregnancies that are spontaneously conceived and the relative amounts of dimeric inhibin-A, B, and alpha inhibin subunit in maternal serum may change throughout gestation (Seifer et al., 1996).

Next study related to evaluation of inhibin A as a marker of persistent ectopic pregnancy was published in 1998 (D'Antona et al., 1998). Results of this study suggest that inhibin A will not be a useful marker for ectopic pregnancy but that it may provide a more accurate preoperative assessment of trophoblast viability than hCG, thereby improving management.

Another study (prospective case control study) performed 3 years ago evaluated whether inhibin A concentrations is a clinically useful marker of ectopic pregnancy (Segal et al., 2008). It was confirmed that inhibin A may be reliable marker for diagnosis of ectopic pregnancy.

There is also report that serum inhibin A levels can be used in the prediction of failing "pregnancy of unknown location" but according to authors this marker is not such reliable as serum hCG levels (Kirk, 2009).

The new concept for diagnose ectopic pregnancy is based on the genomic technology. The attention should be paid on recent discovery that there are differences in function of the decidualized endometrium in tubal ectopic and intrauterine pregnancies of similar gestations. Inhibin/activin β_B subunit expression was related to the degree of decidualization of the endometrium and was reduced in tubal ectopic pregnancies.
Serum inhibin levels have been reported to be lower in spontaneously conceived ectopic pregnancies compared with intrauterine pregnancies (Seifer et al., 1996).
Serum inhibin A levels can be used in the prediction of failing "pregnancy of unknown location" (Kirk et al., 2009).
Segal et al (2010) performed a prospective case-control study to determine whether inhibin A concentrations is a clinically useful marker of ectopic pregnancy (Segal et al., 2010). They confirmed that inhibin A may be reliable marker for diagnosis of ectopic pregnancy.
There are also suggestions that inhibin A will not be a useful marker for ectopic pregnancy but that it may provide a more accurate preoperative assessment of trophoblast viability than hCG, thereby improving management (D'Antona et al., 1998)

3.2 Inhibin B in ectopic pregnancy

There are no reports about inhibin B as useful marker of ectopic pregnancy.

3.3 Total inhibin in ectopic pregnancy

Total inhibin is the sum of precursors, subunits of inhibins and molecules. Estimation of total inhibin may play a role in polycystic ovary syndrome (PCOS) and may serve as a potential marker for ovarian cancer (Tsigkou et al, 2007, 2008).
Inhibins act indirectly through the antagonistic action to activin, which are dimers with protein molecular weight of about 24,000 Da.
There is only one report cited above (Seifert et al., 1996) about role of total inhibin in patients with ectopic pregnancy. This study presents that serum total and dimeric inhibin concentrations in women with ectopic pregnancy were < 60% of the concentrations for women with single intrauterine pregnancies.

4. Activins in ectopic pregnancy

The placenta is the main source of activin A during pregnancy. In the maternal circulation serum activin A concentrations are higher than in nonpregnant women and increase throughout pregnancy until delivery. It is thought that activin A plays an essential role in the endocrine physiology of human pregnancy (Petraglia et al., 1987).
As the embryo moves toward the uterine cavity, the uterine tubes are biologically active, providing an environment that assures fertilization and early embryonic development. There is an embryonic maternal cooperation in which the maternal reproductive tract and the embryo changes to provide embryonic and endometrial maturation. Recently, the expression of activin subunits, type II receptors and follistatin by the premenopausal Fallopian tube was demonstrated. It is suggested that activins are combined with follistatin and play a paracrine and autocrine role in early development and transport of embryo (Bahathiq et al., 2002).
Patients with the diagnosis of ectopic pregnancy are characterized by lower serum activin A concentrations than in patients with first-trimester spontaneous abortion and in patients with intrauterine pregnancy. The findings of low activin A concentrations in ectopic pregnancy are quite recent. It is suggested that an impaired secretion of activin A occurs in the presence of problems related to trophoblast invasion and implantation.

Variations in maternal activin A concentrations occurring in trophoblast diseases are believed to be part of the adaptive response of the placenta to adverse environmental conditions (Florio et al., 2001).

Patients with the diagnosis of ectopic pregnancy demonstrate disturbed activin A release in the placenta, which impairs the endometrium vascularization and subsequently trophoblast implantation not in the uterus (Dimitriadis et al., 2005).

Role of the endometrium which is a pivotal source of activin A is essential in the ground of implantation of ectopic pregnancy. During the secretory phase of the menstrual cycle (at the time of blastocyst implantation), activin A is present in the uterine fluid of cycling women in higher concentrations than during the proliferative phase. Activin A is a well-known regulator of the differentiation of proliferative cytotrophoblast into extravillous invasive trophoblast cells of the anchoring villi (Norwitz et al., 2001). The lack of an adequate endometrial secretion of activin A may be related to the lack of appropriate messages to the placenta for a right implantation. Additionally, activin A levels correlate with endometrial thickness. Such an increase of endometrial activin A and secretion at the time of blastocyst apposition may play an important role in embryo implantation (Caniggia et al., 1997).

The probability of having an ectopic pregnancy may be estimated more precisely and more quickly if activin A measurement is performed.

Single activin A measurement may identify patients at risk of ectopic pregnancy with a high sensibility and specificity. Positive predictive value for ectopic pregnancy (approximately 97%) is possible when low serum activin levels are observed. These procedures may select pregnancies at higher risk of ectopic pregnancy earlier and possibly to prevent unnecessary interventions.

Additionally, activins play an important role in inflammation and are involved in the pathogenesis of inflammatory, fibrotic diseases and early scar formation. Activin A expression has been reported to increase in several inflammatory diseases, such as septicemia, inflammatory bowel disease, rheumatoid arthritis and asthma (Phillips et al., 2001).

Nowadays, there is a suggestion that activin A could play an essential role in chlamydial infection. Refaat B. et al in 2009 performed a study about role of activins in the ectopic pregnancy in patients with or without Chlamydia trachomatis infection (Refaat, 2009).

Infection with Chlamydia trachomatis increases the production of tumor necrosis factor alpha (TGF-α) in human cervical tissue, interleukin-1 in human fallopian tube bearing an ectopic pregnancy, and interleukin-6 in serum from women diagnosed with ectopic pregnancy. Activin A has been reported to modulate the function of B lymphocytes, which play an important role in controlling reinfection with Chlamydia trachomatis. Infection with Chlamydia trachomatis is associated with scar formation. Repeated Chlamydia trachomatis infection of pigtailed macaque fallopian tubes produces a Th1-like cytokine response associated with fibrosis and scarring.

There is an increased activin A expression and its related molecules by human tubal epithelial cells in patients with the diagnosis of ectopic pregnancy. It has been suggested that tubal activins may be involved in the immune response to chlamydia-induced tubal chronic inflammation. This impairment in the activin expression by epithelial cells of fallopian tube may result in tubal pathology and subsequently may be the cause of development of ectopic pregnancy (Roan et al., 2008).

Increased expression of activin βA subunit and type II receptors may lead to impairment of tubal motility, an increase in tubal receptivity, and subsequently the development of ectopic pregnancy. It is said that tubal activin A, its type II receptors could be involved in the microbial-

mediated immune response within the fallopian tube, and their pathological expression may lead to tubal damage and the development of ectopic pregnancy (Refaat, 2009).
The intensity of expression of activin-βA subunit, ActRIIA and ActRIIB and follistatin by the epithelial cells of human Fallopian tubes in patients with ectopic pregnancy is increased. However, the up-regulation of the proteins is accompanied by a down-regulation of the mRNA of these molecules. The mRNA of these molecules is rapidly translated and degraded, resulting in rapid turnover of the mRNA, with depletion of these mRNAs due to the prolonged synthesis of large amounts of activin-A, its receptors, and follistatin. (Refaat et al., 2009).
Epithelial cells of the Fallopian tube have been reported to expressed nitric oxide (NO) and NO synthase. Activin-A stimulates the NO production in a concentration-dependent manner in a variety of tissues and cells. NO is engaged in many female reproductive functions and it has a relaxing effect on smooth muscles of the Fallopian tube. Additionally, Perez in 2000 reported in rat oviduct a significant increase in tubal transport of ova after the local administration of NO synthase inhibitors (Perez, 2000).
Increased activin-A expression by the Fallopian tube epithelial cells may stimulate tubal decidualization and trophoblast invasion within the tube. Furthermore, an increase in activin-A expression by the Fallopian tube epithelial cells may increase the production of NO in a concentration-dependent manner, resulting in pathological relaxation of the tubal smooth muscles, failure of propulsion of the early embryo along the Fallopian tube and the development of ectopic pregnancy.

5. Conclusion

Ectopic pregnancy is really an important clinical problem. Particular aspect is referred to precise and fast diagnosis with the use of serum biomarkers. Activins and inhibins can be regarded as such biomarker candidate. So far the number of reports on the role of activins and inhibins in ectopic pregnancy diagnosis is limited.
Majority of studies on inhibin A (but the number is very limited) indicates that this substance can be consider as possible marker of ectopic pregnancy.
New biomarkers can be based on genomic technology. The attention should be paid on recent discovery the inhibin/activin beta B under-expression in the decidualized endometrium of women with tubal ectopic pregnancies. This kind of discovery can indicate that some secreted proteins associated with uterine decidualization can be useful in the diagnostic process of ectopic pregnancy.
During pregnancy, the human placenta is the main source of maternal activin A and serum concentrations of activin A progressively increase throughout pregnancy until delivery. Impaired secretion of activin A is related to trophoblast invasion and implantation. Patients with the diagnosis of ectopic pregnancy are thought to have low serum activin A concentrations.
There is no doubts that further studies on activins and inhibins in the aspect of ectopic pregnancy are required.

6. Acknowledgment

Address all correspondence and requests for reprints to: Assoc. Professor Blazej Meczekalski, Chairman of the Department of Gynecological Endocrinology, Poznan University of Medical Sciences, Poznan, ul. Polna 33, 60-535 Poznan, Poland.

E-mail: blazejmeczekalski@yahoo.com
Disclosure Statement: The authors have nothing to declare.

7. References

Al-Azemi M, Ledger WL, Diejomaoh M, Mousa M, Makhseed M, Omu A. 2003. Measurement of inhibin A and inhibin pro-alphaC in early human pregnancy and their role in the prediction of pregnancy outcome in patients with recurrent pregnancy loss. *Fertil Steril.* Dec;80(6):1473-9.

Bahathiq AO, Stewart RL, Wells M, Moore HD, Pacey AA, Ledger WL. 2002 Production of activins by the human endosalpinx. *J Clin Endocrinol Metab.* 87:5283–5289.

Burger HG. & Igarashi M. 1988. Inhibin: definition and nomenclature, including related substances. *J Clin Endocrinol Metab.* 66:885-6.

Caniggia I, Lye SJ, Cross JC. 1997. Activin is a local regulator of human cytotrophoblast cell differentiation. *Endocrinology.* 138:3976–3986.

Condous G. 2009. Ectopic pregnancy : challenging accepted management strategies. *Obstet Gynecol.* 49 (4), 246-351.

Centers for Disease Control and Prevention (CDC). 1995. Ectopic Pregnancy: United States, 1990-1992. MMWR Morb Mortal Wkly Rep. 44, 46-48.

Danforth DR, Arbogast LK, Mroueh J, Kim MH, Kennard EA, Seifer DB, Friedman CI. 1998. Dimeric inhibin: a direct marker of ovarian aging. *Fertil Steril.* 70:119-23.

D'Antona D, Mamers PM, Lowe PJ, Balazs N, Groome NP, Wallace EM. 1998. Evaluation of serum inhibin A as a surveillance marker after conservative management of tubal pregnancy. *Hum Reprod.* Aug;13(8):2305-7.

de Kretser DM, Hedger MP, Loveland KL, Phillips DJ. 2002. Inhibins, activins and follistatin in reproduction. *Hum Reprod Update.* 8:529-41.

Develioglu OH, Bilgin T, Yalcin OT, Ozalp S. 2003. Transvaginal ultrasonography and uterine artery Doppler in diagnosing endometrial pathologies and carcinoma in postmenopausal bleeding. *Arch Gynecol Obstet.* Aug;268(3):175-80. Epub 2002 Dec 21.

Dimitriadis E, White CA, Jones RL, Salamonsen LA .2005. Cytokines, chemokines and growth factors in endometrium related to implantation. *Hum Reprod Updat.e* 11:613–630.

Dixit VD, Parvizi N. 2001. Nitric oxide and the control of reproduction. *Anim Reprod Sci.* 65:1–16.

Florio P, Cobellis L, Luisi S, Ciarmela P, Severi FM, Bocchi C, Petraglia F. 2001. Changes in inhibins and activin secretion in healthy and pathological pregnancies. *Mol Cell Endocrinol* 180:123–130.

Florio P, Luisi S, Ciarmela P, Severi FM, Bocchi C, Petraglia F. 2004. Inhibins and activins in pregnancy. *Mol Cell Endocrinol.* 225:93-100.

Florio P, Severi FM, Bocchi C, Luisi S, Petraglia F. 2003. Abruptio placentae and highest maternal serum activin A levels at mid-gestation: a two cases report. *Placenta.* 24:279–280.

Florio P, Severi FM, Bocchi C, Luisi S, Mazzini M, Danero S, Torricelli M, Petraglia F. 2007. Single serum activin a testing to predict ectopic pregnancy. *J Clin Endocrinol Metab.* May;92(5):1748-53. Epub 2007 Mar 6.

Francis M, Arkle M, Martin L, Butler TM, Cruz MC, Opare-Aryee G, Dacke CG, Brown JF. 2003. Relaxant effects of parathyroid hormone and parathyroid hormone-related peptides on oviduct motility in birds and mammals: possible role of nitric oxide. *Gen Comp Endocrinol.* 133:243–251.

Groome NP, Illingworth PJ, O'Brien M, Pai R, Rodger FE, Mather JP, McNeilly AS. 1996. Measurement of dimeric inhibin B throughout the human menstrual cycle. *J Clin Endocrinol Metab.* 81:1401-5.

Hatakeyama D, Sadamoto H, Watanabe T, Wagatsuma A, Kobayashi S, Fujito Y, Yamashita M, Sakakibara M, Kemenes G, Ito E. 2006. Requirement of new protein synthesis of a transcription factor for memory consolidation: paradoxical changes in mRNA and protein levels of C/EBP. *J Mol Biol* 356:569- 577.

Horne AW, Duncan WC, Critchley HO. 2010. The need for serum biomarker development for diagnosing and excluding tubal ectopic pregnancy. *Acta Obstet Gynecol Scand.* Mar;89(3):299-301.

Jones RL, Findlay JK, Farnworth PG, Robertson DM, Wallace E, Salamonsen LA. 2006 Activin A and inhibin A differentially regulate human uterine matrix metalloproteinases: potential interactions during decidualization and trophoblast invasion. *Endocrinology* 147:724–732.

Katsikis I, Rousso D, Farmakiotis D, Kourtis A, Diamanti-Kandarakis E, Panidis D. 2006. Receiver operator characteristics and diagnostic value of progesterone and CA-125 in the prediction of ectopic and abortive intrauterine gestations. *Eur J Obstet Gynecol Reprod Biol.* Apr 1;125(2):226-32. Epub 2005 Nov 21.

Kirk E, Papageorghiou AT, Van Calster B, Condous G, Cowans N, Van Huffel S, Timmerman D, Spencer K, Bourne T. 2009. The use of serum inhibin A and activin A levels in predicting the outcome of 'pregnancies of unknown location'. *Hum Reprod.* Oct;24(10):2451-6. Epub 2009 Jun 23.

Klein NA, Illingworth PJ, Groome NP, McNeilly AS, Battaglia DE, Soules MR. 1996. Decreased inhibin B secretion is associated with the monotropic FSH rise in older, ovulatory women: a study of serum and follicular fluid levels of dimeric inhibin A and B in spontaneous menstrual cycles. *J Clin Endocrinol Metab.* 81:2742-5.

Kriebs JM, Fahey JO. 2006. Ectopic pregnancy. *J Midwifery Womens Health.* 51:431–439.

Lipscomb GH. 2010. Ectopic pregnancy: still cause for concern. *Obstet Gynecol.* Mar;115(3):487-8.

Lozeau AM, Potter B. 2005. Diagnosis and management of ectopic pregnancy. *AM Fam Physician.* 72: 1707-1714.

Lyons RA, Saridogan E, Djahanbakhch O. 2006. The reproductive significance of human Fallopian tube cilia. *Hum Reprod Update.* 12:363–372.

Meczekalski B, Podfigurna-Stopa A. 2009. The role of inhibins in functions and dysfunctions of female reproduction. Part I. *Pol Merkur Lekarski.* Mar;26(153):258-62. Review. Polish.

Meczekalski B, Podfigurna-Stopa A. 2009. The role of inhibins in functions and dysfunctions of female reproduction--Part II. *Pol Merkur Lekarski.* Jun;26(156):676-8. Review. Polish.

Munro KJ, Horne AW, Duncan WC, Critchley HOD. 2008. Features associated with the time to diagnosis and amanagement of ectopic pregnancy. *Scot Med J.* 53, 49.

Muttukrishna S, Child T, Lockwood GM, Groome NP, Barlow DH, Ledger WL. 2000. Serum concentrations of dimeric inhibins, activin A, gonadotrophins and ovarian steroids during the menstrual cycle in older women. *Hum Reprod.* 15:549-56.

Norwitz ER, Schust DJ, Fisher SJ. 2001. Mechanisms of disease: implantation and the survival of early pregnancy. *N Engl J Med.* 345:1400–1408.

Pangas SA, Woodruff TK. 2000. Activin signal transduction pathways. *Trends Endocrinol Metab.* 11:309–314.

Perez Martinez S, Viggiano M, Franchi AM, Herrero MB, Ortiz ME, Gimeno MF, VillalonM. 2000. Effect of nitric oxide synthase inhibitors on ovum transport and oviductal smooth muscle activity in the rat oviduct. *J Reprod Fertil* .118:111–117.

Petraglia F., Zanin E., Faletti A., Reis FM. 1999. Inhibins: paracrine and endocrine effects in female reproductive function. *Curr Opin Obstet Gynecol.* 11:241-7.

Phillips, D. J., K. L. Jones, J. Y. Scheerlinck, M. P. Hedger, and D. M. de Kretser. 2001. Evidence for activin A and follistatin involvement in the systemic inflammatory response. *Mol. Cell. Endocrinol.* 180:155–162.

Practice Committee of the American Society for Reproductive Medicine. 2006. Medical treatment of ectopic pregnancy. *Fertil Steril.* 86, Suppl 1, S96-102.

Refaat BA, Bahathiq AO, Sockanathan S, Stewart RL, Wells M, Ledger WL. 2004. Production and localization of activins and activin type IIA and IIB receptors by the human endosalpinx. *Reproduction.* 128:249–255.

Refaat B, Al-Azemi M, Geary I, Eley A, Ledger W. 2009. Role of activins and inducible nitric oxide in the pathogenesis of ectopic pregnancy in patients with or without Chlamydia trachomatis infection. *Clin Vaccine Immunol.* Oct;16(10):1493-503. Epub 2009 Aug 19.

Roan, N. R., and M. N. Starnbach. 2008. Immune-mediated control of Chlamydia infection. *Cell. Microbiol.* 10:9–19.

Sau M, Sau AK, Roberts JK, Goldthorp W. 2000. Treatment of unruptured ectopic pregnancy with methotrexate.AU.K. experience. *Acta Obstet Gynecol Scand.* 79:790–792.

Segal S, Gor H, Correa N, Mercado R, Veenstra K, Rivnay B. 2008. Inhibin A: marker for diagnosis of ectopic and early abnormal pregnancies. *Reprod Biomed Online.* Dec;17(6):789-94.

Segal S., Mercado R., Rivnay B. 2010. Ectopic pregnancy early diagnosis markers. *Minerva Ginecol.* 62, 49-62.

Seifer DB, Lambert-Messerlian GM, Canick JA, Frishman GN, Schneyer AL. 1996. Serum inhibin levels are lower in ectopic than intrauterine spontaneously conceived pregnancies. *Fertil Steril.* Mar;65(3):667-9.

Tay JI, Moore J, Walker JJ. 2000. Ectopic pregnancy. *BMJ.* 320:916–919.

Tsigkou A., Luisi S., De Leo V. Patton L, Gambineri A, Reis FM, Pasquali R, Petraglia F. 2008. High serum concentration of total inhibin in polycystic ovary syndrome. *Fertil Steril.* Nov;90(5):1859-63.

Tsigkou A., Marrelli D., Reis FM. Luisi S, Silva-Filho AL, Roviello F, Triginelli SA, Petraglia F. 2007. Total inhibin is a potential serum marker for epithelial ovarian cancer. *J Clin Endocrinol Metab.* Jul;92(7):2526-31.

Yamaguchi M-A., Mizunuma H., Miyamoto K., Hasegawa Y, Ibuki Y, Igarashi M. 1991. Immunoreactive inhibin concentrations in adult men: prcsence of a circadian rhythm. *J Clin Endocrin Metab.* Mar;72(3):554-9.

Walker JJ. 2007. Ectopic pregnancy. *Clin Obstet Gynecol.* Mar;50(1):89-99.

Welt CK, Martin KA., Taylor AE., Lambert-Messerlian GM, Crowley WF Jr, Smith JA, Schoenfeld DA, Hall JE. 1997. Frequency modulation of follicle-stimulating hormone (FSH) during the luteal-follicular transition: evidence for FSH control of inhibin B in normal women. *J Clin Endocrinol Metab.* Aug;82(8):2645-52.

Zane SB, Kieke BA Jr, Kendrick JS, Bruce C. 2002. Surveillance in a time of changing health care practices: estimating ectopic pregnancy incidence in the United States. *Matern Child Health J.* Dec;6(4):227-36.

10

Term Extra-Uterine Pregnancy

Ismail A. Al-Badawi[1], Osama Al Omar[1] and Togas Tulandi[2]
[1]King Faisal Specialist Hospital & Research Center
[2]Department of Obstetrics and Gynecology, McGill university, Montreal, Quebec,
[1]Saudi Arabia
[2]Canada

1. Introduction

Extrauterine pregnancies rarely reach third trimester of gestation. However, abdominal pregnancy can result in term delivery. Term cervical pregnancy has also been reported. The most unusual is term tubal ectopic pregnancy.
Our objective is to review cases of term extra-uterine pregnancy and to evaluate its consequences on the mother and the fetus. Due to its ill impact, the best management is early diagnosis and treatment. Prolongation of an ectopic pregnancy should be avoided.

2. Abdominal pregnancy (AP) reaching fetal viability or term

2.1 Introduction/definition/incidence

AP represents a variant of ectopic gestation in which the conceptus is sited in the abdominal cavity, external to the uterus, fallopian tubes and broad ligament (1, 2). Devoid of endometrial support, the placenta may attach to the peritoneum, bowel, uterine serosa and omentum. AP is the rarest form of ectopic pregnancy, with an incidence of 1% of all ectopic gestations (3).
AP is defined as advanced once fetal viability is reached. At this stage AP carries significantly high mortality rates for both mother (0-20%) and fetus/newborn (40-95%) (2, 4). The latter is partly due to a 20-40% rate of congenital fetal malformations (4).

2.2 Diagnosis

A high index of suspicion for this rare and serious condition, complemented by often nonspecific findings in the clinical history and physical examination may lead to a timely correct diagnosis. Recurrent abdominal pain and tenderness, a relatively mobile abdominal mass in an amenorrheic woman of reproductive age, painful fetal movements in the upper abdomen associated with a persistently abnormal lie, fetal heart sounds localized in the upper epigastrium, should raise the possibility of an AP and be followed by an ultrasound examination (5). In early pregnancy the diagnosis of AP might be missed by failure to obtain an image demonstrating continuity of the vagina, cervix and uterus with its pregnancy contents (1). Four ultrasound criteria have been suggested to support the diagnosis of AP: (1) absence of an intrauterine gestational sac, (2) absence of both an evident dilated tube and a complex adnexal mass, (3) a gestational sac surrounded by loops of bowel and separated by peritoneum, (4) a wide mobility similar to fluctuation of the sac particularly evident with pressure of the transvaginal probe toward the posterior cul-de-sac (6). Characteristic sonographic features in an advanced AP are: fetal parts adjacent to the mother's abdominal content, absence of the uterine wall between the maternal urinary bladder and the fetus, a pseudo-placenta previa appearance, oligohydramnios (4). Despite the availability of prenatal ultrasound in developed countries, AP continues to be reported at a late gestation underscoring the difficulty in diagnosing this entity as well as the failure to observe basic ultrasound techniques (1). This would explain a 50-90% diagnostic failure rate and the often unexpected diagnosis of AP during elective Caesarean Sections performed for fetal malpresentation or low-lying placenta (7, 8, 9, 10). Puerperal presentations of a living heterotopic AP have been described, thus underscoring the diagnostic challenge represented by this rare entity (11, 12). In undiagnosed advanced AP cardiovascular shock due to intra-abdominal bleeding and sudden death are more ominous presentations (13). MRI offers, apart from diagnostic reassurance, no additional information to ultrasound assessment and is therefore, as an adjunct imaging modality, not central to the diagnosis of advanced AP (1, 14).

2.3 Management of AP

Management of an AP requires a careful initial evaluation of the fetus in terms of gestational age, the presence of associated fetal anomalies, the amount of amniotic fluid (as a determinant of fetal pressure deformities and pulmonary hypoplasia)(4, 15). This is best accomplished at a referral center with adequate resources: medical imaging and interventional radiology service, blood bank, intensive care unit as well as a surgical team capable of handling possible bowel, vascular, genitourinary complications that might arise. Because of the risk of sudden intra-abdominal haemorrhage due to either placental abruption or vascular invasion, most advise surgical intervention as soon as the diagnosis of AP is confirmed and regardless of the fetal condition (4). A conservative approach may be considered and delivery delayed until fetal maturity is reached, if the gestational age exceeds 20 weeks and the following prerequisites are met: absence of fetal malformations, adequate amniotic fluid volume, absence of maternal medical contraindications, placental implantation site not in the proximity of major vessels, liver or spleen, continuous maternal hospitalization in an appropriate facility, fetal surveillance with daily heartrate monitoring and serial ultrasound assessments, and informed consent from the patient (4).

In the absence of complications, delivery of an advanced AP can be planned for 34 weeks' gestation. Careful preoperative preparations should include: an adequate supply of blood and blood products, appropriate intravenous infusion access, availability of cell-saver and MAST (Military Antishock Trouser) Suit, a multidisciplinary surgical team (4, 7, 10, 15). A midline vertical skin incision should be employed for entry into the abdominal cavity as adequate exposure is paramount. Bleeding could be prevented by incising the amniotic sac in an avascular area, avoiding the proximity of the placenta, as well as by careful removal of the fetus without disturbing the placenta and surrounding membranes (4, 15). Placental management following an advanced AP has shifted towards a non-surgical approach, leaving this organ in situ (16, 17). Although this approach has decreased the high maternal morbidity and mortality associated with attempted surgical removal, leaving the placenta in situ has also potential risks for the mother: a prolonged resorption period, haemorrhage, bowel obstruction and peritonitis (18). The use of methotrexate to accelerate absorption of a retained placenta remains controversial due to the potential severe associated complications

(19). Ultrasound evaluation is of benefit in the follow-up of placental involution after delivery of an advanced AP (14).

2.4 Conclusion

Although still rare, the increasing incidence of AP in both developed and especially developing countries mandates awareness of this diagnosis, particularly in pregnant or postpartum women presenting with abdominal pain (11).

3. Term cervico-isthmic pregnancy

3.1 Introduction

Both cervical and cervico-isthmic pregnancies are rare, life-threatening forms of ectopic gestations. The former is reported to have an estimated incidence of one in 2,500 to one in 18,000 pregnancies, and represents less than 1% of all ectopic gestations (1). A cervical pregnancy (CP) results from the implantation and growth of a blastocyst within the mucosa of the endocervical canal and is located completely within the cervical canal, with no placental tissue above the internal cervical os (2, 3). Currently CP are diagnosed by transvaginal ultrasound early in the first trimester of pregnancy and terminated by conservative, fertility sparing medical and/or surgical management. Most cases are not reported and therefore the exact incidence of CP is unclear. A CP is never viable and is unlikely to progress past 20 weeks of gestation. Previous reports of CP ending in live births are now thought to have been cervico-isthmic pregnancies (CIP) (3, 4, 5). In a CIP the gestational sac implants in the uterine isthmus, between the histologic and anatomic cervical os, and subsequently extends into the lower uterine segment (3, 4). The process of incorporation of the lower uterine segment into the gestational cavity occurs from the cervix upward rather than from the uterine cavity downward, as it happens in a normally implanted pregnancy (4). CIP are even more important clinically because they can grow to advanced gestational age and have significant perinatal complications. The growing gestational sac causes premature cervical effacement and dilatation which result in preterm premature rupture of the amniotic membranes and preterm delivery (6). Trophoblastic invasion of the endocervical and isthmic mucosa and stroma result in placenta accreta, placenta increta or placenta percreta and explain the massive hemorrhage at attempted placental removal (6, 7). Since 1980, when the term CIP was coined (3), the English language literature reported thirteen CIP exceeding 24 weeks, which is considered as the gestational age of neonatal viability (3, 4, 6 – 16). Table 1 summarizes these reports.

3.2 Diagnosis

Diagnostic algorithms and clinical prediction rules for CIP are difficult to validate because of the limited number of reported cases. In five of the thirteen women (38.5%) with advanced CIPs, the correct diagnosis was made at the time of delivery, underscoring the diagnostic challenge of this entity (3, 8, 10, 13, 15).

Several associated clinical signs noted historically should be heeded for a timely diagnosis of CIP. In case of painless vaginal bleeding occurring after 20 weeks of gestation, in a nulliparous woman in the fourth or fifth decade of life, CIP should be considered in the differential diagnosis. Painless vaginal bleeding was the presenting clinical sign in six women diagnosed with CIP reaching fetal viability (46%) (6, 7, 9, 11, 14, 16). Maternal age was 35 years or above in seven of the thirteen CIP (54%) and 54% of women had no prior deliveries.

After an ultrasound examination confirmed normal placental localization in a woman with painless vaginal bleeding, speculum examination could reveal premature cervical

Author, Year Reference	Maternal age Parity	Gestational age at diagnosis	Gestat age at delivery/Outcome	Treatment Blood transfusion in Units
David 1980 (3)	28 years; P0	At delivery	40 weeks/alive	CS + TAH No transfusions
Kalakoutis 1985 (8)	43 years; P1	At delivery	28 weeks/alive	VD + TAH 18 Units
Cohen 1985 (9)	36 years; P0	At 25 weeks	27 weeks/alive	CS + TAH 5 Units
Hoffman 1987 (10)	42 years; P2	At delivery	32 weeks/alive	CS + TAH Not stated
Weyerman 1989 (11)	38 years; P0	16 weeks	26 weeks/ Neonatal death	CS + TAH 4 Units
Jelsema 1992 (12)	30 years; P1	5.5 weeks	38 weeks/ alive	CS + TAH 8 Units
Iloabachie 1993 (13)	26 years; P0	At delivery	37 weeks/twins alive	CS 16 Units
Souter 1995 (14)	27 years; P0	21 weeks	28 weeks/ Alive	CS + TAH 52 Units
Strobelt 2001 (4)	41 years; P2	7 weeks	30 weeks /Alive	CS + TAH 7 Units
Mesogitis 2001 (15)	26 years; P0	At delivery	37 weeks /Alive	VD + TAH 4 Units
Honda 2005 (6)	39 years; P0	6 weeks	32 weeks /Alive	CS + TAH 5 Units
Kayem 2008 (16)	32 years; P2	25 weeks	34 weeks/ Alive	CS + Segmental resection of the uterine wall and placenta; No Transfusions
Avery 2009 (7)	35 years; P2	5 weeks 6 days	38 weeks /Alive	CS + TAH 20 Units

Table 1. Summary of CIP reaching neonatal viability (1980-2009)

effacement and dilatation and a bulging lower uterine segment. These findings are indicative of two impending perinatal complications of CIP: preterm premature rupture of amniotic membranes and preterm birth. Eight of thirteen CIP (61.5%) delivered prematurely. The gestational age range at delivery was 26 to 34 weeks (4, 6, 8-11, 15, 16). Seven out of eight prematurely born babies survived (87.5%). One neonatal death occurred following delivery at 26 weeks of gestation (11).

The diagnosis of CIP is confirmed by medical imaging and intraoperative findings.

Sonography has made early diagnosis of CP and CIP possible and has replaced histologic diagnosis (7). Transvaginal ultrasound has been able to identify CIP at 6 and 7 weeks of gestation in four patients with CIP which reached neonatal viability (4, 6, 7, 12), whereas abdominal ultrasound diagnosed three CIP in mid-trimester (9, 11, 16). Two ultrasound criteria have been proposed to support a diagnosis of CIP and differentiate it from CP: a well-preserved and closed cervical canal, thus ruling out CP and more than half of the uterine cavity above the gestational sac uninvolved by gestational sac implantation (4, 6) Image 3.1. Magnetic Resonance Imaging was useful in distinguishing between CP and CIP (17, 18) Image 3.2.

Intra-operatively the diagnosis of CIP is confirmed by the following findings: a small sized, empty uterine corpus and fundus, an abnormally distended and thin walled lower uterine segment, a placenta implanted below the peritoneal reflection of the anterior and posterior surfaces of the uterus, a densely adherent placenta, placental penetration and neovascularization visible under the serosal surface (6, 7, 12).

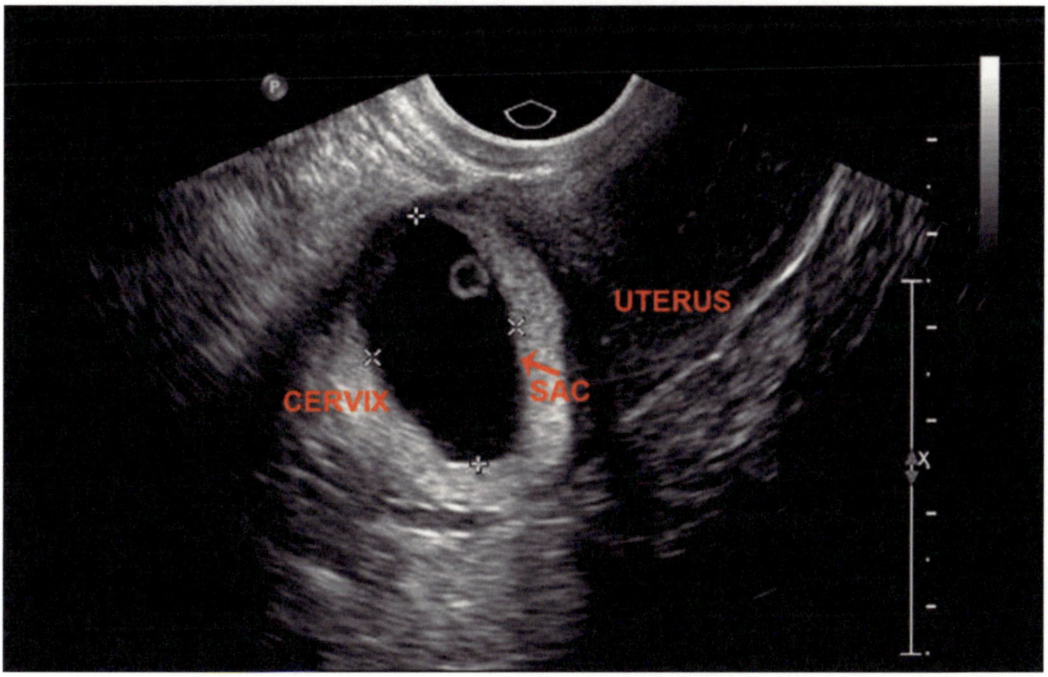

Image 3.1. Ultrasound of Cervical pregnancy

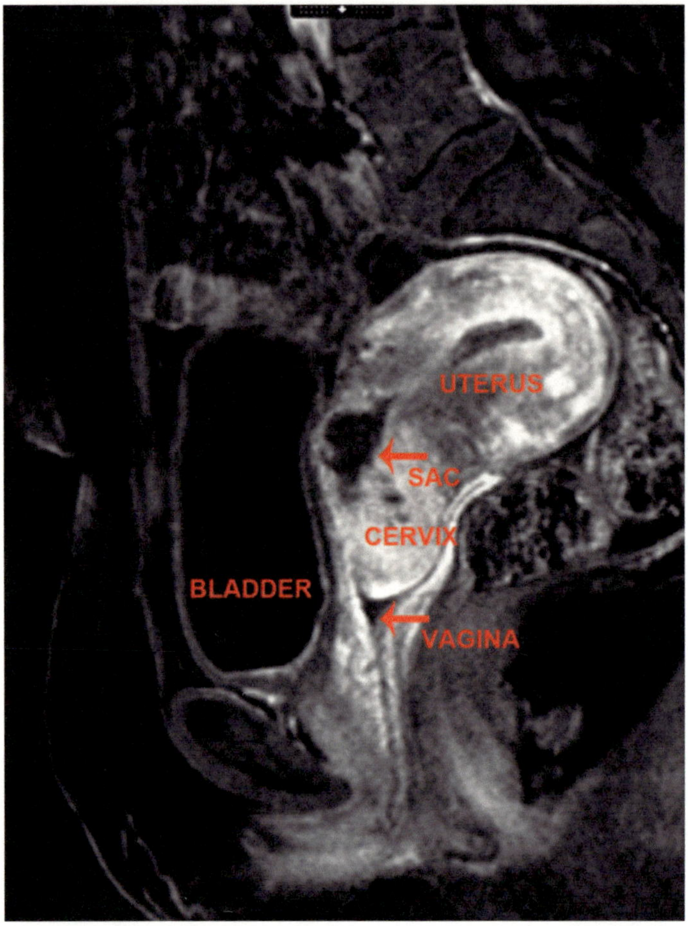

Image 3.2. MRI of Cervical pregnancy

3.3 Treatment

There are no clinical guidelines for the management of CIP as no center has accumulated enough data and experience with the treatment of this rare entity. Individual case reports, despite their inherent shortcomings, serve as reference in formulating management strategies for CIP which attained neonatal viability.

The management of CIP is dictated by the timing of the diagnosis.

If the diagnosis of CIP is made un-expectantly at the time of delivery, as it occurred in 38.5% of the reported advanced CIP, the therapeutic priority is to minimize the risks of catastrophic postpartum hemorrhage. This can be achieved by controlling the bleeding and replacement of the blood loss. Surgical occlusion of the internal iliac and uterine arteries or segmental resection of the uterine wall and attached placenta (16) could be initially employed if continuing fertility is desired and surgical expertise is available. Of the five women diagnosed at the time of delivery four required a total abdominal hysterectomy (3, 8, 10, 15) for control of postpartum hemorrhage, including the two women who were delivered vaginally (8, 15). This underscores the difficulty in controlling massive postpartum hemorrhage in previously unsuspected advanced CIP.

Once a CIP is diagnosed in the first trimester or early mid-trimester, termination of pregnancy should be offered after patient counseling. The latter should emphasize the possibility of severe life-threatening maternal and neonatal morbidity associated with continuation of the pregnancy (preterm delivery, postpartum hemorrhage, and hysterectomy) as opposed to the high success rate of early pregnancy termination by conservative, fertility sparing management (1, 6, 7, 17). If continuing the CIP is the patient's request after informed consent, then careful antenatal and perinatal management planning is imperative. Consideration should be given to timely transfer to a referral center with adequate resources: medical imaging and interventional radiology, extensive blood bank capabilities, adult and neonatal intensive care unit and surgical expertise to control massive postpartum hemorrhage. Continuous maternal hospitalization is advised in women with repeated antepartum bleeding or reduced cervical length (6). Transvaginal cervical length assessments should complement serial fetal ultrasound surveillance and alert the clinician about the possibility of preterm delivery (4, 6, 12). Delivery planning should ensure the availability of a large supply of blood and blood products. Eleven of thirteen women (84.6%) with advanced CIP received intra and/or postpartum blood transfusions (4, 6 - 15). Ten women were transfused 139 units of packed red blood cells, an average of 14 units per patient (4, 6 – 9, 11-15). These figures underscore the life-threatening nature of postpartum bleeding and the need of adequate blood bank services. Cesarean section is considered the safest route of delivery (6). Vaginal delivery remains an option and was accomplished in two women (8, 15). In the absence of a hemorrhagic emergency, placement of hypogastric artery catheters prior to delivery enables immediate internal iliac and uterine artery occlusion by embolization in the event of massive postpartum bleeding. (4).Eleven out of thirteen women with advanced CIP (84.6%) had a total abdominal hysterectomy after delivery of a viable newborn. The high postpartum hysterectomy rate has several reasons: the diagnosis is un-expectantly entertained at the time of delivery, the life-threatening nature of the postpartum hemorrhage and the lack of expertise in conservative operative techniques employed to control postpartum hemorrhage. Despite these challenges, the overall neonatal survival rate was 93%. Thirteen out of fourteen babies survived and one CIP was a twin gestation delivered at term (13).

The subsequent reproductive performance after CP was reassuring in 37 reported gestations: 54% of women had a term delivery, 14% had a premature delivery and 8% experienced a first trimester spontaneous abortion (19). Notwithstanding this argument, recurrent, consecutive CP were reported after use of assisted reproductive technology (20, 21). The subsequent successful obstetric experience after CP, reaffirms the enthusiasm for conservative, fertility sparing treatment enabled by early diagnosis. The reproductive performance after CIP remains elusive as the obstetric experience is limited to a single gestation that occurred in one of the two women whose uterus was preserved after term delivery of a CIP (16).

4. Term tubal pregnancy

4.1 Introduction

Term tubal pregnancy, however is extremely rare. Review of the literature revealed that at least over 13 cases of term tubal pregnancy have been reported. Most of them were published in the nineteen fifties. The most recent article on this subject was published in 2010. So, despite being a rather rare event, it can still be encountered especially in places with limited medical facilities.

4.2 Diagnosis

McElin and Randal (2) established 4 criteria of tubal pregnancy near or at term without rupture of the tube: 1) that comp lete extirpation of the fetal sac and products of conception be achieved by salpingectomy 2) that there be no gross or microscopic evidence of tubal rupture, 3) that ciliated columner epithelium be demonstrated at a few points in the inner lining of the sac and 4) that smooth muscle be found in the sac wall at multiple sites and at considerable distances from normal, undilated tube.

4.3 Conclusion and management

Tubal ectopic pregnancy accounts for approximately 1% of all pregnancies. Term tubal pregnancy, however is extremely rare. Review of the literature revealed that at least over 12 cases of term tubal pregnancy have been reported. Most of them were published in the 1950s [1-11]. The most recent article on this subject was published by us in 2010 [12]. With the recent advances in ultrasound and diagnostic imaging, it would be quite rare for ectopic pregnancy to reach up to term. In the event this would happen, an urgent laparotomy and salpingectomy with the removal of the affected fallopian tube would be the recommended option. Figure 1 and 2 demonstrate term tubal ectopic pregnancy with normal uterus and dilated fallopian tube after surgically opening it (figure 4.1). Then the term macerated fetus inside the tube (figure 4.2).

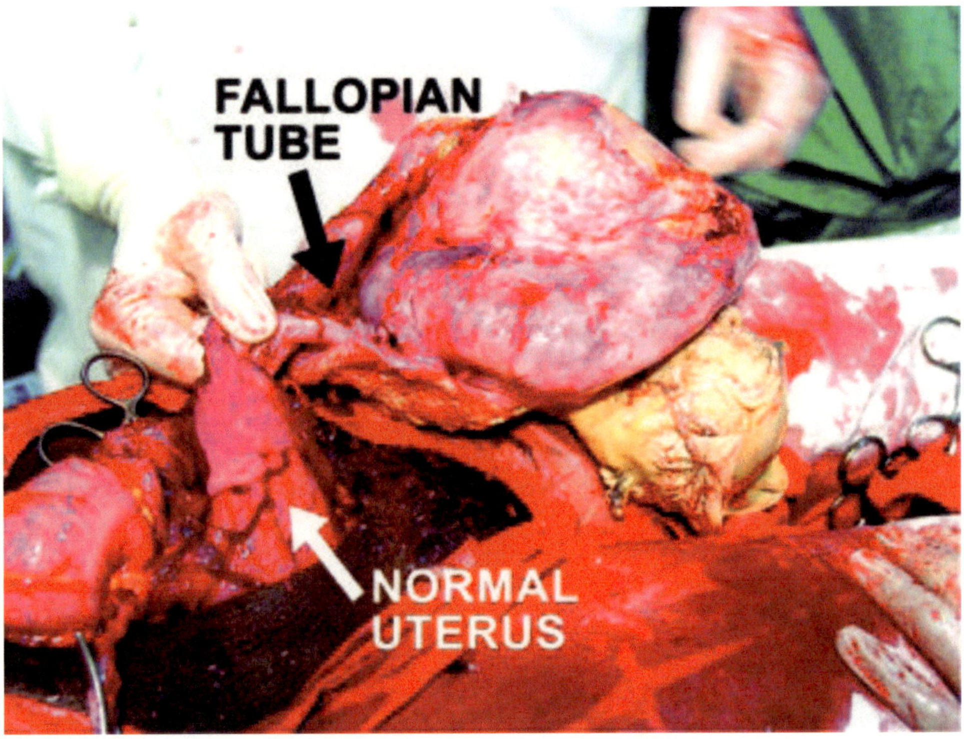

Fig. 4.1. Reatained term tubal pregnancy

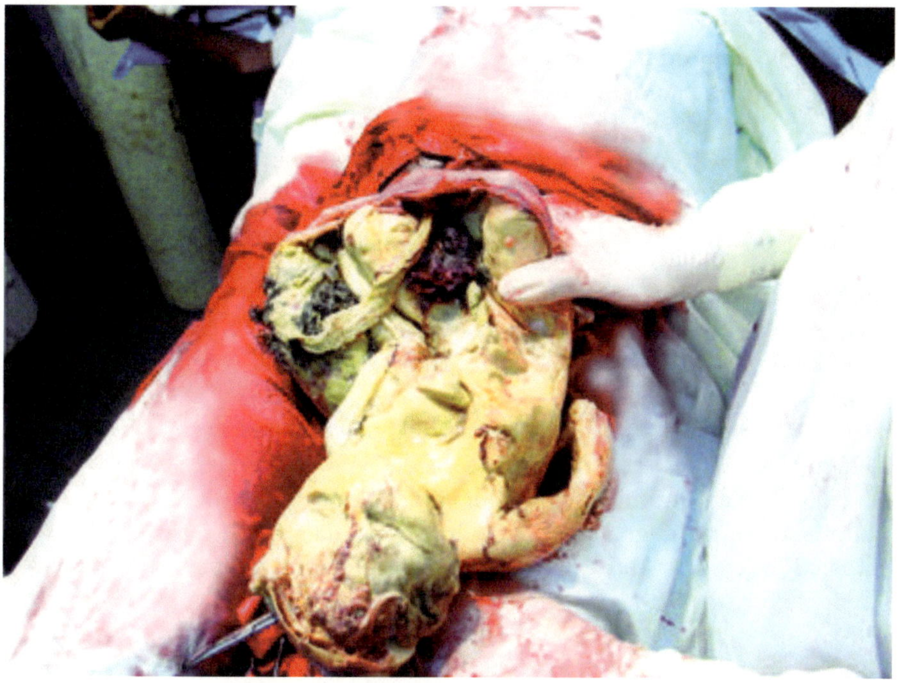

Fig. 4.2. Reatained term tubal pregnancy

5. References

Abdominal Pregnancy - References

[1] Roberts RV, Dickinson JE, Leung Y, et al. Advanced abdominal pregnancy: still an occurrence in modern medicine. Austral New Zealand J Obstet Gynaecol. 2005; 45: 518-521.

[2] Varma R, Mascrenhas L, James D. Successful outcome of advanced abdominal pregnancy with exclusive omental insertion. Ultrasound Obstet Gynecol 2003; 21: 192-194.

[3] Bouyer J, Coste J, Fernandez H et al. Sites of ectopic pregnancies: a 10 year population-based study of 1800 cases. Hum Reprod 2002;17: 3224-3230.

[4] Bertrand G, Le Ray C, Simard-Emond L, et al. Imaging in the management of abdominal pregnancy: a case report and review of the literature. J Obstet Gynaecol Can 2009;31(1): 57-62.

[5] Zeck W, Kelters I, Winter R, et al. Lessons learned from four advanced abdominal pregnancies at an East African Health Center. J Perinat Med 2007; 35: 278-281.

[6] Gerli S, Rosetti D, Baiocchi G, et al. Early ultrasonographic diagnosis and laparoscopic treatment of abdominal pregnancy. Eur J Obstet Gynaecol Reprod Biol 2004;113: 103-105.

[7] Ramachandran K, Kirk P. Massive haemorrhage in a previously undiagnosed abdominal pregnancy presenting for elective Cesarean delivery. Can J Anaesth 2004; 51(1): 57-61.

[8] Faller E, Kauffmann E, Chevriere S, et al. Full term abdominal pregnancy. J Gynecol, Obstet Biol Reprod 2006; 35(7): 732-735.
[9] Brasso K, Strom KV. Abdominal pregnancy with a living infant. Ugeskrift for Laeger. 1991; 153 (22): 1593-1594.
[10] Helmer JF, Perrier JF, Vedel M, et al. Hemorrhagic delivery in a full-term abdominal pregnancy with a live infant. Annales Francaises d'Anesthesie et de Reanimation 1986; 5(4):450-452.
[11] Crabtree KE, Collet B, Kilpatrick SJ. Puerperal presentation of a living abdominal pregnancy. Obstet Gynecol 1994; 84(4Pt2):646-648.
[12] Ludwig M, Kaisi M, Bauer O, et al. The forgotten child - a case of heterotopic, intra-abdominal and intrauterine pregnancy carried to term. Hum Reprod 1999; 14(5):1372-1374.
[13] Atrash HK, Friede A, Hogue CJR. Abdominal pregnancy in the United States. Frequency and maternal mortality. Obstet Gynecol 1987; 69: 333-337.
[14] Valenzano M, Nicoletti L, Odicino F, et al. Five-year follow-up of placental involution after abdominal pregnancy. J Clin Ultrasound 2003; 31: 39-43.
[15] Costa SD, Presley J, Bastert G. Advanced abdominal pregnancy. Obstet Gynecol Surv. 1991; 46(8): 515-525.
[16] Bajo JM, Garcia-Frutos A, Huertas MA. Sonographic follow-up of a placenta left in situ after delivery of the fetus in an abdominal pregnancy. Ultrasound Obstet Gynecol 1996; 7: 285-288.
[17] Martin JN, Sessums JK, Martin RW, et al. Abdominal pregnancy: Current concepts of management. Obstet Gynecol 1988; 71: 549-557.
[18] Rahaman J, Berkovitz R, Mitty H et al. Minimally invasive management of an advanced abdominal pregnancy. Obstet Gynecol 2004; 103: 1064-1068.
[19] Rahman MS, Al Suleiman SA, Rahman J et al. Advanced abdominal pregnancy - observation in 10 cases Obstet Gynecol 1982; 59: 366-372.

Term Cervical Pregnancy-References

[1] Chetty M, Elson J. Treating non-tubal ectopic pregnancy. Best Practice Research Clinical Obstetrics and Gynecology.2009; 23: 529-538.
[2] Paalman RJ, McElin TW. Cervical pregnancy. Am J Obstet Gynecol. 1959; 77: 1261-1270.
[3] David MP, Bergman A, Delighdish L. Cervico-isthmic pregnancy carried to term. Obstet Gynecol 1980; 56 : 247-252.
[4] Strobelt N, Locatelli A, Ratti M, et al. Cervico-isthmic pregnancy: A case report, critical reappraisal of the diagnostic criteria, and reassessment of the outcome. Acta Obstet Gynecol Scand 2001;80: 586-588.
[5] Jelsema RD, Zuidema L. First-trimester diagnosed cervico-isthmic pregnancy resulting in term delivery. Obstet Gynecol 1992; 80: 517-519.
[6] Honda T, Hasegawa M, Nakahori T, et al. Perinatal management of cervicoisthmic pregnancy. J Obstet Gynaecol Res. 2005; 31(4): 332-336.
[7] Avery DM, Wells MA, Harper DM. Cervico-isthmic corporeal pregnancy with delivery at term: a review of the literature with a case report. Obstet Gynecol Survey. 2009;64(9): 335-344.

[8] Kalakoutis GM, Lilford RJ. Cervical pregnancy ending in a live vaginal birth. Eur J Obstet Gynecol Reprod Biol 1985; 20: 319-323.
[9] Cohen I,Atras M, Siegal A, et al. Cervico-isthmic pregnancy ending with delivery of a liveborn infant in late second trimester. Eur J Obstet Gynecol Reprod Biol. 1985; 20:61-64.
[10] Hoffmann HMH, Urdl W, Hofler H, et al. Cervical pregnancy: case report and current concepts in diagnosis and treatment. Arch Gynecol Obstet 1987;241:63-69.
[11] Weyerman PC, Verhoeven AT, Alberda AT. Cervical pregnancy after in vitro fertilization and embryo transfer. Am J Obstet Gynecol 1989;161:1145-1146.
[12] Jelsema RD, Zuidema L. First-trimester diagnosed cervico-isthmic pregnancy resulting in term delivery. Obstet Gynecol. 1992;80: 517-519.
[13] Iloabachie GC, Igwegbe AQ, Izuora KL. Cervico-isthmic twin pregnancy carried to 37 weeks. Int J Gynaecol Obstet 1993;40: 59-61.
[14] Souter DJ, Roberts AB, Stables S. Cervico-isthmic pregnancy with placenta percreta ending in a livebirth. Aust NZ J Obstet Gynaecol 1995;35: 453-456.
[15] Mesogitis SA, Daskalakis GJ, Doublis DG, et al. Cervico-isthmic pregnancy: An extremely rare case diagnosed during labor. Eur J Obstet Gynecol Reprod Biol 2001; 98: 251-252.
[16] Kayem G, Deis S, Estrade S, et al. Conservative management of a near-term cervico-isthmic pregnancy followed by a successful subsequent pregnancy: a case report. Fert Steril 2008; 89(6): 1826.e13-1.
[17] Oyelese Y, Elliott TB, Asomani N, et al. Sonography and Magnetic Resonance Imaging in the diagnosis of cervico-isthmic pregnancy. J Ultrasound Med 2003;22: 981-983.
[18] Itakura A, Okamura M, Ohta T, et al. Conservative treatment of a second trimester cervicoisthmic pregnancy diagnosed by Magnetic Resonance Imaging. Obstet Gynecol 2003;101: 1149-1151.
[19] Ushakov FB, Elchalal U, Aceman PJ, et al. Cervical pregnancy: Past and Future. Obstet Gynecol Survey. 1996;52(1): 45-59.
[20] Qasim SM, Bohrer MK, Kemmann E. Recurrent cervical pregnancy after assisted reproduction by intrafallopian transfer. Obstet Gynecol 1996;87: 831-832.
[21] Radpour CJ, Keenan JA. Consecutive cervical pregnancies. Fert Steril 2004; 81(1): 210-213.

Term Tubal Pregnancy - References

[1] Waltz JH (1950) Term tubal pregnancy. A case report. North Carolina. Med J 11:634–637
[2] McElin TW, Randall LM (1951) Intratubal term pregnancy without rupture: review of the literature and presentation ofdiagnostic criteria. Am J Obstet Gynecol 61:130
[3] O'Connell CP (1952) Full-term tubal pregnancy. Am J Obstet Gynecol 63:1305–1311
[4] Frachtman KG (1953) Unruptured tubal term pregnancy. Am JSurg 85:161
[5] Gustafson GW, Bowman HE, Stout FE (1953) Extrauterine pregnancy at term. Obstet Gynecol 2:17
[6] Vaish R (1959) Term tubal pregnancy with survival of mother and infant. Am J Obstet Gynecol 77:1309–1311
[7] Kent JF (1963) Term tubal pregnancy. Aust NZ J Obstet Gynaecol 41:139–141

[8] Marais OA (1962) Full-term tubal pregnancy with retention of skeleton for ten months. S Afr Med J 36:327–328

[9] Schokman CM (1966) Advanced tubal pregnancy: a case of survival of mother and baby. Aust NZ J Obstet Gynaecol 6:171, 13

[10] Maas DA, Slabber CF (2007) Diagnosis and treatment of advanced extrauterine pregnancy. S Afr Med J 1975:49

[11] Augensen K (1983) Unruptured tubal pregnancy at term with survival of mother and child. Obstet Gynecol 61:259–260

[12] Al-Badawi IA, Tulandi Tugas (2010) Retained Term Tubal Ectopic Pregnancy. Gyneco Surgery

Part 4

Management of Ectopic Pregnancy

11

Clinical Treatment of Unruptured Ectopic Pregnancy

Julio Elito Junior
Obstetrics Department of the Federal University of São Paulo
Brazil

1. Introduction

Ectopic pregnancy is a major public health problem worldwide. The incidence of ectopic pregnancy (EP) has been increasing recently. Currently, approximately up to 2% of pregnancies are ectopic (CDC, 1995). It is a leading cause of mortality in the first trimester of pregnancy (Berger et al., 2003). Furthermore, it is an important cause of morbidity and a high percentage of these patients may become infertile. For all these reasons efforts should be made to perform an early diagnosis before the occurrence of rupture. However, there can be misdiagnosis because the clinical presentation of ectopic pregnancy can simulate a variety of other pelvic diseases. Therefore, the physician must keep a high index of suspicion. Diagnosis has improved with the evaluation of the levels of beta-human choriongonadotropin hormone (beta-hCG) and through transvaginal ultrasound. Consequently, ectopic pregnancies can often be diagnosed before the patient's condition has deteriorated, which has changed the former clinical picture of a life-threatening disease into a more benign condition in frequently asymptomatic patients. As a result, early detection through non-invasive diagnosis makes it possible to perform conservative treatment, such as expectant management or medical treatment with methotrexate (MTX).

Additionally, atypical localization of ectopic pregnancies is associated with greater morbidity. In these situations medical treatment with systemic MTX and in cases with embryonic cardiac activity treatment with direct injection of potassium chloride or MTX has been used effectively. Clinical treatment avoids surgeries such as hysterectomy that end up being required in great number of cases of unusual localization.

In this chapter, it will be discussed aspects related to the conservative treatment of ectopic pregnancy, mainly clinical treatment with expectant management and medical treatment of methotrexate. The chapter will point out features of the selection criteria, methotrexate protocols, predictive factors of success and reproductive future.

2. Expectant mangement

Ectopic pregnancy is associated with life-threatening risk and is considered to be a dangerous disease. Fear of tubal rupture caused by the uncertainty of this clinical situation induces gynecologists to take rapid decisions to solve the problem. However, knowledge of this disease has demonstrated that patients present a broad spectrum of symptoms. Thus, ectopic pregnancy does not always end in tubal rupture. In some cases, even without intervention ectopic pregnancies may progress to abortion from their tubal implantation with minimal bleeding or even be reabsorbed. The great challenge is to identify the cases in which intervention is unnecessary.

2.1 History

Lund (1955) was the first to describe expectant management in women with ectopic pregnancy. This retrospective study compared expectant management (119 cases) versus open surgery (85 patients). Women with a typical course of ectopic pregnancy and a positive pregnancy test without hemoperitoneum on admission formed the group of expectant management. These patients were hospitalized until the pregnancy test became negative and pain ceased, whereas the other group of women was operated. Surprisingly, expectant management was successful in 57% of women. In 20% an operation was carried out for signs of intra abdominal hemorrhage, while in 23% of women an operation was performed after a four weeks stay in the hospital with no signs of the disease becoming quiescent.

All subsequent studies of expectant management selected patients with unruptured ectopic pregnancy with declining titers of beta-hCG. In 1982, Mashiach et al. observed and treated a series of five cases with tubal pregnancy diagnosed by laparoscopy with serum beta-hCG concentrations $\leq$250 mIU/mL or decreasing, based on the knowledge that the natural course of many early ectopic pregnancies will result in tubal abortion or reabsorption. Expectant management was successful in four patients (80%).

Based on these works, some case series have been published describing expectant management in selected patients.

2.2 Inclusion criteria

As expectant management has been practiced based on the acknowledgement that the natural course of many early EPs is a self-limiting process. One important point is to select the best cases for this treatment.

The inclusion criteria for expectant management are: hemodynamically stable patients, beta-hCG $\leq$ 1500 mUI/ml, decline of the titers of beta-hCG in an interval of 24/48h, extraovarian adnexal mass $\leq$ 3.5cm without fetal cardiac activity (Table 1). The exclusion criteria are patients with a viable ectopic pregnancy, signs of tubal rupture and active intra abdominal bleeding. The main inclusion criterion is the decrease of the levels of beta-hCG in an interval of 24/48h, because it represents that the pregnancy is in regression (Elito et al., 2008).

The maximum value of beta-hCG to adopt this management is controversial. The majority of studies recommend the treatment when the titers of beta-hCG is equal or less than 1500 mIU/mL (Hajenius et al., 1995). However, others perform the observation with beta-hCG > 1500 mIU/mL (Lang et al., 1997). Elito and Camano (2006) demonstrated that the mean values of beta-hCG were 648.8 ± 754.7 mIU/ml in the expectant management compared to 2642.7 ± 2315.1 mIU/mL in the methotrexate treatment. Another interesting observation in this study is the period of amenorrhea that was longer in the expectant management group (8.87 ± 1.71 weeks) compared to the MTX treatment (6.81 ± 1.88 weeks). Therefore, women diagnosed with ectopic pregnancy may be categorized into two groups: those with an early diagnosis, and those with a late diagnosis. Early diagnosis is characterized by a shorter time since the last menstrual period, serum beta-hCG levels increasing or maintained over 24 and 48-hour intervals, higher beta-hCG levels, rapid growth, and higher probability of tubal rupture. For that reason, these cases require medical treatment with methotrexate or surgery. Late diagnosis is characterized by a longer time since the last menstrual period, beta-hCG levels decreasing over 24 and 48-hour intervals, lower beta-hCG levels, a latent prolonged clinical course, and lower chance of tubal rupture. Consequently, these cases require expectant management.

Expectant Management
Hemodynamically stable patients
Decline of the titers of beta-hCG < 15% in an interval of 24/48h
Beta-hCG < 1,500 mUI/ml
Extraovarian adnexal mass < 3.5 cm
Adnexal mass without embryonic cardiac activity
Desire of future fertility
Informed consent obtained

Table 1. Inclusion Criteria for Expectant Management (Elito et al, 2008)

2.3 Follow-up

Beta-hCG levels are followed up weekly to ensure that concentrations decline gradually until it becomes undetectable. Complete resolution of an ectopic pregnancy usually takes 20 days (range from 4 to 67 days). Kamrava et al. (1983) described that the serum clearance of beta-hCG may take at least up to 24 days after surgery. The same time necessary to complete resolution of an ectopic pregnancy managed expectantly. When declining beta-hCG levels rise again, there is a diagnosis of a persistent ectopic pregnancy. Success rates in several studies vary between 47.7% and 100% (van Mello et al., 2009) (Table 2). Transvaginal ultrasound is not required as a routine during the period of declining beta-hCG levels. However, patients with severe pain or pain that is prolonged should be evaluated by transvaginal ultrasound and hematocrit. Although the ultrasound findings are not helpful in the majority of patients, it can be use to reassure patient and physician that there ectopic pregnancy has not ruptured. It is important to realize that cul-de-sac fluid is very common, and the amount of fluid may increase if a tubal abortion occurs. For this reason, a surgical intervention is not necessary unless the patient has a typical clinical presentation of tubal rupture.
The period for the regression of the adnexal mass at ultrasound is approximately of 3 months. During this period patients are asked not to become pregnant. When the tubal mass is not recognized at ultrasound the patient should be submitted to hysterosalpingography.

Authors	Cases	Success
Ylostalo et al, 1992	83	57 (68.7%)
Korhonen et al, 1994	118	77 (65.3%)
Cacciatore et al, 1995	71	49 (69%)
Trio et al, 1995	67	49 (73.1%)
Shalev et al, 1995	60	28 (47.7%)
Lui et al, 1997	17	17 (100%)
Han et al, 1999	70	69 (98.6%)
Olofsson et al, 2001	17	14 (82.4%)
Elson et al, 2004	107	75 (70.1%)

Table 2. Results of Studies of Expectant Management for Tubal Pregnancy

2.4 Predictive factors of success

The most commonly identified predictors of success of expectant management are beta-hCG levels decreasing over 24 and 48-hour intervals, lower initial beta-hCG levels, absence of gestational sac at ultrasound and longer time since the last menstrual period (Han et al, 1999; Elito e Camano, 2006). The mean levels of beta-hCG in the cases with success of the expectant management was 374mUI/ml, however when there was a failure the mean value was of 741 mUI/ml. Élson et al. (2004) observed that the success rate of the expectant management was 88% when beta-hCG levels was less than 200 mUI/ml, on the other hand the failure occur in 75% of the cases with beta-hCG > 2000 mUI/ml. Whereas the prognosis for successful expectant management has been demonstrated repeatedly to correlate with the initial hCG level, no consensus on a threshold value that best predicts success or failure has been established.

2.5 Randomized trials

Only two randomized controlled trials have been published on expectant management for ectopic pregnancy (Egarter et al., 1991; Karhonen et al., 1996).

Egarter et al. (1991) compared expectant management and local and systemic prostaglandins including 23 women with an unruptured ectopic pregnancy and a serum beta-hCG concentration <2,500 mIU/ml. This trial shows that expectant management was significantly less successful than prostaglandin therapy (RR 0.12, 95% CI 0.02 to 0.81).

Karhonen et al. (1996) compared expectant management versus systemic methotrexate. In this double blind placebo controlled trial, expectant management was compared with oral methotrexate in a low dosage (2.5 mg/day during five days) in 60 hemodynamically stable women with a small tubal ectopic pregnancy (<4 cm) without fetal cardiac activity and a serum hCG concentration <5,000 mIU/ml. This study virtually represents a comparison between two placebo treatments as is demonstrated in similar success rates of 77% in both treatment groups (RR 1.0, 95% CI 0.76 to 1.3). The mean serum hCG concentrations were low, i.e., 211 mIU/ml (range 20 to 1,343 mIU/ml) in the expectant group and 395 mIU/ml (range 61 to 4,279 mIU/ml) in the methotrexate group.

An evaluation of expectant management for tubal ectopic pregnancy cannot be adequately made with these trials. Recently, there is a well-designed trial that will evaluate expectant management in the treatment of ectopic pregnancy. In a double blinded setting, single dose intramuscular methotrexate is compared with placebo in selected women with an ectopic pregnancy and a serum hCG concentration < 1500 mIU/ml. Therefore, nowadays the efficacy of expectant management for tubal ectopic pregnancy cannot be adequately evaluated (Hajenius et al., 2007).

2.6 Reproductive future

The fertility of women managed expectantly for an unruptured ectopic pregnancy can be determined by hysterosalpingography (HSG) or a spontaneous pregnancy (Rantala e Mäkinen, 1997; Debby et al., 2000). In spite of the inconveniences and interpretation doubts, HSG is considered a good examination to evaluate the tube patency (Gladstein et al., 1997).

Hysterosalpingography is an important diagnostic method after conservative treatment of an ectopic pregnancy (Mol et al., 1997). If HSG demonstrates tubal patency, there is a possibility of spontaneous pregnancy; and in cases revealing obstruction in both tubes; the treatment is fertilization *in vitro*. Hysterosalpingography usually is performed 3 months after expectant management, when the adnexal mass usually disappears on ultrasound examination.

Elito et al. (2005a) showed a patency rate of 78% in the ipsilateral tube in women managed expectantly, which was similar to the rates reported in other studies (Stovall et al., 1991; Debby et al., 2000). The patency rate of the contralateral tube was 92% in women managed expectantly, which is also similar to the rates in other reports (Stovall et al., 1991; Zohav et al., 1996; Mass et al., 1997).

When clinical treatment is chosen for unruptured ectopic pregnancy and tubal patency is evaluated via HSG, doubts arise: Could the tubal obstruction precede the ectopic pregnancy, or could it be a consequence of the treatment? To answer this question the obstruction of the contralateral tube has to be determined. Elito et al. (2005a) demonstrated that it occurred in 8% of the women managed expectantly. These results suggest that some of the women probably had an obstruction of the contralateral tube before the ectopic pregnancy, probably caused by salpingitis. The obstruction rate of the ipsilateral tube was 22% in the expectant management. Comparing these rates with those for contralateral tube obstruction (8%) shows that the difference between the obstruction rates for the ipsilateral and contralateral tubes could be a consequence of the tubal pregnancy treatment. Thus, the contralateral tube may give a picture of the tubal status previous to the tubal pregnancy. The difference between the obstruction rates of the ipsilateral and the contralateral tubes after clinical treatment may demonstrate which women experience tubal obstruction as a sequel of the nonsurgical treatment.

The spontaneous healing of EP should not harm the tube and should result in a good long-term fertility outcome. However, normal radiologic findings show nothing about tubal function, since a disturbance can also be a cause for ectopic pregnancy. On the other hand, if the HSG demonstrates obstruction of the tubes, these results reduce the possibility of a spontaneous pregnancy and the patients should be offered *in vitro* fertilization.

3. Medical treatment

3.1 Systemic treatment

Systemic methotrexate for the treatment of gestational trophoblastic disease has been used since 1956 (Li et al., 1956). MTX is a folic acid antagonist. Folic acid normally is reduced to tetrahydrofolate by the enzyme dihydrofolate reductase (DHFR), a step in the synthesis of DNA and RNA precursors. MTX inhibits DHFR, causing depletion of cofactors required for DNA and RNA synthesis. When multiple doses of MTX are used, side effects may occur, such as gastric distress, nausea, vomiting, ulcerative stomatitis, dizziness and some rare situations like severe neutropenia, reversible alopecia and pneumonitis. Folinic acid is an antagonist to MTX that can help reduce side effects, particularly when multiple doses of MTX are used (Barnhart et al., 2001). Long-term follow-up of cases treated with MTX for gestational trophoblastic disease shows no increase in congenital malformation or spontaneous abortions. Therefore, none would be expected after treatment of ectopic pregnancy because a smaller dose is required and shorter treatment duration is used.

3.1.1 History

At first, methotrexate was used for the treatment of placenta left in situ after laparotomy for an abdominal pregnancy. Tanaka et al. (1982) during a laparotomy identified an advanced but unruptured interstitial pregnancy in a young patient. The authors to avoid the surgery that could compromise the reproductive future opted for a medical treatment with multiple doses of intramuscular MTX. Since the beginning of the medical treatment of ectopic pregnancy, starting in 1982 with Tanaka et al., it has represented an important alternative for the treatment of ectopic pregnancy. Several authors have been studying this therapeutic treatment (Stovall et al., 1989; Elito et al., 1999a; Lipscomb et al., 2000). One important study to consider is that performed by Stovall et al. In 1989, it individualized the methotrexate dosage to improve patient compliance, to minimize side effects, and to reduce overall costs, which ultimately led to a single-dose regimen of 50 mg/m^2 body surface area intramuscular without folinic acid.

3.1.2 Selection criteria

Selection criteria for the systemic treatment with MTX are: hemodynamic stability, extraovarian adnexal mass $\leq$ 3.5cm, beta-hCG $\leq$ 5000 mUI/ml, no severe or persistent abdominal pain, commitment to follow-up until the ectopic pregnancy has resolved, and desire of future pregnancy (Table 3). The exclusion criteria are: intrauterine pregnancy, presence of free fluid in peritoneal cavity, adnexal mass with embryonic cardiac activity detected by transvaginal ultrasonography, decline of more than 15% in the levels of beta-hCG in an interval of 24 h prior to the treatment, hepatic dysfunction, blood dyscrasia, renal disease, evidence of immunodeficiency, sensitivity to MTX, active pulmonary or peptic ulcer disease and refusal to accept blood transfusion (Elito et al., 2008) (Table 4 and 5).

Prior to the treatment, women should be screened with a complete blood count, liver function tests, serum creatinine and blood type and Rh (prescribe Rhogam if patient is Rh negative). Patients having a history of pulmonary disease should also have a chest x-ray (ASRM Practice Committee, 2008).

- Hemodynamic stability
- Extraovarian adnexal mass < 3.5cm
- No severe or persistent abdominal pain
- Desire of future pregnancy
- Commitment to follow-up until the ectopic pregnancy has resolved
- Informed consent obtained

Table 3. Inclusion Criteria for Systemic Methotrexate (Elito et al, 2008; ASRM Practice Committee, 2008)

- Intrauterine pregnancy
- Evidence of immunodeficiency
- Moderate to severe anemia
- Leukopenia (Leukocytes < 2000 Cel/Mm3)
- Thrombocytopenia (Platelets < 100000)
- Sensitivity to Methotrexate
- Active pulmonary disease
- Active peptic ulcer disease
- Clinically important hepatic or renal dysfunction
- Breast feeding

Table 4. Absolute Contraindications for Systemic Methotrexate (Elito et al, 2008; ASRM Practice Committee, 2008)

- Embryonic cardiac activity detected by transvaginal ultrasonography
- High initial hCG concentration (>5,000mIU/mL)
- Decline of the titers of beta-hCG > 15% in an interval of 24/48h
- Refusal to accept blood transfusion
- Inability to participate in follow-up

Table 5. Relative Contraindications for Systemic Methotrexate (Elito et al, 2008; ASRM Practice Committee, 2008)

3.1.3 Methotrexate protocols (single and multiple doses)

There are two commonly used MTX treatment protocols: single dose and multiple doses (Barnhart, 2009). The single dose MTX treatment uses a $50mg/m^2$ intramuscular dose (Stovall et al., 1993; Elito et al., 1999a). Body surface area is calculated based in height and weight conformed Table 6. As a follow-up beta-hCG levels are tested on days 1, 4 and 7 after MTX injection. The protocol stipulated that any patient who did not have a 15% decline in the beta-hCG levels between days 4 and 7, should be given a second intramuscular dose of MTX ($50mg/m^2$) one week after the first dose. Patients with declining beta-hCG levels > 15% between days 4 and 7 were monitored weekly until the beta-hCG levels decreased below 5 mIU/ml. The term "single dose" is actually misleading. Whereas it describes the number of MTX injections planned, the treatment may include additional doses of MTX (maximum 3 doses) when the response is inadequate (Stovall et al., 1993; Barnhart, 2009).

Height cm / Weight kg	150	155	160	165	170	175	180
40	1,30	1.33	1.37	1.40	1.43	1.46	1.49
45	1.37	1.40	1.44	1.47	1.50	1.53	1.56
50	1.43	1.47	1.50	1.54	1.57	1.60	1.64
55	1.49	1.53	1.56	1.60	1.63	1.67	1.70
60	1.55	1.59	1.62	1.66	1.70	1.73	1.77
65	1.60	1,.64	1.68	1.72	1.75	1.79	1.83
70	1.65	1.69	1.73	1.77	1.81	1.85	1.89
75	1.70	1.74	1.78	1.82	1.86	1.90	1.94
80	1.75	1.79	1.83	1.87	1.92	1.96	2.00
85	1.80	1.84	1.88	1.92	1.97	2.01	2.05
90	1.84	1.88	1.93	1.97	2.01	2.06	2.10

Table 6. Calculation Body Surface Area ($\log BSA = 0.425 \log W + 0.725 \log H - 2.1436$) (Du Bois, Du Bois, 1916).

The multiple-dose protocol alternates 4 intramuscular doses of MTX (1mg/kg) with 4 intramuscular doses of leucovorin (0,1 mg/kg). The patients are followed up with beta-hCG levels in the day of MTX injection. MTX is continued until beta-hCG falls by 15% from its peak concentration. Approximately 50% of patients will not require the full 8-day regimen (Pisarka et al., 1998). A meta-analysis of nonrandomized studies showed success rates of 93% for multiple-dose treatment and 88% for single-dose therapy (Barnhart et al., 2003). The odds ratio for failure of single-dose therapy as compared with multiple-dose therapy was

2.0 after adjustment for the beta-hCG value and 4.8 after adjustment for the presence of fetal cardiac activity. As compared with the multiple-dose treatment, the single-dose protocol is more simple, commonly used, requires fewer visits and has fewer side effects. For all this reasons it should be the first option in cases of tubal pregnancy with levels of beta-hCG less than 5000 mIU/mL (Elito et al, 1999a). On the other hand, in cases of non-tubal pregnancy with high levels of beta-hCG more than 5000 mIU/mL, the best choice is the protocol of multiple-dose of MTX.

Recently, an alternative protocol of MTX was described. In this protocol women received 2 doses of methotrexate 50mg/m^2 IM (Barnhart et al., 2007). The initial day of treatment was designated day 0. Patient returned on day 4 and received the second dose of MTX, and the beta-hCG level was measured. On day 7, the beta-hCG level was measured and compared with the level on day 4. If there was a decline of at least 15%, the treatment was considered successful. These patients were monitored weekly until the beta-hCG levels decreased below 5 mIU/ml. The protocol stipulated that any case who did not have a 15% decline in the beta-hCG levels between days 4 and 7, should be given a third intramuscular dose of MTX (50mg/m^2) on day 7. Patients then returned on day 11 for another beta-hCG measurement. If the beta-hCG level declined by at least 15% between day 7 and 11, the treatment was deemed successful and weekly beta-hCG levels were verified until the results were negative. If not, a fourth dose of MTX was administered, and a beta-hCG level was checked on day 14. If the beta-hCG titers declined at least 15% between days 11 and 14, the treatment was considered successful. Otherwise, the patient was referred for surgical treatment. The two-dose regimen was designed to increase the likelihood of successful therapy without more visits than are required with a single-dose regimen, but it has not been directly compared with the other regimens. One important consideration is that two-dose protocol should be indicated in cases with increase beta-hCG levels on day 4 after MTX.

When the criteria for MTX treatment are fulfilled, treatment success rates are comparable to those achieved with conservative surgery (Hajenius et al., 1997). Numerous open-label studies have been published demonstrating the efficacy of MTX protocols. One review concluded that MTX treatment was successful in 78%-96% of selected patients (Lipscomb et al., 2000).

3.1.4 Follow-up

Patients with declining beta-hCG levels after MTX protocols (single or multiple-dose) are monitored weekly until the beta-hCG levels are negative. Elito et al. (1998) evaluated the interval of time for beta-hCG levels to become negative. It took 15 days in 50% of the cases, 15 to 30 days in 38.8% and more than 30 days in 11.2% of the cases. Complete resolution of an ectopic pregnancy usually takes between 2 and 3 weeks but can take as long as 6 to 8 weeks when pre-treatment beta-hCG levels are in higher ranges (Elito et al, 1999a; Pisarka et al, 1998; Barnhart et al, 2003). When declining beta-hCG levels rise again, the diagnosis of a persistent trophoblastic tissue is made. Another important consideration is that the period for the regression of the tubal mass at ultrasound range from 3 to 6 months (Brown et al., 1991). Elito et al. (1996) evaluated the period necessary for the complete resolution of the tubal mass at ultrasound and observed that it took more than 30 days in 62.5% of the cases. Therefore, serial ultrasonographic examinations after MTX treatment are unnecessary because ultrasonographic findings cannot demonstrate or predict treatment failure, unless evidence of recent tubal rupture is observed (Atri et al., 1992).

Although several treatment protocols have been developed, it is prudent to inform the patient some instructions for the follow-up after the systemic treatment with MTX. Patients should avoid: sexual intercourse until beta-hCG levels is negative, sun exposition to minimize the risk of dermatitis after MTX, alcohol use, nonsteroidal antiinflammatory drugs (in cases of pain prescribe acetaminophen), foods and multivitamins containing folic acid, become pregnant for at least 3 months (risk of teratogenicity).

MTX is a safe treatment for an unruptured ectopic pregnancy. Life-threatening complications rarely have been reported with MTX (Isaacs et al., 1996). Approximately 40% of the patients feel pain between 3 and 7 days after MTX injection, but such pain normally resolves within 4 to 12 hours (Lipscomb et al., 1999). In cases of acute pain, it is important to rule out tubal rupture. Therefore, it is prudent to evaluate the patient's vital signs and hematocrit, and if rupture is suspected, surgery should be performed.

Signs of treatment failure or suspected rupture are indications to abandon medical treatment and to proceed with surgical treatment. Signs suggesting treatment failure or possible rupture include hemodynamic instability; increasing abdominal pain, regardless of trends in beta-hCG levels; and rapidly increasing beta-hCG concentrations after methotrexate treatment (ASRM Practice Committee, 2008).

More commonly encountered treatment effects of MTX are increase in abdominal girth, increase in beta-hCG during initial therapy, vaginal bleeding or spotting and abdominal pain. The commonly side effects encountered are gastric distress, nausea and vomiting, stomatitis, dizziness, and other rare conditions such as severe neutropenia, reversible alopecia and pneumonitis (ASRM Practice Committee, 2008).

Sexual intercourse is allowed when the beta-hCG titer is negative. At this moment, patients are instructed to begin contraceptive methods until the regression of the adnexal mass at ultrasound. Patients are asked not to become pregnant for at least 3 months following the completion of treatment so that a hysterosalpingography can be performed.

3.1.5 Predictive factors of success

Although the failure of the treatment is not very high, when the tubal rupture occurs after a few days, a doubt arises: Would it not been better to perform a conservative surgery at the moment of the early diagnosis? To reduce the failure of the treatment several authors studied the predictive factors for the success of MTX treatment. Initial level of beta-hCG is one of the most important variables in the prediction of therapeutic response to MTX in patients with an ectopic pregnancy. The evolution of ectopic pregnancy depends on the degree of trophoblast invasion. Intense trophoblastic activity is more frequently associated with tubal rupture, while lesser activity is associated with a lower capacity of invasion and a greater likelihood of success with MTX treatment. The invasion of the trophoblastic tissue in patients with an ectopic pregnancy may be calculated from their serum beta-hCG level. In studies carried out in fallopian tubes affected by ectopic pregnancy, Natale et al. (2003) used histopathology to demonstrate that the concentration of beta-hCG was proportional to the degree of invasion of the tubal wall. Therefore, the higher is the beta-hCG level, the greater is the invasion of the trophoblast and the lesser the likelihood of therapeutic success with MTX (Menon et al., 2007). If the beta-hCG level is low, then the likelihood of therapeutic success is high; however, if beta-hCG is high, surgery would be preferable. Lipscomb et al. (1999) noted that the failure rate of single-dose treatment was 13% (6/45) for initial beta-hCG values between 5,000 IU/L and 9,999 IU/L, 18% (4/22) for concentrations between

10,000 IU/L and 14,999 IU/L, and 32% (7/22) when beta-hCG values exceeded 15,000 IU/L. Elito et al. (1999) have reported failure rates of 62% when the initial beta-hCG concentration is over 5,000 IU/L. Systematic review combining all published data yields an odds ratio for failure of 5.45 (95% CI, 3.04–9.78) when the initial beta-hCG value above 5,000 IU/L compared with that observed when beta-hCG concentrations are below that threshold (Menon et al., 2007). Because the failure rate rises with the pre-treatment beta-hCG concentration, the single-dose MTX treatment regimen may be better reserved for patients with a relatively low initial beta-hCG level (Elito et al., 1999a; Barnhart et al., 2003; Potter et al., 2003).

Attempting to improve the selection of patients for the medical treatment with MTX and reduce the likelihood of therapeutic failure, some authors evaluated an additional predictive variable: the increment in beta-hCG levels in the 48-h interval prior to administration of MTX (Dudley et al., 2004; da Costa Soares et al., 2008). The hypothesis is that the increase in beta-hCG levels in the 48-h period prior to treatment would represent a dynamic assessment of the degree of evolution of the ectopic trophoblastic tissue and, consequently, of its invasion and its probable response to treatment. Moreover, this variable is easily obtainable. Da Costa Soares et al. (2008) demonstrated that the average increment in beta-hCG levels in the 48-h period prior to treatment was greater in the patients with therapy failure when compared to the cases of therapeutic success (36.28 vs. 13.15%, respectively). One important point to consider is that when initial beta-hCG level is low but its increment in the 48-h period is high, this is indicative of an ectopic trophoblastic tissue with a high degree of invasion, and the risk of tubal rupture is high so surgical treatment is preferable. Furthermore, when beta-hCG is elevated, this parameter alone is sufficient to serve as a guideline for treatment, with good sensitivity and specificity. Nevertheless, in cases of early diagnosis (the ideal situation for non-surgical treatment), baseline beta-hCG is generally low and in this situation the increment in beta-hCG values in the 48-h period prior to treatment is of great importance, since depending on the evolution of beta-hCG, the predicted response to nonsurgical treatment may be better assessed, leading to increased specificity and sensibility with respect to the success of treatment. Dudley et al. (2004) reported that the increase in beta-hCG prior to diagnosis and the increase in beta-hCG following MTX therapy were more accurate predictors of tubal rupture than beta-hCG on the day of MTX therapy. These results suggest that the changes in beta-hCG prior to and following MTX administration represent independent risk factors for subsequent tubal rupture.

Another important consideration is the aspect of the image at ultrasound (hematosalpinx, tubal ring and live embryo) (Figure 1 and 2). Elito et al. (1999a) observed better results with hematosalpinx image and worse results with live embryo. Several authors considered relative contraindications for systemic treatment with MTX the presence of embryonic cardiac activity detected by transvaginal ultrasonography (Lipscomb et al., 1999; Tawfiq et al., 2000).

Other variables that may be predictive of therapeutic response to MTX in cases of ectopic pregnancy are: size and volume of the gestational mass ($\leq$ 3.5 cm), absence of free peritoneal blood an endometrial thickness (<7mm) (Elito et al., 1999a; Soares et al., 2004; da Costa Soares et al., 2008).

Therefore, factors that are associated with failure of medical management include initial beta-hCG values greater than 5000 mIU/mL, ultrasonographic detection of a moderate or large amount of free peritoneal fluid, the presence of embryonic cardiac activity, and a pretreatment increase in the serum hCG level of more than 50% over a 48-hour period (ASRM Practice Committee, 2008).

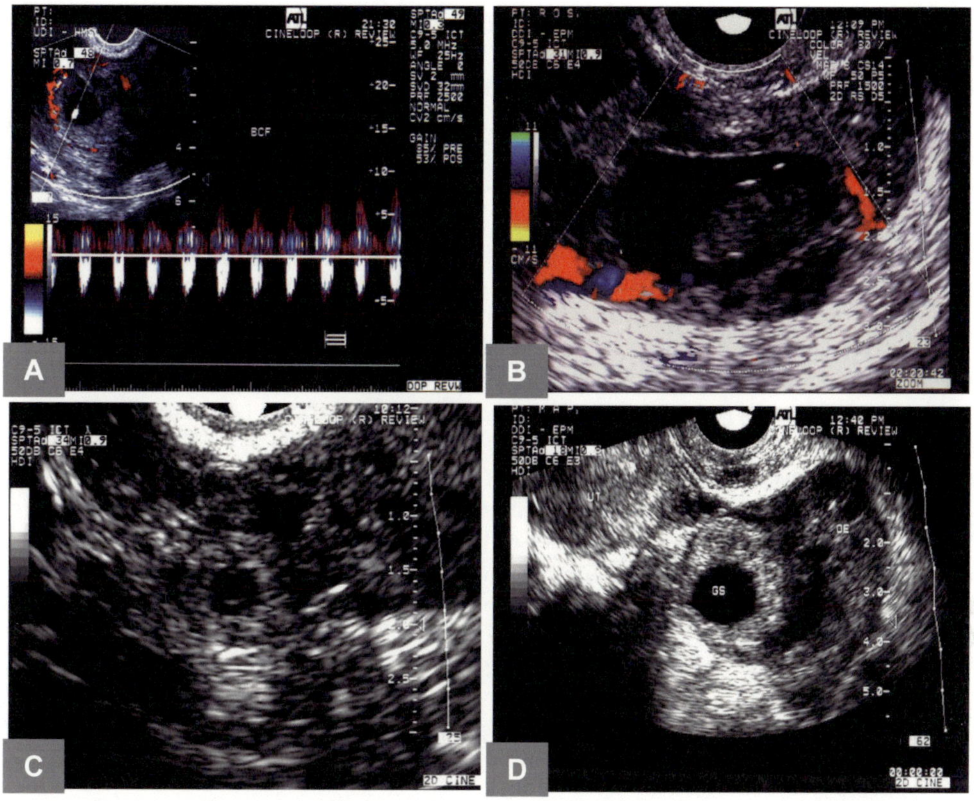

Fig. 1. Ultrasound of ectopic pregnancy with tubal ring: A) extra-uterine gestational sac with live embryo. B) gestational sac with absence of embryonic cardiac activity. C) gestational sac with yolk sac. D) gestational sac without yolk sac or fetal pole (Elito, Camano, 2010a).

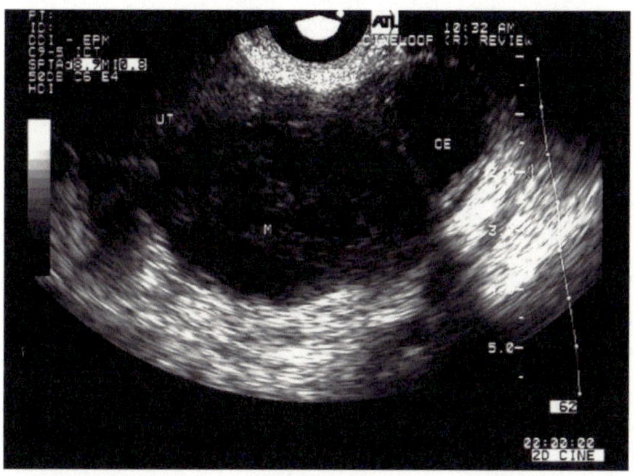

Fig. 2. Ultrasound of tubal pregnancy with hematosalpinx (Elito, Camano, 2010a).

3.1.6 Reproductive future

The fertility outcome of patients treated conservatively with MTX for unruptured EP can be evaluated by means of hysterosalpingography (HSG) or future pregnancy (Debby et al.,

2000). Elito et al. (2005b) showed that 84% of the diseased tubes were pervious after MTX treatment for ectopic pregnancy by HSG, similar to the rates in other reports that demonstrated post-treatment hysterosalpingography documented tubal patency in 78% of cases (Lipscomb et al., 2000; Stovall et al., 1991). This high rate of radiologically normal tubes after clinical treatment proves that the spontaneous regression of EP does not result in an increased harm or damage to the tube - i.e. the risk of repeating EP is rather low. However, the radiologically normal findings show nothing about the tubal function, when a disturbance can also be a cause of EP. On the other hand, if the results of HSG demonstrate obstruction of the tubes, the possibility of a spontaneous pregnancy will be reduced and should be treated with *in vitro* fertilization. Elito et al. (2005b) showed that beta-hCG levels were directly related to the obstruction of the tube. The increase in beta-hCG levels was followed by an enhancement in tubal obstruction risk. The explanation for these events is probably that in patients with high level of beta-hCG there is more invasion of the trophoblast tissue at the serosa of the tube, which increases damage to the tube.

The parameter considered most important for MTX treatment of unruptured EP is beta-hCG. Several authors have demonstrated its importance (Elito et al., 1999a; Lipscomb et al., 1999) and shown that the higher the level of beta-hCG, the lower the chances of successful treatment. Patients with indication for clinical treatment of EP usually have an important desire for future pregnancy. It is important to have a parameter, such as the levels of beta-hCG, in order to predict the tube sequel.

Lipscomb et al. (2000) demonstrated that 65% of patients who attempted subsequent pregnancies succeeded, and the incidence of recurrent ectopic pregnancy was a relatively low 13% (Stovall et al., 1989; Lipscomb et al., 2000).

3.2 Local treatment

Methotrexate can be administered locally in the tube. Efforts to attain maximal efficacy and minimize adverse effects of systemic MTX resulted in various protocols for local medical treatment administered into the gestational sac transvaginally under sonographic or under laparoscopic guidance. Drugs that have been used for local treatment are methotrexate 1mg/kg (Feichtinger, Kemeter, 1987; Pansky, Bubowski, 1989; Fernandez et al., 1993), KCL, prostaglandins, and hyperosmolar glucose.

3.2.1 History

Feichtinger and Kemeter (1987) described the first case where local treatment with MTX was administered into the gestational sac transvaginally under sonographic. The authors used the same technique used for retrieval of the oocytes from the ovary using a transvaginal technique involving an ultrasound-guided needle utilized for in vitro fertilization. The gestational sac of the tubal pregnancy was puncture and injected 10 mg of MTX. The case was treated successful and without side effects.

In 1989, Panski et al. presented another via to puncture the tubal pregnancy by laparoscopy. The gestational sac of 27 patients was punctured and injected 12,5 mg of MTX. The success rate was 88,9%, there are no side effects and tubal patency was 90.5%.

3.2.2 Selection criteria

Local treatment is indicated in ectopic pregnancies with embryonic heart activity, especially in cases of non-tubal ectopic pregnancies (Elito et al., 2008). One important point to consider is that in cases of ectopic pregnancy with absence of embryonic cardiac activity, there is no reason to submit the patient to ultrasound-guided injection. In these cases the systemic treatment with MTX is considered to be the best choice. Although local injection appears to be relatively safe and as effective as systemic methotrexate, this approach requires an additional procedure and a certain degree of expertise and added cost. A further consideration is that the appropriate dose of local MTX is yet to be determined. Several doses of MTX have been described (Benifla et al., 1996; Sagiv et al., 2001; Lin et al., 2007). The most used is a dose of 1 mg/kg body weight and this is the dose selected for the study (Fernandez et al., 1993)). However, other doses including 100 mg single dose (Lin et al., 2007), 50mg/m^2 body surface (Lim et al., 2007) and an unadjusted dose of 12.5 mg have been used (Sagiv et al., 2001). Transvaginal ultrasound is the preferred mode for guidance and laparoscopic guidance has a limited role. The procedures were carried out under general anesthesia. The patient was placed in the lithotomy position. Methotrexate was injected under transvaginal ultrasound guidance, a 22-gauge, 15 cm Wallace needle was inserted via vaginal route into the embryonic heart and 1 ml (2 mEq/ml) KCL solution was injected. Following the cessation of embryonic cardiac activity, the tip of the needle was directed into the gestational sac and some amniotic fluid was aspirated. Then, a 1 mg/kg dose of MTX was injected into the gestational sac. The transvaginal administration of methotrexate under sonographic guidance requires visualization of an ectopic gestational sac and specific skills and expertise of the physician. Compared to the local treatment, systemic methotrexate is practical, easier to be administered, and less dependent from clinical skills. In combination with non-invasive diagnosis, systemic methotrexate offers the option of a totally non-invasive outpatient management. Therefore, the local treatment is restricted to the cases of non-tubal ectopic pregnancy with live embryo (Chetty et al., 2009).

3.2.3 Follow-up

Patients are followed up with beta-hCG levels on days 4 and 7 after MTX injection. The protocol stipulates that any patient, who did not have a 15% decline in the beta-hCG levels between days 4 and 7, would be given an intramuscular dose of MTX (50 mg/m^2). In cases of ectopic pregnancy with high levels of beta-hCG the use of only ultrasound-guided injection seems to be less effective and the combination of systemic treatment of MTX could improve the results. On the other hand, patients who present a decline of more than 15% in the beta-hCG levels in this period are monitored weekly until the beta-hCG levels are below 5 mUI/ml. Follow up also includes clinics visits and repetition of transvaginal ultrasound if necessary. After approximately 3 months of treatment when the ectopic pregnancy disappeared at transvaginal ultrasound, a hysterosalpingography is performed.

4. Atypical ectopic pregnancies

The main localizations of atypical ectopic pregnancies are: cervical, caesarean scar, ovarian, interstitial, cornual and abdominal. This group represents less than 10% of all ectopic pregnancies but is associated with greater morbidity (Jourdain et al., 2003). Traditionally these pregnancies have been lately diagnosed and managed by open surgery. Advances in ultrasound technology have led to an increase in the early diagnosis of non-tubal ectopic pregnancies. This means that management of these rare cases of ectopic pregnancy has now progressed from open surgical management to the use of minimally invasive access techniques and the exploration of medical and conservative treatments either alone or as adjuvant therapies.

4.1 Interstitial pregnancy

Interstitial pregnancy is an ectopic pregnancy that implanted in the interstitial portion of the fallopian tube. The interstitial portion is constricted, with its lumen being as narrow as 0.1mm to 0.7 mm in diameter and 1-2 cm in length, this relatively thick section of the tube has a significantly greater capacity to expand before rupture than do the distal tubal segments (Eddy, Pauerstein, 1980). For this reason, in some cases the interstitial pregnancy may remain asymptomatic until 7-16 weeks of gestation, at which time rupture can result in important hemorrhage (Lau, Tulandi, 1999). Because of the rich vascular anastomosis of the uterine and the ovarian arteries in this region there can be accentuated hemorrhage. Therefore, early diagnosis is essential to reduce morbidity and mortality.

Interstitial pregnancies are an uncommon form of ectopic pregnancy, account for only 2-4% of tubal pregnancies or approximately 1 in 2500-5000 live births (Damario et al., 2003). Despite their rarity, the mortality rate is as high as 2.5%, a rate that is 7 times greater than that of ectopic pregnancies in general (Walker, 2007). This is because the difficult diagnose that often presents late with rupture and hemorrhage.

Interstitial pregnancy sometimes is incorrectly confused with cornual and angular pregnancies. It is important to make a distinction among these conditions because their behavior, management, and outcomes are different. In contrast to interstitial pregnancy, an angular pregnancy refers to a viable intra-uterine pregnancy that is implanted in one of the lateral angles of the uterine cavity, medial to the uterotubal junction. During laparoscopy, angular pregnancy appears as an asymmetric protuberance in one of the uterine angles, medial to the round ligament. On the other hand, interstitial pregnancy appears lateral to the round ligament.

Cornual pregnancy refers to a pregnancy in a horn of a bicornuate uterus. The clinical outcome of cornual pregnancy varies greatly, depending on the size and expansile nature of the affected horn.

Traditional treatments for interstitial ectopic pregnancy have ranged from exploratory laparotomy with cornual wedge resection to total abdominal hysterectomy. However, the development of high-resolution ultrasound evaluation and rapid quantitative beta-hCG exams has advanced the detection of interstitial gestations before rupture, which, in turn, has made possible more conservative treatment options for the patient whose condition is hemodynamically stable. Risk factors for interstitial pregnancy are tubal damage from previous ectopic pregnancy, previous ipsilateral or bilateral salpingectomy, conception after *in vitro* fertilization, and history of sexually transmitted disease (Tulandi, Al-Jaroudi, 2004). The most common symptoms of interstitial pregnancy are abdominal pain and vaginal bleeding in the first trimester of pregnancy. On physical examination, an asymmetric uterine enlargement may be palpable. Signs of acute abdomen may be elicited in cases of cornual rupture and hemoperitoneum; in severe cases, tachycardia and subsequent hypotension may be evident. Early diagnoses of interstitial pregnancies are often discovered in asymptomatic patients during transvaginal ultrasound that is performed in the first trimester. Ultrasonographic criteria for diagnosis is an empty uterine cavity, an eccentricity of the gestational sac, a chorionic sac separate and at least 1 cm from the lateral edge of the uterine cavity, and a presence of a myometrial tissue that surrounds the gestational sac with a thickness of □5 mm (Timor-Tritsch et al., 1992; Ackerman et al., 1993) (figure 3).

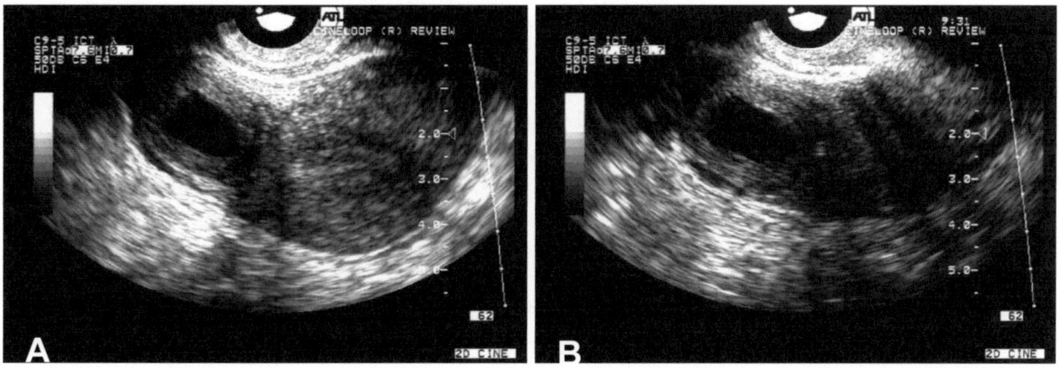

A) Transversely oriented transvaginal ultrasound. B) Longitudinally oriented transvaginal ultrasound.

Fig. 3. Interstitial ectopic pregnancy: presence of an eccentric gestational sac with myometrial tissue that surrounds the gestational sac with a thickness of 2 mm (Elito, Camano, 2010).

Despite the advent of conservative strategies, the most appropriate technique for treatment of interstitial pregnancy and treatment of these patients during subsequent pregnancies remains controversial. Treatment options depend on the extent of uterine wall trauma, whether rupture has occurred and the patient's desire for future pregnancy. If the diagnosis is made before rupture, minimally invasive surgery and nonsurgical treatment options can be used. Conservative options include methotrexate administration (local and systemic), expectant management and minimally invasive surgical techniques that include resection of the involved tube and pregnancy alone with preservation of the uterine architecture. The potential advantage of clinical treatment is to avoid a surgical scar on the uterus and the risks that are associated with surgery.

Expectant management that has been practiced based on the natural course of many early EPs is a self-limiting process (Zalel et al., 1994). The inclusion criteria for this management are hemodynamically stable patients, beta-hCG $\leq$ 1500 mUI/ml, decline of the titers of beta-hCG in an interval of 24/48h, small interstitial pregnancy mass without fetal cardiac activity. The most important disadvantage of expectant management is the risk of rupture and associated maternal morbidity and death.

Systemic methotrexate treatment was used for the first time in an interstitial pregnancy. In 1982, Tanaka et al. treated successfully an interstitial pregnancy with multiple dose of methotrexate. Ectopic interstitial pregnancies without embryonic cardiac activity and beta-hCG $\leq$ 5000 mUI/ml should be treated with single dose of MTX 50 mg/m^2 IM. Cases with beta-hCG > 5000 mUI/ml should be treated with multiple doses of MTX. On the other hand, cases with embryonic heart activity should be treated with transvaginal administration of MTX and KCL under sonographic guidance. The major risk for patients after treatment of interstitial pregnancy is uterine rupture during subsequent pregnancy and the risk of recurrent interstitial pregnancy. Careful prenatal with a planned cesarean delivery at term appears to be the safest approach (Moawad et al., 2010).

4.2 Cervical pregnancy

Cervical pregnancy is an atypical localization and represents less than 1% of all ectopic pregnancies (Pisarka, Carson, 1999). It is a high-risk condition because of the possibility of

severe hemorrhage. Baptiste (1953) said: "The great majority of certified obstetricians will never see a cervical pregnancy. The minority who do happen to encounter this complication will probably wish they had not".
The endocervix is eroded by the trophoblast that invade the fibrous cervical wall. If the trophoblast invasion is severe, the greater is the risk of hemorrhage.
Some pre-disposing factors for cervical implantation described in the literature are previous abortion, uterine curettage, previous cesarean section, uterine fibroids, use of intrauterine devices and assisted reproduction with embryo transfer (Pisarka, Carson, 1999; Hsieh et al., 2004).
The diagnosis is based on the history of vaginal bleeding after a period of amenorrhea and physical exam demonstrating a cervical enlargement with vascular congestion and a thin-walled cervix with a partially dilated external os (Figure 4).

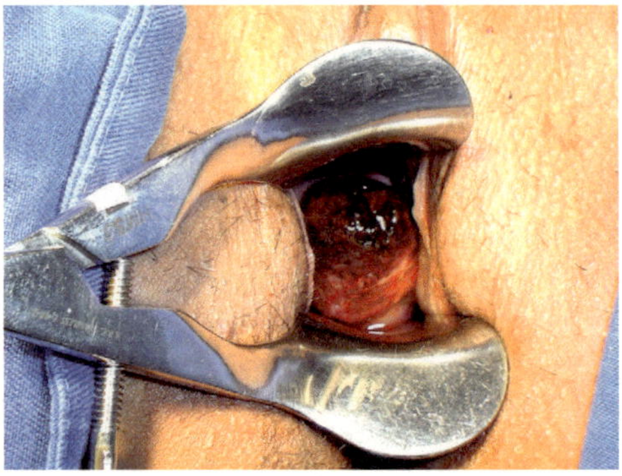

Fig. 4. Physical exam demonstrating a cervical enlargement with vascular congestion (Elito, Camano, 2010a).

The confirmation is made by ultrasound showing an empty uterine cavity and a gestational sac below the level of a closed internal os within the cervix (Dialani, Levine, 2004). The main ultrasonographic criteria for cervical pregnancy are: empty uterine cavity or the presence of a pseudo gestational sac, decidual transformation of the endometrium with dense echo structure, diffuse uterine wall structure, hourglass uterine shape, ballooned cervical canal, gestational sac in the endocervix, placental tissue in the cervical canal and closed internal os (Hofmann et al., 1987) (figure 5).
The classical treatment for cervical pregnancy is the hysterectomy. This modality of treatment compromises the reproductive future of the patient and is associated with significant morbidity. This procedure has a high risk of hemorrhage and trauma of the urinary tract because the enlargement of the cervix. The vaginal bleeding can be also treated with conservative surgical management such as curettage, local haemostatic sutures, intracervical balloon tamponade and arterial embolization (De La Veja et al., 2007; Xu et al., 2007). However, the majority of conservative surgical treatments are ineffective and lead to a hysterectomy.
The early diagnosis in asymptomatic cases has made a more conservative management of cervical pregnancy feasible. Medical treatment especially with methotrexate (MTX) can be administered systemically or locally with ultrasound guidance (Monteagudo et al., 2005; Mesogitis et al., 2005). The presence of embryonic heart activity is a relative contraindication for the systemic treatment with MTX. The predictive factors for failure in the systemic MTX

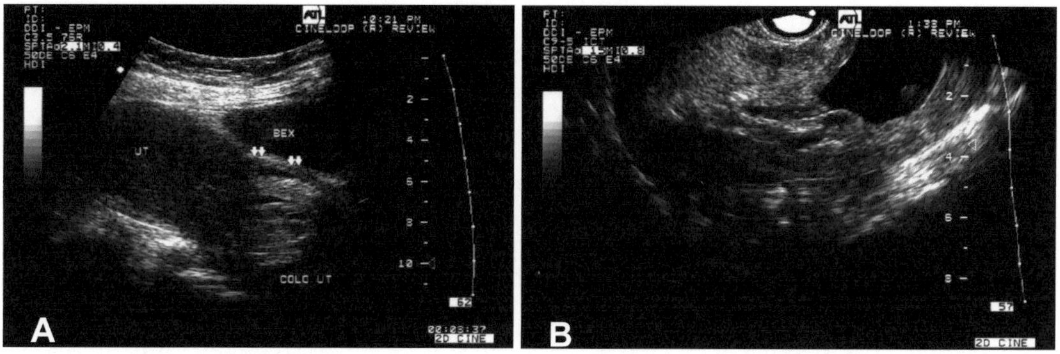

Fig. 5. A) Longitudinally oriented transabdominal ultrasound of cervical pregnancy showing an empty uterine cavity, hourglass uterine shape, placental tissue in the cervical canal and closed internal os. B) Longitudinally oriented transvaginal ultrasound showing an empty uterine cavity, hourglass uterine shape, gestational sac in the endocervix and closed internal os (Elito et al., 1999b).

treatment of cervical pregnancy were described as being gestational age > 9 weeks, beta-hCG levels > 10,000 mIU/ml, crown-rump length >10 mm, and embryonic cardiac activity (Bai et al., 2002). These situations have been shown to be associated with a higher risk of primary failure of treatment of cervical ectopic pregnancy with systemic methotrexate and combination therapy with intra-amniotic injection seemed to increase the chance of successful treatment.

For this reason in cases with live embryo the preferable therapeutic is the ultrasound-guided local injection of MTX and potassium chloride (Jeng et al., 2007). KCl is injected under transvaginal ultrasound guidance into the embryonic heart. Following the cessation of fetal cardiac activity, the tip of the needle is directed into the gestational sac and gestational tissues and some amniotic fluid was aspirated. Then, a 1 mg/kg dose of MTX is injected into the gestational sac. Patients are followed up with beta-hCG levels on days 4 and 7 after MTX injection. The protocol stipulated that any patient who does not have a 15% decline in the beta-hCG levels between days 4 and 7, would be given an intramuscular dose of MTX (50 mg/m^2). On the other hand, patients who present a decline of more than 15% in the beta-hCG levels in this period are monitored weekly until the beta-hCG levels are below 5 mUI/ml. Follow up also include clinics visits and repeated transvaginal ultrasound if necessary. After approximately 3 months of treatment when the cervical pregnancy at transvaginal ultrasound disappears, a hysterosalpingography is performed.

A total of 15 patients with cervical pregnancy were referred to our institution. Embryonic heart activity was detectable in 7 cases (46,7%), which were treated with ultrasound-guided injection. The assessment of the demographic characteristics of these patients demonstrated that 4 patients had a history of previous abortion with uterine curettage and the other 3 cases had a previous cesarean section. The gestational age ranged from 8 to 11 weeks and the initial beta-hCG levels ranged from 3013 to 71199 mUI/ml. In 3 cases the titers of beta-hCG had not declined 15% between days 4 and 7 after MTX and the patient received a single intramuscular dose of MTX (50 mg/m2). All patients evolved with clinical success and in none of the cases hysterectomy or any further intervention were required. None of cases needed blood transfusion. In our series in only one case there was a complication. The patient evolved after 7 days of the treatment with fever and the cervical examination demonstrated purulent secretion. The patient was hospitalized and received intravenous antibiotics. She recovered without the necessity of any further intervention. Another case submitted to local and systemic MTX presented with stomatitis, a minor side effect of MTX. The interval of time for the levels of beta-hCG to become negative ranged from 2 to 12 weeks. The period for the regression of the cervical pregnancy at ultrasound ranged from 3 to 14 weeks. Two patients of our series had an intrauterine pregnancy after the treatment. One patient had placenta previa and was submitted to a cesarean section at 37 weeks. The other case evaluated to a vaginal delivery at 39 weeks (Elito et al., 1999b).

4.3 Cesarean scar pregnancy

Implantation of a pregnancy within a cesarean scar is an uncommon form of ectopic pregnancy and constitutes a life-threatening condition (Fylstra et al., 2002). A cesarean scar pregnancy is considered to be more aggressive than placenta accreta because of its early invasion of the myometrium in the first trimester and the risk for uterine rupture (Seow et al., 2000). Rotas et al. (2006) and Ash et al. (2007) describe an increasing incidence of cesarean scar pregnancies of about 1:2000 pregnancies. This is likely to increase, as does the cesarean delivery rate. Its true incidence, however, has not been determined because so few cases have been reported in the literature: only 18 cases appeared in the literature between 1978 and 2001 (Fylstra, 2002; Seow et al., 2004).

One of the theories to explain the occurrence of cesarean scar pregnancy is that the blastocyst enters into the wall through a microscopic dehiscent tract consequence of a cesarean or uterine surgery.

Clinical diagnosis of an early cesarean scar pregnancy is challenge, it may occasionally be delayed until the uterus ruptures and the patient experiences life-threatening bleeding (Seow et al., 2000, 2004; Weimin and Wenqing, 2002; Maymon et al., 2004). Thus, a prompt and accurate diagnosis is crucial. Diagnosis should be based on history and clinical manifestations, such as abdominal pain and vaginal bleeding, but up to 40% of women are asymptomatic, and the diagnosis is made during routine ultrasound exam (Rotas et al., 2006).

Ultrasonography can detect an enlargement of the cesarean scar in the lower segment and a gestational sac that is attached to it. The most common sonographic criteria for a pregnancy in scar diagnosis are: an empty uterus, an empty cervical canal, the gestational sac being located in the anterior part of the isthmic portion of the uterus with a diminished myometrial layer between the bladder and the sac and a discontinuity in the anterior wall of the uterus being demonstrated on a sagittal view of the uterus when the direction of the ultrasound beam runs through the amniotic sac (Vial et al., 2000) (Figure 6). These criteria assist in distinguishing this type of pregnancy from other diagnostic options, such as cervicoisthmic implantation, cervical pregnancy and spontaneous abortion in progress (Godin et al., 1997; Fylstra, 2002). Magnetic resonance imaging may also provide a more reliable way to identify this condition (Figure 7).

With the limited experience on cesarean section scar pregnancies in the first trimester, it is difficult to conclude on the optimal management for individual cases. Management depends on the gestation and includes expectant management, medical and surgical treatment. The mode of treatment in some cases is dictated by the clinical presentation, with laparotomy and hysterectomy being the most appropriate treatment for the patients who present with haemoperitoneum and hypovolaemic shock. In a haemodynamically stable patient, two

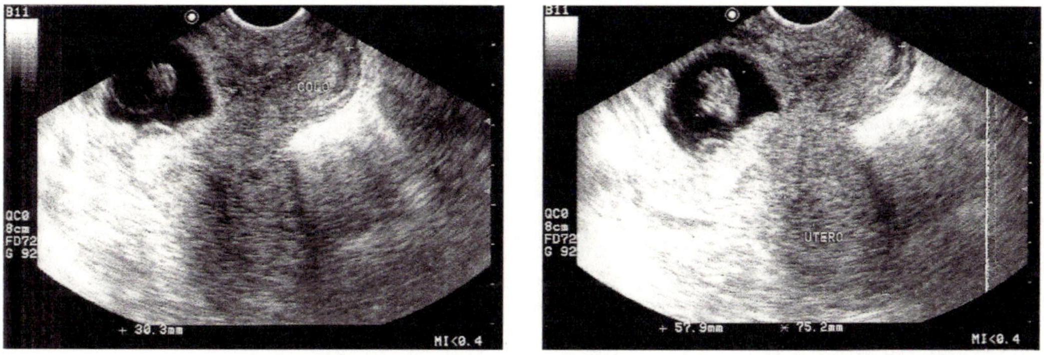

Fig. 6. Longitudinally oriented transvaginal ultrasound of the uterus demonstrating an empty uterus, an empty cervical canal, the gestational sac being located in the anterior part of the isthmic portion of the uterus with a diminished myometrial layer and a discontinuity in the anterior wall of the uterus (Elito, Camano, 2010a).

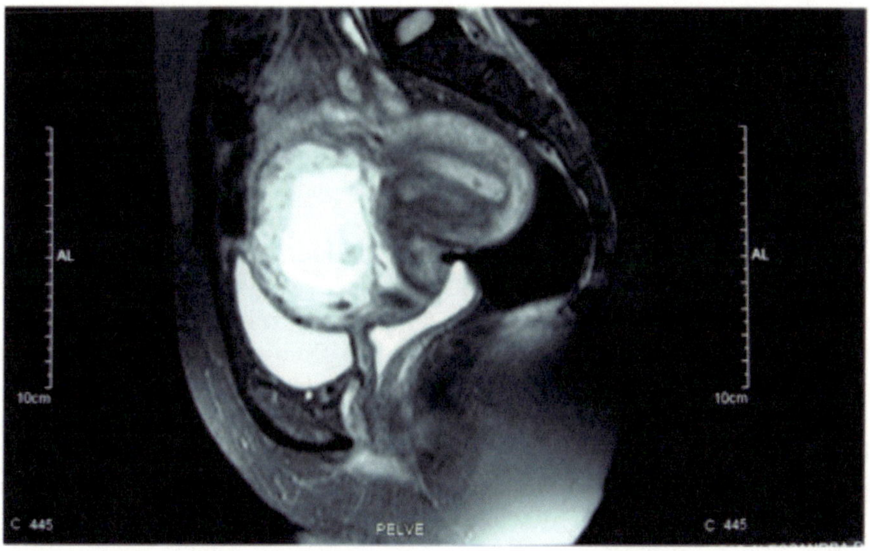

Fig. 7. Magnetic resonance imaging of the same case (Elito, Camano, 2010a).

principle management options may be considered, clinical or surgical, both aimed to eliminate the gestational sac and retain the patient's fertility. In cases where the diagnosis is made early and the patient is haemodynamically stable, assessment of the thickness of the anterior uterine wall is essential because a non-surgical procedure is the most appropriate option when the trophoblast reaches the vesico-uterine space on the bladder wall, thereby obviating an extended operation. There are few reported cases of cesarean section scar pregnancies managed expectantly in the literature. Two of these required additional treatment with methotrexate (Godin et al., 1997; Jurkovic et al., 2003) and two had emergency hysterectomies (Herman et al., 1995; Jurkovic et al., 2003). Expectant management does not therefore seem to be an appropriate choice, with the majority of cases reported requiring medical or surgical intervention.

Medical treatment consists of methotrexate administered systemically, locally or combined. Medical management with local injection of methotrexate has been more successful, with success rates of 70–80% when used as the initial treatment option (Jurkovic et al., 2003). This involves the direct injection of methotrexate into the pregnancy, performed transvaginally under ultrasound guidance. Local injections of potassium chloride have also been reported and were used prior to local methotrexate where embryonic cardiac activity was detected. Methotrexate has also been used systemically. The risk of cesarean scar rupture and heavy bleeding may occur following medical treatment. This has led some authors to propose that the medical approach should be combined with either bilateral uterine artery embolization or vasopressin intracervical injection combined with 18 Foley catheter balloon tamponade (Chuang et al., 2003), thus avoiding such complications (Ghezzi et al., 2002).

4.4 Ovarian pregnancy

Ovarian pregnancy represents the most common type of atypical localization of ectopic pregnancy.

In primary ovarian pregnancy the ovum is not guided into the tube but is fertilized in the peritoneal cavity and then implants onto the ovary. It causes the same symptoms as a tubal pregnancy and severe internal bleeding will eventually occur. In the secondary type, there is a tubal abortion with secondary implantation of the embryo on the tubal surface. Ovarian pregnancy is a rare form of ectopic gestation with estimates of frequency ranging from 1 in 2100 to 1 in 7000 pregnancies (Hage et al., 1994). It represents 0.5-3% of all ectopic pregnancies (Bouyer, Coste, 2002). Risk factors include previous pelvic inflammatory disease, IUD use, endometriosis, and assisted reproductive technologies (Marret et al., 1997).

Spiegelberg (1878) suggested four criteria to diagnose an ovarian pregnancy: the fallopian tube with its fimbria should be intact and separate from the ovary, the gestational sac should occupy the normal position of the ovary, the gestational sac should be connected to the uterus by the ovarian ligament and ovarian tissue must be present in the specimen attached to the gestational sac.

The diagnosis is difficult and a continuous challenge to the gynecologist. The presentation of ovarian pregnancy is commonly indistinguishable from tubal pregnancy, except for the predisposition to early rupture. The diagnosis of an ovarian ectopic pregnancy is seldom made before surgery. Transvaginal ultrasound is an important tool in the diagnosis of this condition. At ultrasound ovarian pregnancies show as a cyst with a wide echogenic outside ring. A yolk sac or embryo is less commonly seen and the appearance of the sac contents tends to lag in comparison to gestational age. However, it can be mistaken for a hemorrhagic corpus luteum or ovarian cyst. Misdiagnoses range from 35% (Hallat, 1982) to 75% (Herbertsson et al., 1987). Thick-walled ovarian cysts in the patient with an empty uterus and a serum beta-hCG level above the discriminatory zone should be investigated with particular care (Bontis et al., 1997). Most commonly symptoms are abdominal pain and light vaginal bleeding and diagnostic laparoscopy is often required to make the diagnosis of an ovarian pregnancy which is later confirmed by histological examination of the specimen (De Seta et al., 2001). Intraoperatively, ovarian ectopic pregnancies often resemble haemorrhagic cysts.

With early diagnosis laparoscopic surgery is the main method of treatment for ovarian ectopic pregnancies. Early detection of an ovarian pregnancy prior to rupture of the gestational sac and to onset of active bleeding permits laparoscopic surgery and removal of the ectopic pregnancy without excessive removal of healthy ovarian tissue (figure 8).

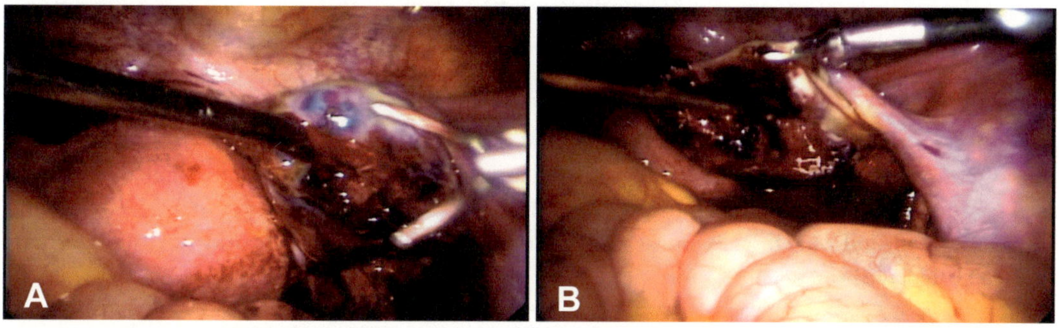

Fig. 8. Laparoscopic conservative surgery with removal of trophoblast tissue of the ovarian pregnancy (Elito, Camano, 2010b).

The medical treatment with methotrexate could be used in selected patients. It avoids surgical complications such as intraoperative hemorrhage, oophorectomy and pelvic adhesions.

Systemic methotrexate has been successfully used to treat ovarian ectopic pregnancy. There may be a place for medical management of carefully selected cases of ovarian ectopic pregnancy but selection criteria are not defined. Methotrexate may also be useful in the treatment of persistent trophoblastic tissue after laparoscopy (Einenkel et al., 2000). Though, if the initial diagnosis of an ectopic pregnancy is made during laparoscopy, it is preferable to remove it at the procedure. Nowadays, with early diagnosis and improvement of surgical techniques the ovarian tissue is preserved with minimal pelvic adhesions.

In the majority of cases ovarian pregnancies are diagnosed definitively at the time of surgical exploration. Therefore, MTX is not a first- line treatment for this condition.

4.5 Abdominal pregnancy

Abdominal pregnancy is one of the rarest form of ectopic pregnancy at 1.3% (Bouyer, Coste, 2002). It is described as primary or secondary where a tubal pregnancy aborts through the fimbrial end and implants in the peritoneal cavity. The vast majority of abdominal pregnancies are secondary. Most abdominal pregnancies are confined to the lower abdomen limited to the adnexa or the broad ligament (Holzhacker et al., 2008). However, abdominal pregnancies have been reported on the spleen, liver and diafragm. Early diagnosis is very important in this situation. Treatment is easier in the first trimester of pregnancy. Clinical signs of early abdominal pregnancy are similar to those of other ectopic pregnancies. However, in advanced abdominal pregnancy frequent symptoms are abdominal pain, nausea, vomiting, diarrhea, painful fetal movement and fetal movements high in the abdomen. Ultrasound is the diagnostic procedure of choice. The following ultrasound criteria have been suggested as being diagnostic: an empty uterus, absence of both an evident dilated tube and a complex adnexal mass, a gestational cavity surrounded by loops of bowel and separated by peritoneum, a wide mobility similar to fluctuation of the sac particularly evident with pressure of the transvaginal probe toward the posterior cul-de-sac. MRI may also provide a more reliable way to identify this condition (figure 9). Early diagnosis allows for optimization of surgical conditions, including pre-operative arterial embolization, availability of blood products, bowel prepare and multidisciplinary surgery team. The traditional management involves a laparotomy with removal of the fetus with or without placental tissue (Ayinde et al., 2005). Recently, there have been several reports of laparoscopic management (Shaw et al., 2007). One of the problems associated with the removal of abdominal pregnancies after the first trimester is the risk of massive blood loss from the placental bed. Adjuvant treatment with methotrexate alongside selective arterial embolization has been suggested to control this (Oki et al., 2008). There are also case reports of early abdominal pregnancies being treated successfully with systemic methotrexate and ultrasound guided injection of potassium chloride, leading to reabsorption of the products of conception without the need for further surgery (Mitra, Le Quire, 2003).

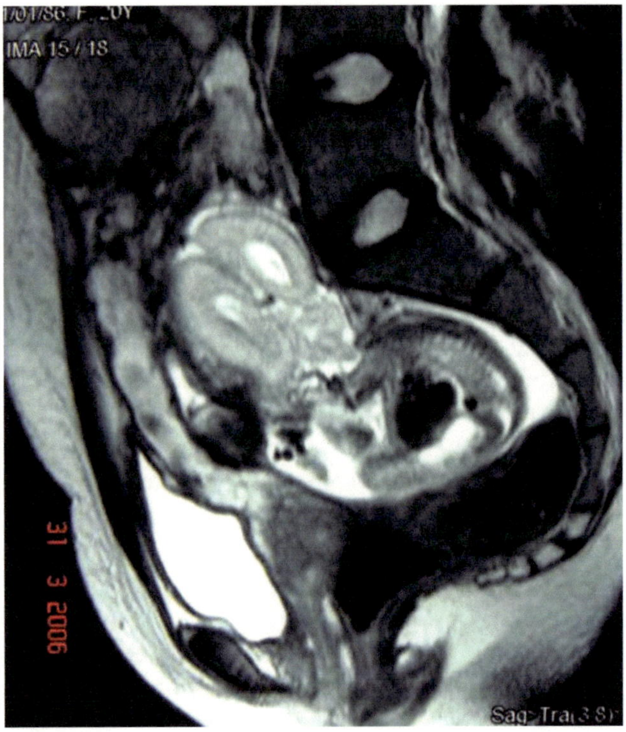

Fig. 9. MRI of advanced intraligamentar abdominal pregnancy (Holzhacker et al., 2008)..

4.6 Heterotopic pregnancy

Heterotopic pregnancy is defined by coexisting intrauterine and extrauterine pregnancies (figure 10). The increase of assisted reproduction resulted in a rise of heterotopic pregnancy. Nowadays approximately 1% of pregnancies resulting from assisted reproduction are heterotopic pregnancies. Unfortunately, approximately 50% of heterotopic pregnancies present symptoms of tubal rupture. Surgery is usually required and MTX is contraindicated (Chin et al., 2004; Fernandez et al., 2004). In cases of heterotopic pregnancy with an association of intra-uterine pregnancy and non-tubal pregnancy with embryonic cardiac activity, an alternative treatment could be local injection of KCL under ultrasound guidance. One important drawback for medical treatment in heterotopic pregnancy is the follow-up. Usually, the follow-up after medical treatment is made by the evaluation of the levels of beta-hCG. In heterotopic pregnancies this parameter cannot be used and ultrasound is a poor method to follow the patient. Therefore, medical treatment of heterotopic pregnancy should be restricted to cases with an association of atypical localization and intrauterine pregnancy, because in this situation the surgical treatment of choice is the hysterectomy. Other uncommon presentation of heterotopic pregnancy is the association of two extra-uterine pregnancies, such as tubal pregnancy and interstitial pregnancy or both tubal pregnancies. In these cases of heterotopic pregnancies without a viable intrauterine pregnancy medical treatment can be performed following the same rules of other ectopic pregnancies.

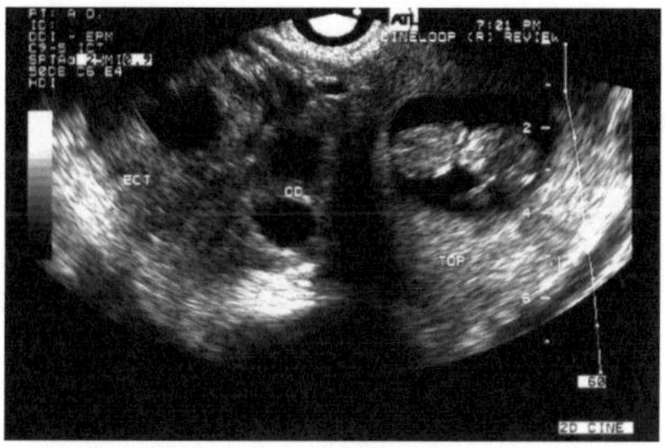

Fig. 10. Transvaginal ultrasound of heterotopic pregnancy showing at left side the tubal ring pregnancy and at right side the intrauterine pregnancy, between both the ovarian with two corpus luteum (Elito, Camano, 2010a).

4.7 Management in atypical ectopic pregnancies

There are many different approaches to the management of unusual ectopic pregnancies. Cases with embryonic cardiac activity should be treated with transvaginal administration of MTX and KCL under sonographic guidance. Ectopic pregnancies without embryonic cardiac activity and beta-hCG $\leq$ 5000 mUI/ml should be treated with single dose of MTX 50 mg/m^2 IM. Cases with beta-hCG > 5000 mUI/ml should be treated with multiple doses of MTX (Elito et al., 2008). It seems reasonable to treat some of these pregnancies with a combination of local and systemic MTX, in particular cases with high levels of beta-hCG. Adjunctive techniques for controlling hemorrhage (cervical cerclage, uterine artery embolization) should also be considered and a plan made for urgent assistance.

Surgery remains the main way for treatment of ovarian and abdominal ectopic pregnancies (Holzhacker et al., 2008).

5. Reproductive future

5.1 Hysterosalpingography

The fertility outcome of patients with unruptured EP treated conservatively with either MTX or expectant management can be evaluated indirectly through the hysterosalpingography (HSG) and directly by means of future pregnancy (Debby et al., 2000; Elito et al., 2006). The HSG represents important diagnosis methods after the treatment of EP, in spite of the inconveniences and doubts about the interpretation of this examination. The tubal patency after MTX is 84% and after expectant management is 78% (Elito et al., 2005a). This high rate of radiologically normal tubes after clinical treatment proves that the spontaneous regression of EP does not result in an increased harm or damage to the tube. However, the radiologically normal findings show nothing about the tubal function, when a disturbance can also be the cause of EP. On the other hand, if the results of HSG demonstrate obstruction of the tubes, the possibility of a spontaneous pregnancy will be reduced and should be treated with *in vitro* fertilization. The tubal obstruction is increased in cases with high beta-hCG levels (Elito et al., 2005b). The explanation for higher incidence of tubal obstruction is that in patients with higher levels of beta-hCG there is more invasion of the trophoblast tissue at the tube's serosa, what increases the damage to the tube.

5.2 Future pregnancy

After medical treatment 65% of patients who attempted subsequent pregnancies succeeded, and the incidence of recurrent ectopic pregnancy was relatively low at 13% (Stovall et al., 1989; Lipscomb et al., 2000). Systemic MTX in a single-dose regimen compared with laparoscopic salpingostomy of four trials (Fernandez et al., 1998; Saraj et al., 1998; Sowter et al., 2001; El-Sherbiny et al., 2003), involving 265 haemodynamically stable women with a small unruptured tubal EP, showed no significant differences in the number of IUPs (RR 1.01, 95% CI 0.66–1.54), whereas there was a non-significant trend towards a lower incidence of repeat EPs (RR 0.63, 95% CI 0.14–2.77) (Mol et al., 2008). Systemic MTX in a fixed multiple dose regimen compared with laparoscopic salpingostomy observed that fertility outcome was no significant different for IUP (RR 0.88, 95% CI 0.49–1.60) as well as for repeat EP (RR 0.88, 95% CI 0.21–3.67) (Dias Pereira et al., 1999).

6. Cost analysis

Serial serum beta-hCG measurements and transvaginal ultrasound examination can provide early diagnosis of most ectopic pregnancies allowing medical treatment with methotrexate. Approximately 40% of women diagnosed with ectopic pregnancy are candidates for medical management (Barnhart et al., 2003), and 90% of those can be treated successfully without surgery (Lipscomb et al., 2000). Whereas the costs of surgery and outpatient medical management vary widely, many cost-effectiveness analyses have favored MTX therapy. Systemic MTX in a single-dose regimen resulted in significant savings in direct costs compared with laparoscopic surgery: mean direct costs per patient were € 756 and € 1585, respectively, with a mean difference of € 829 (95% CI 599–1060). Furthermore, systemic MTX resulted in significant savings in indirect costs: mean indirect costs per patient were € 587 and € 977, respectively, with a mean difference of € 390 (95% CI 142–638). However, in women with initial serum hCG concentrations >1500 IU/l the difference in indirect costs was lost due to the prolonged follow-up and a higher rate of surgical re-interventions

(Sowter et al., 2001). Therefore, medical treatment is less expensive than surgery, except in cases with higher levels of beta-hCG (Sowter et al., 2001).

7. Conclusion

The early non-invasive diagnosis of ectopic pregnancy, before there is tubal rupture, can be made through transvaginal ultrasonography and with the dosage of the beta-fraction of the chorionic gonadotrophin. After the diagnosis, range of treatments may be used. Either a surgical intervention or a clinical treatment (expectant management or methotrexate therapy) may be taken into consideration. Expectant management should be indicated in cases of decline in the beta-hCG titers within 48 hours before the treatment, and when the initial titers are under 1,500 mUI/mL. The use of methotrexate (MTX) is a safe clinical procedure and in some cases could be indicated as the first option for treatment. The main criteria for MTX indication are hemodynamic stability, beta-hCG <5,000 mUI/mL, adnexal mass ≤3,5 cm, and no embryonic cardiac activity. It is preferable to administer a single intramuscular dose MTX (50 mg/m²) because it is easier, more practical and with less side effects (diagram 1). Protocol with multiple doses should be restricted for the cases with atypical localization (interstitial, cervical, caesarean section scar and ovarian) with values of beta-hCG >5,000 mUI/mL and no fetal heart activity. Indication for local treatment with an injection of MTX (1 mg/kg) and KCl guided by transvaginal ultrasonography should occur in cases of embryonic cardiac activity but with an atypical localization (Elito et al., 2008).

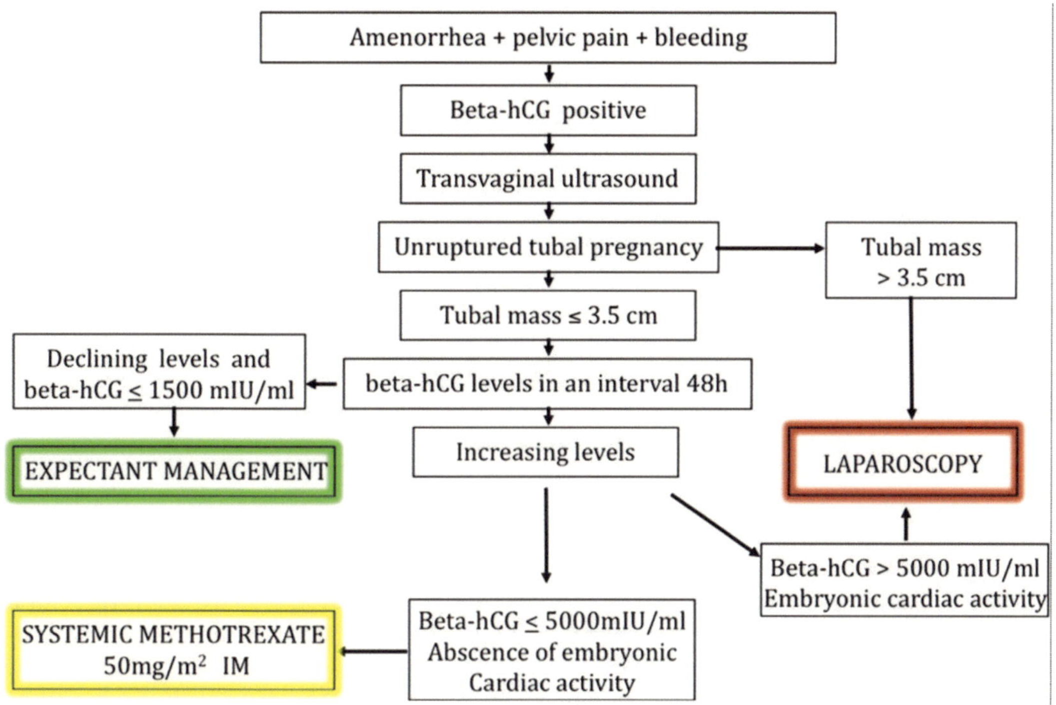

Diagram 1. Recommendation for Treatment of Unruptured Tubal Pregnancy (Elito et al., 2008)

8. References

Ackerman TE, Levi CS, Dashefsky SM, Holt SC, Lindsay DJ. Interstitial line: sonographic finding in interstitial (cornual) ectopic pregnancy. Radiology 1993;189:83-7.

Ash A, Smith A, Maxwell D. Caesarean scar pregnancy. BJOG. 2007 Mar;114(3):253-63.

Atri M, Bret PM, Tulandi T, Senterman MK. Ectopic pregnancy: evolution after treatment with transvaginal methotrexate. Radiology 1992;185:749–53.

Ayinde OA, Aimakhu CO, Adeyanju OA et al. Abdominal pregnancy at the University College Hospital, Ibadan: a ten-year review. Afr J Reprod Health 2005; 9: 123–127.

Bai SW, Lee JS, Park JH, Kim JY, Jung KA, Kim SK, Park KH. Failed methotrexate treatment of cervical pregnancy. Predictive factors. J Reprod Med. 2002; 47:483-8.

Baptiste A. Cervical pregnancy. Obstet Gynecol 1953; 1:353.

Barnhart K, Coutifaris C, Esposito M. The pharmacology of methotrexate. Expert Opin Pharmacother 2001;2:409–17.

Barnhart KT, Gosman G, Ashby R, Sammel M. The medical management of ectopic pregnancy: a meta-analysis comparing "single dose and multidose" regimens. Obstet Gynecol 2003;101:778–84.

Barnhart K, Hummel AC, Sammel MD, Menon S, Jain JK, Chakhtoura NA.Use of "2-dose" regimen of methotrexate to treat ectopic pregnancy. Fertil Steril 2007;87:250-6.

Barnhart KT. Clinical practice. Ectopic pregnancy. N Engl J Med. 2009 Jul 23;361(4):379-87.

Benifla JL, Fernandez H, Sebban E, Darai E, Frydman R, Madelenat P. Alternative to surgery of treatment of unruptured interstitial pregnancy: 15 cases of medical treatment. Eur J Obstet Gynecol Reprod Biol 1996;70:151-6.

Berg CJ, Chang J, Callaghan WM, Whitehead SJ. Pregnancy-related mortality in the United States, 1991–1997. Obstet Gynecol 2003;101: 289–96.

Bontis J, Grimbizis G, Tarlatzis BC et al. Intrafollicular ovarian pregnancy after ovulation induction/intrauterine insemination: pathophysiological aspects and diagnostic problems. Hum Reprod 1997; 12(2): 376–378.

Bouyer J, Coste J, Ferrnandez H et al. Sites of ectopic pregnancy; a 10 year population-based study of 1800 cases. Hum Reprod 2002; 17: 3224–3230.

Brown DL, Felker RE, Stovall TG, Emerson DS, Ling FW. Serial endovaginal sonography of ectopic pregnancies treated with methotrexate. Obstet. Gynecol., 77: 406-9, 1991.

Cacciatore B, Korhonen J, Stenman UH, Ylostalo P. Transvaginal sonography and serum hCG in monitoring of presumed ectopic pregnancies selected for expectant management. Ultrasound Obstet Gynecol 1995; 5: 297-300.

Centers for Disease Control and Prevention (CDC). Ectopic pregnancy - United States, 1990-1992. MMWR Morb Mortal Wkly Rep. 1995;44(3):46-8.

Chetty M, Elson J. Treating non-tubal ectopic pregnancy. Best Pract Res Clin Obstet Gynaecol. 2009 Aug;23(4):529-38.

Chin HY, Chen FP, Wang CJ, Shui LT, Liu YH, Soong YK. Heterotopic pregnancy after in vitro fertilization-embryo transfer. Int J Gynaecol Obstet 2004;86:411–6.

Chuang J, Seow KM, Cheng WC, Tsai YL, Hwang JL. Conservative treatment of ectopic pregnancy in a caesarean section scar. BJOG. 2003 Sep;110(9):869-70.

da Costa Soares R, Elito J Jr, Camano L. Increment in beta-hCG in the 48-h period prior to treatment: a new variable predictive of therapeutic success in the treatment of ectopic pregnancy with methotrexate. Arch Gynecol Obstet. 2008 Oct;278(4):319-24.

Damario MA, Rock JA. Ectopic pregnancy.In: Rock JA, Jones HW III, eds. Te Linde's operative gynecology. Philadelphia: Lippincott, Williams & Wilkins; 2003:507-36.

Debby A, Golan A, Sadan O, Zakut H, Glezerman M. Fertility outcome following combined methotrexate treatment of unruptured extrauterine pregnancy. BJOG 2000; 107: 626–30. 3.

De La Veja GA, Avery C, Nemiroff R, Marchiano D. Treatment of early cervical pregnancy with cerclage, carboprost, curettage and balloon tamponade. Obstet Gynecol. 2007; 109:505-7.

De Seta F, Baraggino E, Strazzanti C et al. Ovarian pregnancy: a case report. Acta Obstet Gynecol Scand 2001; 80: 661–662.

Dialani V, Levine D. Ectopic pregnancy: a review. Ultrasound 2004; 20:105-117.

Dias Pereira G, Hajenius PJ, Mol BW, Ankum WM, Hemrika DJ, Bossuyt PM, van der Veen F. Fertility outcome after systemic methotrexate and laparoscopic salpingostomy for tubal pregnancy. Lancet. 1999 Feb 27;353(9154):724-5.

DuBois D, DuBois EF. A formula to estimate the approximate surface area if height and weight be known. Arch Intern Med 1916; 17: 863–871

Eddy CA, Pauerstein CJ. Anatomy and physiology of the fallopian tube. Clin Obstet Gynecol. 1980, 23:1177.

EgarterC,KissH&HussleinP.Prostaglandinversusexpectantmanagementinearlytubalpregnancy.ProstaglandinsLeukot Essent Fatty Acids 1991; 42: 177–179.

Einenkel J, Baier D, Horn L-C et al. Laparoscopic therapy of an intact primary ovarian pregnancy with ovarian hyper- stimulation syndrome. Hum Reprod 2000; 15(9): 2037–2040.

Elito Jr J, Uchiyama M, Camano L. O metotrexato no tratamento sistêmico da prenhez ectópica íntegra. Rev Bras Ginecol Obstet. 1996; 18(7):537-41.

Elito Jr J, Uchiyama M, Camano L. Evolução dos níveis de beta-hCG após tratamento sistêmico da prenhez ectópica íntegra. Rev Assoc Med Bras. 1998; 44 (1):11-5.

Elito J Jr, Reichmann AP, Uchiyama MN, Camano L. Predictive score for the systemic treatment of unruptured ectopic pregnancy with a single dose of methotrexate. Int J Gynaecol Obstet 1999a;67:75–9.

Elito Jr J, Uchiyama M, Camano L. Gravidez ectópica cervical com embrião vivo: relato de quatro casos. Rev Bras Ginecol Obstet. 1999b; 21(6):347-50.

Elito Jr J, Camano L. Unruptured tubal pregnancy: different treatments for early and late diagnosis. São Paulo Med J. 2006 Nov 7;124(6):321-4.

Elito Jr J, Han KK, Camano L. Tubal patency after clinical treatment of unruptured ectopic pregnancy. Int J Gynaecol Obstet. 2005a; 88(3):309-13.

Elito Jr J, Han KK, Camano L. Values of beta-human chorionic gonadotropin as a risk factor for tubal

obstruction after tubal pregnancy. Acta Obstet Gynecol Scand. 2005b; 84(9):864-7.

Elito Jr J, Han KK, Camano L. Tubal patency following surgical and clinical treatment of ectopic pregnancy. Sao Paulo Med J. 2006 Sep 7;124(5):264-6.

Elito Jr J, Montenegro NA, Soares RC, Camano L. Unruptured ectopic pregnancy: diagnosis and treatment. State of art. Rev Bras Ginecol Obstet. 2008 Mar;30(3):149-59.

Elito Jr J, Camano L. Hemorragias no primeiro trimestre de gestação: prenhez ectópica. In Pastore AR, Cerri GG. "Ultrassonografia em Ginecologia e Obstetrícia". 2a Edição. Livraria e Editora Revinter, 2010.pg:114-133.

Elito Jr J; Camano L. Gestação ectópica. In: Moron AF; Camano L; Kulay Jr L. Obstetrícia - UNIFESP/ EPM. 1a Ed, Editora Manole, São Paulo, 2010; pg 151-168.

El-Sherbiny MT, El G I, Mera IM. Methotrexate verus laparoscopic surgery for the management of unruptured tubal pregnancy. Middle East Fertil Soc J 2003;8:256-262.

Elson J, Tailor A, Banerjee S, Salim R, Hillaby K, Jurkovic D. Expectant management of tubal ectopic pregnancy: prediction of successful outcome using decision tree analysis. Ultrasound Obstet Gynecol 2004; 23: 552-556.

Feichtinger, W.; Kemeter, P.- Conservative treatment of ectopic pregnancy by transvaginal aspiration under sonographic control and MTX injection. Lancet. 1987; 1: 381-92.

Fernandez, H.; Benifla, J. A.- Metotrexate treatment of ectopic pregnancy - 100 cases treated by primary transvaginal injection under sonographic control. Fertil. Steril. 1993; 59: 773-7.

Fernandez H, Yves Vincent SC, Pauthier S, Audibert F, Frydman R. Randomized trial of conservative laparoscopic treatment and methotrexate administration in ectopic pregnancy and subsequent fertility. Hum Reprod. 1998 Nov;13(11):3239-43.

Fernandez H, Gervaise A. Ectopic pregnancies after infertility treatment: modern diagnosis and therapeutic strategy. Hum Reprod Update 2004;10:503–13.

Fylstra DL. Ectopic pregnancy within a cesarean scar: a review. Obstet Gynecol Surv. 2002 Aug;57(8):537-43.

Glatstein IZ, Sleeper LA, Law Y, Simon A, Adoni A, Laufer N, et al. Observer variability in the diagnosis and management of the hysterosalpingogram. Fertil Steril 1997;67:233–7

Godin PA, Bassil S, Donnez J. An ectopic pregnancy developing in a previous caesarian section scar. Fertil Steril. 1997 Feb;67(2):398-400.

Ghezzi F, Lagana D, Franchi M, Fugazzola C, Bolis P. Conservative treatment by chemotherapy and uterine arteries embolization of a cesarean scar pregnancy. Eur J Obstet Gynecol Reprod Biol. 2002 Jun 10;103(1):88-91.

Hage PS, Arnouk IF, Zarou DM et al. Laparoscopic management of ovarian pregnancy. J Am Assoc Gynecol Laparosc 1994; 1: 283–285.

Hallat J. Primary ovarian pregnancy. A report of twenty-five cases. Am J Obstet Gynecol. 1982; 143: 50-60.

Hajenius PJ, Mol BWJ, Ankum WM et al. Suspected ectopic pregnancy: expectant management in patients with negative sonographic findings and low serum hCG concentrations. Early Pregnancy: Biol Med 1995; 1: 258–262.

Hajenius PJ, Engelsbel S, Mol BW, Van der Veen F, Ankum WM, Bossuyt PM, et al. Randomised trial of systemic methotrexate versus lap- aroscopic salpingostomy in tubal pregnancy. Lancet 1997;350:774–9.

Hajenius PJ, Mol F, Mol BW, Bossuyt PM, Ankum WM, van der Veen F. Interventions for tubal ectopic pregnancy.Cochrane Database Syst Rev. 2007 Jan 24;(1):CD000324.

Han KK; Elito Jr J, Camano L. Conduta expectante para gravidez tubária íntegra. Rev Bras Ginecol Obstet. 1999; 21(8):465-70.

Herbertsson G, Magnusson SS, Benediktsdottir K. Ovarian pregnancy and IUCD use in a defined complete population. Acta Obstet Gynecol Scand 1987;66:607.

Herman A, Weinraub Z, Avrech O et al. Follow up and outcome of isthmic pregnancy located in a previous caesarean section scar. Br J Obstet Gynaecol 1995; 102: 839–841.
Hsieh BC, Lin YH, Huang JW, Chang JZ, Seo WKM, Pan HS, Hwang JL. Cervical pregnancy after in vitro fertilization and embryo transfer successfully treated with methotrexate and intracervical injection of vasopressin. Acta Obstet Gynecol Scand 2004; 83:112-4.
Hofmann HMH, Urdl W, Hofler H. Cervical pregnancy: Case reports and current concepts in diagnosis and treatment. Arch Gynecol Obstet. 1987; 241:63.
Holzhacker S, Elito Jr J, Santana RM, Hisaba W. Advanced intraligamentary abdominal pregnancy - case report. Rev Assoc Med Bras. 2008 Sep-Oct;54(5):387-9.
Isaacs JD, Mcgehee RP, Cowan BD. Life-threatening neutropenia fol- lowing methotrexate treatment of ectopic pregnancy: a report of two cases. Obstet Gynecol 1996; 88:694–6.
Jeng CJ, Ko ML, Shen J. Transvaginal ultrasound-guided treatment of cervical pregnancy. Obstet Gynecol. 2007; 109:1076-82.
Jourdain O, Fontanges M, Schiano A, Rauch F, Gonnet JM. Management of other ectopic pregnancies (cornual, interstitial, angular, ovarian).J Gynecol Obstet Biol Reprod (Paris) 2003;32:S93–100.
Jurkovic D, Hillaby K, Woelfer B et al. First-trimester diagnosis and management of pregnancies implanted into the lower uterine segment cesarean section scar. Ultrasound Obstet Gynecol 2003; 21: 220–227.
Kamrava MM, Taymor ML, Berger MJ, Thompson IE, Seibel MM. Disappearance of human chorionic gonadotropin following removal of ectopic pregnancy. Obstet Gynecol. 1983 Oct;62(4):486-8.
KorhonenJ,StenmanU&YlostaloP.Lowdoseoralmethotrexatewithexpectantmanagementofectopicpregnancy.Obstet Gynecol 1996; 88: 775–778.
Korhonen J, Stenman UH & Ylo¨ stalo P. Serum human chorionic gonadotropin dynamics during spontaneous resolution of ectopic pregnancy. Fertil Steril 1994; 61: 632–636.
Lang PF, Makinen JI, Irjala KM et al. Laparoscopic instillation of hyperosmolar glucose vs. expectant management of tubal pregnancies with serum hCG < or ¼ 2500 mIU/mL. Acta Obstet Gynecol Scand 1997 Sep; 76(8): 797–800.
Lau S, Tulandi T. Conservative medical and surgical management of interstitial ectopic pregnancy. Fertil Steril 1999;72:207-15.
Li MC, Hertz R, Spencer, DB. Effect of methotrexate therapy upon choriocarcinoma and chorioadenoma. Proc. Sci. Exp. Biol. Med., 93: 361-9, 1956.
Lim JE, Kim T, Lee NW, et al. Ultrasonographic endometrial features in tubal pregnancy: are they predictive factors of successful medical treatment? Ultrasound Med Biol 2007; 33:714-9.
Lin YS, Chen CL, Yuan CC, Wang PH. Successful rescue of an early interstitial pregnancy after failed systemic methotrexate treatment: a case report. J Reprod Med 2007;52:332-4.
Lipscomb GH, Puckett KJ, Bran D, Ling FW. Management of separation pain after single-dose methotrexate therapy for ectopic pregnancy. Obstet Gynecol 1999;93:590–3.

Lipscomb GH, McCord ML, Stovall TG, Huff G, Portera SG, Ling FW. Predictors of success of methotrexate treatment in women with tubal ec- topic pregnancies. N Engl J Med 1999;341:1974–8.

Lipscomb GH, Stovall TG, Ling FW. Nonsurgical treatment of ectopic pregnancy. N Engl J Med 2000;343:1325–9.

Lui A, D'Ottavio G, Rustico MA, Conoscenti G, Fischer Tamaro F, Meir YJ, Maieron A, Mandruzzato GP. [Conservative management of ectopic pregnancy.] Minerva Ginecol 1997; 49: 67-72.

Lund, JJ.- Early ectopic pregnancy treated nonsurgically. J. Obstet. Br. Empire, 62: 70-6, 1955.

Marret H, Hamamah S, Alonso AM et al. Case report and review of the literature: primary twin ovarian pregnancy. Hum Reprod 1997; 12(8): 1813–1815.

Mashiach S, Carp HJA & Serr DM. Non operative management of ectopic pregnancy: a preliminary report. J Reprod Med 1982; 27: 127Lipscomb GH, Stovall TG, Ling FW. Nonsurgical treatment of ectopic pregnancy. N Engl J Med 2000;343:1325–9.

MassJW,EversJL,RietG,KesselsAG. Pregnancy rate following normal versus abnormal hysterosalpingography findings: a meta-analysis. Gynecol Obstet Invest 1997;43:79– 83.

Maymon R, Halperin R, Mendlovic S, Schneider D, Vaknin Z, Herman A, et al. Ectopic pregnancies in Caesarean section scars: the 8 year experience of one medical centre. Hum Reprod. 2004 Feb;19(2):278-84.

Mesogitis S, Pilalis A, Daskalakis G, Papantoniou N, Antsaklis A. Management of early viable cervical pregnancy. BJOG 2005; 112:409-11.

MitraAG&LeQuireMH.Minimallyinvasivemanagementof14.5weekabdominalpregnancywit houtlaparotomy:anovel approach using percutaneous sonographically guided feticide and systemic methotrexate. J Ultrasound Med 2003; 22: 709–714.

Moawad NS, Mahajan ST, Moniz MH, Taylor SE, Hurd WW. Current diagnosis and treatment of interstitial pregnancy (2010) Am J Obstet and Gynecol, 202 (1), pp. 15-29.

Mol BW, Swart P, Bossut PM, Van Der Veen F. Hysterosalpingography an important tool in predicting fertility outcome? Fertil Steril 1997;67:663–9.

Mol F, Mol BW, Ankum WM, van der Veen F, Hajenius PJ. Current evidence on surgery, systemic methotrexate and expectant management in the treatment of tubal ectopic pregnancy: a systematic review and meta-analysis. Hum Reprod Update. 2008 Jul-Aug;14(4):309-19.

Monteagudo A, Minior VK, Stephenson C, Monda S, Timor-Tritsch E. Non-surgical management of live ectopic pregnancy with ultrasound-guided local injection: a case series. Ultrasound Obstet Gynecol 2005; 25:282-8.

Natale, A., Candiani, M., Merlo, D., Izzo, S., Gruft, L., Busacca, M. Human chorionic gonadotropin level as a predictor of trofoblastic infiltration into the tubal wall in ectopic pregnancy: a blinded study. Fertil. Steril. 2003, 79, 981-986.

Olofsson JI, Poromaa IS, Ottander U, Kjellberg L, Damber MG. Clinical and pregnancy outcome following ectopic pregnancy; a prospective study comparing expectancy, surgery and systemic methotrexate treatment. Acta Obstet Gynecol Scand 2001; 80: 744-749.

Oki T, Baba Y, Yoshinaga M et al. Super-selective arterial embolization for uncontrolled bleeding in abdominal pregnancy. Obstet Gynecol 2008; 112: 427–429.
Pansky, M.; Bubowsky, I.- Local methotrexate injection: a nonsurgical treatment of ectopic pregnancy. Am. J. Obstet. Gynecol. 1989; 161: 363-8.
Pisarska MD, Carson SA, Buster JE. Ectopic pregnancy. Lancet 1998;351:1115–20.
Pisarska M, Carson S. Incidence and risk factors for ectopic pregnancy. Clin Obstet Gynecol 1999; 42:2-8.
Potter MB, Lepine LA, Jamieson DJ. Predictors of success with methotrexate treatment of tubal ectopic pregnancy at Grady Memorial Hospital. Am J Obstet Gynecol 2003;188:1192–4.
Practice Committee of American Society for Reproductive Medicine. Medical treatment of ectopic pregnancy.(2008) Fertility and Sterility, 90 (5 SUPPL.), pp. S206-S212.
Rantala M, Ma¨kinen J. Tubal patency and fertility outcome after expectant management of ectopic pregnancy. Fertil Steril 1997;68:1043–6.
Rotas MA, Haberman S, Levgur M. Cesarean scar ectopic pregnancies: etiology, diagnosis, and management. Obstet Gynecol. 2006 Jun;107(6):1373-81.
Sagiv R, Golan A, Arbel-Alon S, Glezerman M. Three conservative approaches to treatment of interstitial pregnancy. J Am Assoc Gynecol Laparosc 2001;8:154-8.
Saraj AJ, Wilcox JG, Najmabadi S, Stein SM, Johnson MB, Paulson RJ. Resolution of hormonal markers of ectopic gestation: a randomized trial comparing single-dose intramuscular methotrexate with salpingostomy. Obstet Gynecol. 1998 Dec;92(6):989-94.
Seow KM, Cheng WC, Chuang J, Lee C, Tsai YL, Hwang JL. Methotrexate for cesarean scar pregnancy after in vitro fertilization and embryo transfer. A case report. J Reprod Med. 2000 Sep;45(9):754-7.
Seow KM, Huang LW, Lin YH, Lin MY, Tsai YL, Hwang JL. Cesarean scar pregnancy: issues in management. Ultrasound Obstet Gynecol. 2004 Mar;23(3):247-53.
Shalev E, Peleg D, Tsabari A, Romano S, Bustan M. Spontaneous resolution of ectopic tubal pregnancy: natural history. Fertil Steril 1995; 63: 15-19.
Shaw SW, Hsu JJ, Chueh HY et al. Management of primary abdominal pregnancy: twelve years of experience in a medical centre. Acta Obstet Gynecol Scand 2007; 86(9): 1058–1062.
Spiegelberg 0-Zur. Cauistik der Ovarial schwangerschaft. Arch E Gynak. 1878; 13: 73
Soares, RC; Elito Jr J, Han KK, Camano L. Endometrial thickness as an orienting factor for the medical treatment of unruptured tubal pregnancy. Acta Obstet Gyn Scand, 2004:83(3): 289-92.
Sowter MC, Farquhar CM, Gudex G. An economic evaluation of single dose systemic methotrexate and laparoscopic surgery for the treatment of unruptured ectopic pregnancy. BJOG 2001;108:204–12.
Stovall TG, Ling FW, Buster JE. Outpatient chemotherapy of unruptured ectopic pregnancy. Fertil Steril 1989;51:435–8.
Stovall TG, Ling FW, Gray LA, Carson SA, Buster JE. Methotrexate treatment of unruptured ectopic pregnancy: a report of 100 cases. Obstet Gynecol 1991;77:749– 53.
Stovall TG, Ling FW. Single-dose methotrexate: an expanded clinical trial. Am J Obstet Gynecol 1993;168:1759-65

Tanaka T, Hayashi H, Kutsuzawa T, Fujimoto S, Ichinoe K. Treatment of intersticial ectopic pregnancy with methotrexate: report of a successful case. Fertil Steril 1982;37:851-5.

Tawfiq A, Agameya AF, Claman P. Predictors of treatment failure for ec- topic pregnancy treated with single-dose methotrexate. Fertil Steril 2000;74:877–80.

Timor-Tritsch IE, Monteagudo A, Matera C, Veit CR. Sonographic evolution of cornual pregnancies treated without surgery. Obstet Gynecol 1992;79:1044-9.

Trio D, Strobelt N, Picciolo C, Lapinski RH, Ghidini A. Prognostic factors for successful expectant management of ectopic pregnancy. Fertil Steril 1995; 63: 469-72.

Tulandi T, Al-Jaroudi D. Interstitial nancy: results generated from the Society of Reproductive Surgeons Registry. Obstet Gynecol 2004;103:47-50.

van Mello NM, Mol F, Mol BW, Hajenius PJ. Conservative management of tubal ectopic pregnancy. Best Pract Res Clin Obstet Gynaecol. 2009 Aug;23(4):509-18.

Vial Y, Petignat P, Hohlfeld P. Pregnancy in a cesarean scar. Ultrasound Obstet Gynecol. 2000 Nov;16(6):592-3.

Xu B, Wang YK, Zhang YH, Wang S, Yang L, Dai SZ. Angiographic uterine artery embolization followed immediate curettage: an efficient treatment for controlling heavy bleeding and avoiding recurrent bleeding in cervical pregnancy. J Obstet Gynaecol Res 2007; 33:190-4.

Ylostalo P, Cacciatore B, Sjoberg J, Kaariainen M, Tenhunen A, Stenman UH. Expectant management of ectopic pregnancy. Obstet Gynecol 1992; 80: 345-348.

Walker JJ. Ectopic pregnancy. Clin Obstet Gynecol 2007;50:89-99.

Weimin W, Wenqing L. Effect of early pregnancy on a previous lower segment cesarean section scar. Int J Gynaecol Obstet. 2002 Jun;77(3):201-7.

Zalel Y, Caspi B, Insler V. Expectant management of interstitial pregnancy. Ultrasound Obstet Gynecol 1994;4:238-40.

Zohav E, Gemer O, Segal S. Reproductive outcome after expectant management of ectopic pregnancy. Eur J Obstet Reprod Biol 1996;66:1–2.

12

MTX Could Be First-Line Therapy Even in Cases Where hCG Level is Greater than 5,000 IU/ml

Yoshiki Yamashita et al.*
Department of Obstetrics and Gynecology, Osaka Medical College
Japan

1. Introduction

Ectopic pregnancy (EP) accounts for approximately 75% of deaths in the first trimester, and 9% of all pregnancy-related deaths are the result of EP.
Recently, EP can be diagnosed accurately at a very early stage using transvaginal ultrasound and serum hCG measurement (1). Methtorexate (MTX) is in a class of drugs known as folic acid antagonists, and folic acid is an essential component in the synthesis of DNA precursors such as purines and thymidylate. MTX was originally used to treat cancer, trophoblastic disease, psoriasis, and rheumatoid arthritis; however, since 1982, it has been used to successfully treat EP (2). Treatment with MTX now reportedly achieves results comparable to surgery for the treatment of appropriately selected ectopic pregnancies and is now commonly used (3). The American Society of Reproductive Medicine (ASRM) introduced the relative and absolute contraindications to MTX therapy, as indicated in Table 1 and 2 (4, 5). Lipscomb et al reported that the rate of success with MTX is relatively low in cases where serum hCG levels are higher than 5,000 IU/ml (Table 3) (6), however, MTX treatment has recently been favored in cost-effectiveness analyses. In this study, we reviewed EP cases treated with MTX regardless of high initial-hCG levels (>5,000 IU/ml) and evaluated the effectiveness of MTX by comparing them with cases where hCG levels were less than 5,000 IU/ml.

1. Embryonic cardiac activity detected by transvaginal ultrasonography
2. High initial hCG concentration (5,000>mIU/ml)
3. Ectopic pregnancy >4 cm in size as imaged by transvaginal ultrasonography
4. Refusal to accept blood transfusion
5. Inability to participate in follow-up

Table 1. Relative contraindication to MTX

*Sousuke Katoh, Yoko Yoshida, Satoe Fujiwara, Sachiko Kawabe, Mika Hayashi, Atsushi Hayashi, Yoshito Terai and Masahide Ohmichi

1. Intrauterine pregnancy
2. Evidence of immunodeficiency
3. Moderate to severe anemia, leukopenia or thrombocytopenia
4. Sensitivity to MTX
5. Active pulmonary disease
6. Active peptic ulcer disease
7. Clinically important hepatic dysfunction
8. Clinically important renal dysfunction
9. Breast feeding

Table 2. Absolute contraindication to MTX

Initial serum hCG level(mIU/ml)	Success (n=30)	Failure (n=14)	Success rate %
<1000	118	2	98
1000-1999	40	3	93
2000-4999	90	8	92
5000-9999	39	6	87
10,000-14,999	18	4	82
≧15,000	15	7	68

Table 3. Initial hCG level and success rate

2. Materials and method

We performed MTX treatment in 44 cases, 14 of which were high-hCG EP cases with initial serum hCG levels greater than 5,000 IU/ml. In our department, diagnosis of EP was confirmed, as shown in Figure 1. After getting informed consent for the possibility of additional surgical intervention, we administered MTX IM at a dosage of 50 mg/m^2. If a decline of more than 15% was not identified between days 4 and 7, an additional 50 mg/m^2 of MTX was administered. Weekly MTX treatment was stopped when hCG levels declined to less than 25 IU/ml (Table 4). Alteration to surgical intervention was adopted according to the patients' requirements.

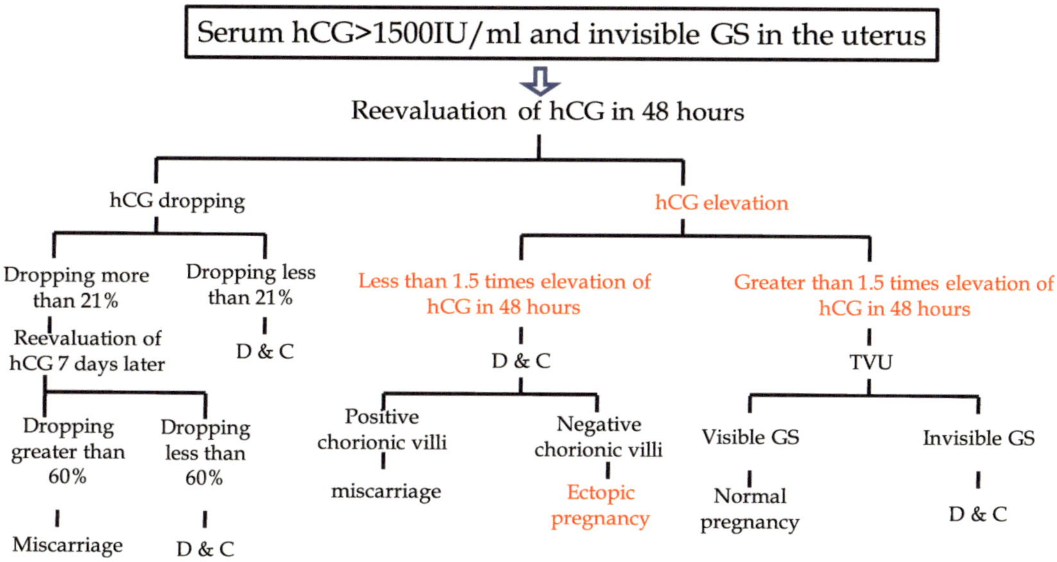

Fig. 1.

Serum hCG (mIU/ml)	Ampurally	Interstitial	Cervical
<1000	12	-	-
1000-1999	7	-	-
2000-4999	11	-	-
5000-9999	6	2	-
10000-14999	-	-	1
>15000	1	4	-

Table 4. Initial serum hCG and pregnancy site

3. Results

Fourteen cases of ectopic pregnancy, with initial hCG levels >5,000 IU/ml were treated with MTX. Of those 14 cases, 1 had IVF treatment, 1 undertook ovulation induction, and 12 were spontaneous pregnancies. It took 3.85 days from the initial visit to confirm the diagnosis of EP, and the average gestational week was 7.31 weeks. Hospitalization days were 13.57 days,

and MTX was administered 1.35 times. Implantation sites were 7 ampullary, 6 interstitial, and 1 cervical (Table 5). The range of initial hCG was from 5,713 to 92,670 IU/ml, and the average was 19619.7 IU/ml. More than two administrations of MTX were necessary in 2 cases, one of which was a case of persistent EP. In that case, additional dactinomycin was given. Laparoscopic surgery was adopted in one case of ampullary pregnancy, where initial hCG was 8952 IU/ml (Table 6).
In the following, we present one successful case and one difficult case where additional Actynomycin D was necessary.

Serum hCG (mIU/ml)	Success (%)	Multiple dose	Failure (%)
<1000	11(91.6)	2	1(8.4)
1000-1999	6(85.7)	0	1(14.3)
2000-4999	7(63.6)	2	4(34.6)
5000-9999	7(87.5)	2	1(12.5)
10000-14999	1(100)	0	0(0)
>15000	5(100)	2	0(0)

Table 5. Clinical outcomes

	Regimen
Multiple dose	Methotrxate 1 mg per kg intramusculrarly, alternate days (days 1, 3, 5, 7) +leucovorin 0.1mg per kg intramuscularly, alternate days (days 2, 4, 6, 8). Continue until beta-hCG falls >15% in 48h or four doses methtorexate. If beta-hCG concentration not <40% of initial value on day 14.
Single dose	Methotrxate 50 mg per m^2 intramusculrarly. If beta-hCG is not <15% between days 4 and 7, repeat dose. Up to 4 doses can be given if beta-hCG does not decline by 15% every week.

Table 6. Regiment of MTX

Case I

In the first case, a patient was referred to our hospital for a suspected right interstitial pregnancy. Initial serum hCG was 5979 IU/ml and clinical findings were consistent with the criteria for the diagnosis of an interstitial pregnancy. The patient selected MTX treatment because of her past history with a left salpingectomy for a right ampullary pregnancy.

Therefore, a single dose of MTX was administered. Serum hCG was followed up according to routine, and hCG declined within the normal range after a triple administration (Figure 2).

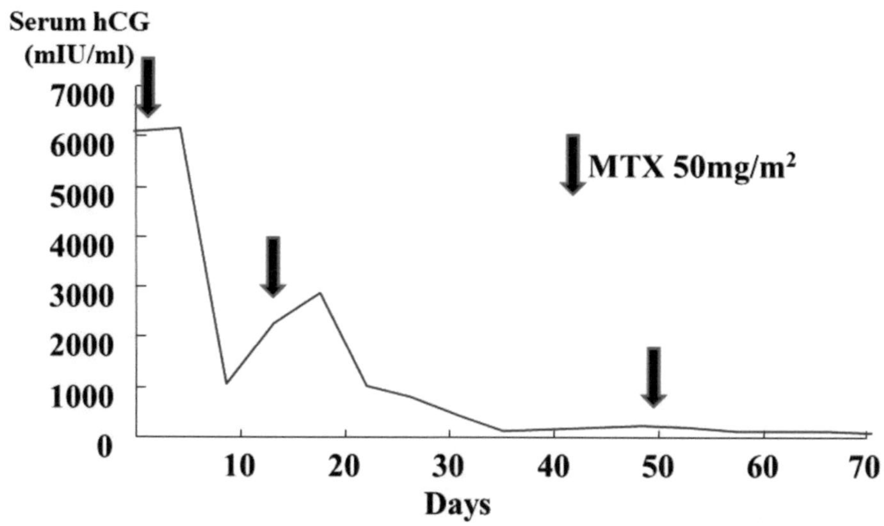

Fig. 2. Time-course of serum hCG level in Case I

Case II

In the second case, the diagnosis of a right interstitial pregnancy was confirmed by MRI and a and high serum hCG level of 26128 IU/ml. Twice before, the patient experienced ectopic pregnancy followed by surgical intervention so, therefore, therefore MTX treatment was started. However, her serum hCG level elevated to 172 IU/ml following three administrations of MTX following the usual single-dose regiment. Therefore, Actinomycin D at a dosage of 12 μg/kg was administered, and an MTX-resistant ectopic pregnancy was suspected (Figure 3). Post-treatment was uneventful, and the side effect of Actinomycin D and MTX was slight nausea alone.

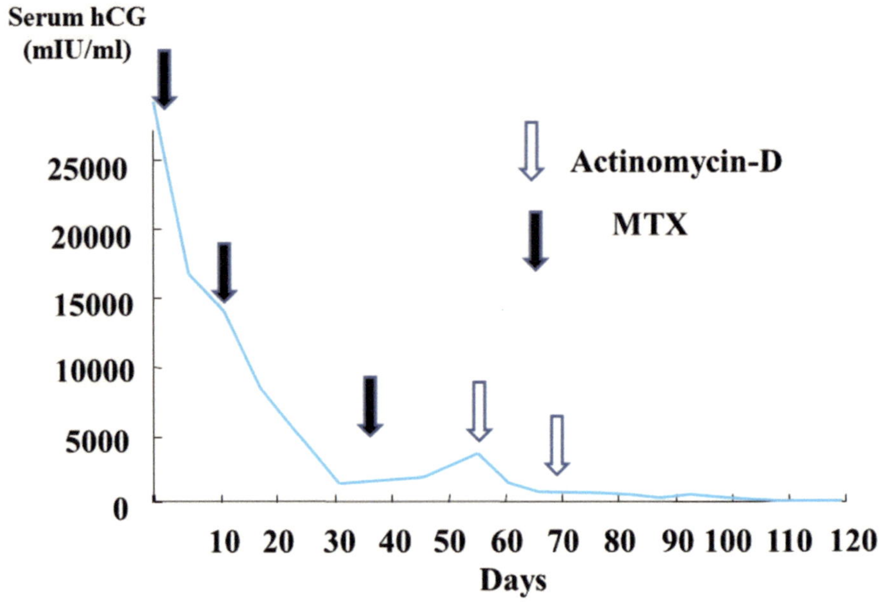

Fig. 3. Time-course of serum hCG level in Case II

4. Discussion

The treatment of EP with MTX was established in the late 1980s and has become an alternative to surgical intervention. Recently, cost-effectiveness analysis has put a priority on the patient's subsequent fertility, rather than on detection and/or complication rates, as previously reported (7-9). Effort should be made to confirm the diagnosis of ectopic pregnancy definitively before starting MTX treatment; otherwise, complication rates or costs could rise on the contrary. Seror et al reported that MTX treatment appeared to be cost-effective in EP cases where the preservation of fertility was important (10). About 40% of women with ectopic pregnancy are treated medically (11), and 90% of them are successfully treated without any surgical intervention at all (12). Medical treatment can be carried out on an outpatient basis, thus making MTX cheaper than the cost of surgical treatment. Surgical intervention is generally adopted when a high possibility of failure and a prolonged time of resolution is predicted. A particularly high serum hCG level or the presence of fetal heart movement results in medical treatment (13).

It is actually difficult to diagnose interstitial pregnancy correctly because of the slight difference between cornual implantation and interstitial pregnancy. Cornual implantation is usually identified in the upper and lateral uterine cavity, whereas interstitial ectopic pregnancy is within the proximal intramural portion of the tube. Therefore, the accurate diagnosis of an interstitial pregnancy requires precise ultrasound imaging (14). Two regimens are commonly used for the administration of MTX (15) (Table 3). The first contains the administration of MTX and leucovorin on alternate days until beta-hCG concentrations begin to drop. This regimen has a success rate of 93%. The second regimen involves the administration of a single dose of MTX, followed by repeated doses every week if beta-hCG concentrations do not fall by 15% within days 4 and 7. It has been reported that at least 13% of women require two doses, and 1% need more than two; however, more than 90% of women who need a second administration avoid surgical intervention (12). The initial level of hCG is the best prognostic indicator of the need for MTX; however, it is still controversial as to what IU should be the cut-point in deciding whether the administration of MTX is necessary. Lipscomb et al. reported that 94% of 350 women whose initial hCG was less than 10,000 IU/ml had success with MTX treatment, therefore suggesting that an initial hCG level greater than 10,000 IU/ml was a factor in the failure of the treatment (12). On the other hand, Gamzu et al. stated that the cut-point to determine the effectiveness of MTX should be lowered to between 2000 mIU/ml and 3000 mIU/ml (16). The hCG incremental rate both before and after MTX represents an independent risk factor for subsequent tubal rupture. Pre-diagnosis concentrations of hCG which increase at least 66% over 48 hours, followed by persistently rising hCG concentrations after treatment with MTX, may lower the threshold for surgical intervention (17).

It is widely accepted that above the discriminatory zone of 1,500 IU/l-2500 IU/l, a normal intrauterine pregnancy (IUP) should be visible via TVU. At our clinic, we consider an initial hCG greater than 1500 IU/ml and an invisible GS clear indicators of a possible ectopic pregnancy, and an elevation of hCG greater than 1.5 times in 48 hours without GS confirms the diagnosis. Orivieto et al. reported that single-dose MTX treatment for EP does not have a negative effect on ovarian function nor on the outcome of following IVF-ICSI (18). Paul et al. reported that when hCG is >4000 IU/ml, the failure rate of MTX treatment is 65% (17). In this study, the MTX-failure rate of 14 cases where initial hCG was >5000 IU/ml was 7.1% (1/14); however, the failure rate of low hCG cases <5000 IU/ml was 16.6%. In tubal pregnancy, EP become less vascularized as it invades the tubal serosa, and tubal rupture is likely to occur, compared with that in interstitial pregnancy, before MTX treatment can solve the EP. Compared with cases of tubal pregnancy, the difficulty in diagnosing interstitial pregnancy is thought to be the reason why hCG levels are higher at the time of confirming the diagnosis. However, in our study, 14 cases consisted of 7 ampullary, 6 interstitial and one cervical pregnancy, indicating that tubal pregnancy does not always rupture in high-hCG cases. Therefore, more study is necessary to determine the cut-off for MTX treatment.

Recently the cost-effectiveness of treatment has been considered in attempts to save on health insurance costs. Seror reported that, although frequent diagnostic ultrasound is necessary, MTX is cost-effective compared with surgical intervention (10). However, subsequent pregnancies should be followed with extreme caution, and elective cesarean section should be considered as an alternative.

In conclusion, a serum hCG level greater than 5,000 IU/ml is not necessarily resistant to MTX treatment, and interstitial pregnancy is a particularly good candidate for conservative treatment, even if initial hCG is higher than 5,000 IU/ml. However, MTX failure and tubal rupture was identified irrespective of an initial hCG level of 800 IU/ml in tubal pregnancy. Emergent access to surgical intervention must be made available. As well, the patient's awareness of risk and her availability for admission and surgery are equally important. Therefore, preparation for surgical intervention for emergent situations, even after conservative treatment is determined, is essential.

5. References

[1] Satoe Fujiwara, Yoshiki Yamashita, Sachiko Kawabe, Hideki Kamegai, Yoshito Terai, Masahide Ohmichi. A case of a methotrexate-resistant ectopic pregnancy in which

dactinomycin was effective as a second-line chemotherapy. Fertil Steril 2009;91:929. e13-15.
[2] Tanaka T, Hayashi H, Kutsuzawa T, Fujimoto S, Ichinoue K. Treatment of interstitial ectopic pregnancy with methotrexate : report of a successful case. Fertil Steril 1982;37:851-2.
[3] Havenius PJ, Engelsbel S, Mol BW, et al. Systemic methtorexate versus laparoscopic salpingostomy in tubal pregnancy: a randomized clinical trial. Lancet 1997; 350:774-79.
[4] Stovall TG, Ling FW, Buster JE. Outpatient chemotherapy of unruptured ectopic pregnancy. Fertil Steril 1989;51:435-8.
[5] Pisarska MD, Crason SA, Buster JE. Ectopic pregnancy. Lancet 1998;351:115-20.
[6] Lipscomb GH, Stovall TG, Ling SW. Nonsurgical treatment of ectopic pregnancy. N Engl J Med 2000;343:1325-9.
[7] The practice committee of the ASRM. Medical treatment of ectopic pregnancy. Fertil Steril 2008;Supply 3:S206-212.
[8] Morlock RJ, Lafata JE, Eisenstein D. Cost-effectiveness of single-dose methotrexate compared with laparoscopic treatment of ectopic pregnancy. Obstet Gynecol 2000;95:407-12.
[9] Dourston WE, Carl ML, Guerra W, Eaton A, Ackerson LM. Ultrasound availability in the evaluation of ectopic pregnancy in the ED: comparison of quality and cost-effectiveness with different approaches. Am J Emerg Med 2000;18:408-17.
[10] Sowter MC, Farquhar CM, Gudex G. An economic evaluation of single dose systemic methotrexate and laparoscopic surgery for the treatment of unruptured ectopic pregnancy. BJOG 2001;108:204-12.
[11] Seror V, Gelfucci F, Gerbaud L, Pouly JL, Fernandez H, Job-Spira N, Bouyer J, Coste J. Care pathways for ectopic pregnancy: a population-based cost-effectiveness analysis. Fertil Steril 2007;87:737-748.
[12] Barnhart KT, Gosman G, Ashby R, Sammel M. The medical management of ectopic pregnancy: meta-analysis comparing "single dose and multidose" regimens. Obstet Gynecol 2003;101:778-84.
[13] Lipscomb GH, McCord ML, Stovall TG, Huff G, Portera SG, Ling FW. Predictors of success of methotrexate treatment in women with rubal ectopic pregnancies. New Engl J Med 1999;341:1974-8
[14] Morlock RJ, Lafata JE, Eisenstein D. Cost-effectiveness of single-dose methotrexate compared with laparoscopic treatment of ectopic pregnancy. Obstet Gynecol 2000;95:407-12.
[15] Malinowski A, Bates SK. Semantics and pfitfalls in the diagnosis cornual/interstitial pregnancy. Fertil Steril 2006;86:e11-14.
[16] Farquhar CM. Ectopic pregnancy. Lancet 2005;366:583-591.
[17] Gamezu R, Almog B, Levin Y, Amiram a, Jaffa A, Lessing J, Baram A. Efficacy of methotrexate treatment in extrauterine pregnancies defined by stable or increasing human gonadotropin concentrations. Fertil Steril 2002;77:761-765.
[18] Dudley PS, Heard MJ, Sangi-Haghpeykar H, Carson SA, Buster JE. Characterizing ectopic pregnancies that rupture despite of treatment with methotrexate. Fertil Steril 2004;82:1374-1378.
[19] Orivieto R, Kruchkovich J, Zohav E, Rabinson J. Does methotrexate treatment for ectopic pregnancy influence the patient's performance during a subsequent in vitro fertilization/embryo transfer cycle? Fertil Steril 2007;88:1685-86.

13

The Treatment of Ectopic Pregnancy with Laparoscopy-Assisted Local Injection of Chemotherapeutic Agents

Ching-Hui Chen[1], Peng-Hui Wang[2], Li-Hsuan Chiu[3] and Wei-Min Liu[1*]
[1]*Department of Obstetrics and Gynecology, Taipei Medical University Hospital and Taipei Medical University, Taipei*
[2]*Department of Obstetrics and Gynecology, Taipei Veterans General Hospital and National Yang-Ming University, Taipei*
[3]*Graduate Institute of Medical Sciences, Taipei Medical University, Taipei*
Taiwan

1. Introduction

Laparoscopy-assisted local injection of chemotherapeutic agents is not yet considered as a standard treatment for ectopic pregnancy. Herein, we demonstrated cases of cesarean scar pregnancy and ovarian ectopic pregnancy successfully treated with trans-vaginal sonography-guided local injection of etoposide. Furthermore, we evaluated the efficacy of laparoscopic local injection of etoposide compared with methotrexate on tubal pregnancy treatment. With the aid of laparoscopic injection, local etoposide treatment offers a precise localization and minimally invasive approach to the management of ectopic pregnancies. Compared to the conventional way to treat ectopic pregnancy using methotrexate, local injection of etoposide is considered to be a high-success rate, low-risk, and less-limitation option for such types of ectopic pregnancies with careful selection of cases.

2. Current opinion and therapeutic strategy on ectopic pregnancies

Ectopic pregnancy is a complication of pregnancy in which the fetus implants outside the endometrial cavity, which ultimately ends in death of the fetus. It constitutes 1.6% of all pregnancies (Lurie, 1992). Most ectopic pregnancies are located in the fallopian tube, but the implantation can also occur in the cervix, ovaries, abdomen, and even cesarean scars. Ectopic pregnancy is usually not viable. If left untreated, half of ectopic pregnancies will resolve without treatment and presents as the tubal abortions. Ectopic pregnancies are considered as a dangerous health problem for women of childbearing age because of the internal bleeding as a common complication. In fact, maternal mortality is 0.14% in cases of ectopic pregnancy (Lurie, 1992; Te Linde, Rock, & Thompson, 1997).

Within various forms of ectopic pregnancies, cesarean scar pregnancy is a rare form of ectopic implantation. The pathogenesis is thought to be a normal fertilization followed by implantation at the ecchymotic lesion site which is bulging from the uterine wall at the

* Corresponding Author

cesarean scar. If a caesarean scar pregnancy continues developing to second or third trimesters, there might be risks of uterine rupture or catastrophic hemorrhage which may cause serious maternal morbidity and loss of fertility. Differential diagnosis and early diagnosis of such an ectopic pregnancy is now more feasible because of the use of high-resolution transvaginal sonography and the availability of sensitive β-hCG assay.

Primary ovarian pregnancy is also considered as an uncommon form of ectopic implantation and represents 0.5%–3% of all ectopic pregnancies. The pathogenic mechanism is thought to be fertilization occurring outside the tube, followed by implantation within the ovary. Differential diagnosis of an ovarian pregnancy from a tubal pregnancy has been a challenge in the past. However, due to the improvement of high-resolution transvaginal sonography and the availability of sensitive β-hCG assay, an early diagnosis of an ovarian pregnancy is now more feasible.

Once diagnosed, the conventional treatment of ectopic pregnancy is surgical approach. The traditional method for management of a cesarean scar pregnancy is surgical removal of the ectopic pregnancy (Arslan, et al., 2005; C. B. Wang & Tseng, 2006; Y. L. Wang, Su, & Chen, 2006). There have been few reports showing that cesarean scar pregnancies were successfully treated by local injection of methotrexate (Hwu, Hsu, & Yang, 2005; Ravhon, Ben-Chetrit, Rabinowitz, Neuman, & Beller, 1997). Similarly, the traditional management mean for ovarian pregnancy is surgical removal of the ectopic site, either by ipsilateral oophorectomy or wedge resection by laparotomy or laparoscopy(Yen & Wang, 2004). There has been sporadic case reports showing that ovarian pregnancy was successfully treated by systemic methotrexate injection (Chelmow, Gates, & Penzias, 1994; Field & Faraj, 2005; Habbu & Read, 2006).

Methotrexate is not yet a first-line treatment for ovarian pregnancy or cesarean scar pregnancy even in candidates who meet the criteria for medical treatment (Bagga, Suri, Verma, Chopra, & Kalra, 2006; Medical treatment of ectopic pregnancy," 2006). However, the use of systemic methotrexate treatment has considered being an option to preserve potential fertility in ectopic pregnancy patients (Hung, Jeng, Yang, Wang, & Lan, 1996; Marcovici, Rosenzweig, Brill, Khan, & Scommegna, 1994; Timor-Tritsch, et al., 1994). Several risk factors have to be evaluated while systemic methotrexate is indicated for the treatment of ectopic pregnancy. The patient should be hemodynamically stable, have no severe contraindications to methotrexate. Furthermore, the size of the gestation sac should not exceed 3 cm under ultrasound measurement, and the serum β-hCG level should not exceed 2000 mIU/mL. In cases of tubal ectopic pregnancy, the presence of an embryonic cardiac activity was generally considered to be a contraindication to methotrexate therapy (Ory, 1992). Ushakov et al. reported that the side effects of systemic methotrexate treatment occurred 15% of the time, which include bone marrow depression, stomatitis, anorexia, nausea, vomiting, and diarrhea (Floridon & Thomsen, 1994; Ushakov, Elchalal, Aceman, & Schenker, 1997). These contraindications and side effects have become the limitations of systemic treatment of methotrexate on ectopic pregnancy.

AS a result, considering the highly vascularized tissues involved in the surgical procedure and the contraindications of systemic therapy, local injection of the chemotherapeutic agents is then suggested. There have been few reports showing that ectopic pregnancies were successfully treated by local injection of methotrexate or etoposide (C. H. Chen, Wang, & Liu, 2009; Hwu, et al., 2005; Juan, Wang, Chen, Ma, & Liu, 2008; Ravhon, et al., 1997). With laparoscopic local injection, the chemotherapeutic agent such as methotrexate or etoposide could be precisely injected into the ectopic implantation. These procedures lead to a significant decline in side effects and contribute to the preservation of the patients' reproductive potential. However, comparing to methotrexate, etoposide is not yet a widely used treatment for ectopic pregnancy, and there are still no criteria established. Even in cases of all kinds of ectopic pregnancy, the uses of etoposide were reported in less than ten cases since 1990 (C. L. Chen, Wang, Chiu, Yang, & Hung, 2002; Juan, et al., 2008; Mantalenakis, et al., 1995; Seki, Kuromaki, Takeda, & Kinoshita, 1997; Takashima, et al., 1995). Herein we demonstrated various cases including ovarian, CS scar, and tubal pregnancies successfully treated by laparoscopic local injection of etoposide with trans-vaginal sonography -assisted localization. Furthermore, since etoposide and methotrexate have been applied locally to treat ectopic pregnancy, we evaluated the clinical efficacies of local treatment of these two chemotherapeutic agents.

3. Cases: The treatment of cesarean scar and ovarian pregnancies with laparoscopy-assisted local injection of etoposide

Case I: A 37 year-old-female, gravida 5, para 2 (cesarean section twice), abortion 2, had presented with a 8-week history of gestational amenorrhea. She accidentally found herself pregnancy and asked for an elective abortion in a local clinic. Her general condition was fair. She was considered intra-uterine pregnancy at local clinic and uterine curettage had been performed 3 times since she kept suffering from vaginal bleeding after first curettage. She came to our hospital for second opinion due to persistent vaginal bleeding. trans-vaginal sonography revealed an empty uterus and suggested an ectopic sac of 1.9 x 1.7 cm in diameter between anterior wall of uterus and bladder on previous cesarean scar. β-hCG level was measured at 572.2 mIU/mL. Based on these findings, a cesarean pregnancy was suspected.
A laparoscopy was then performed while an ecchymotic lesion (2cm) found bulging from the uterine wall at the previous cesarean scar area. The two fallopian tubes and two ovaries were intact and normal. Confirmed with trans-vaginal sonography, the mass was indicated

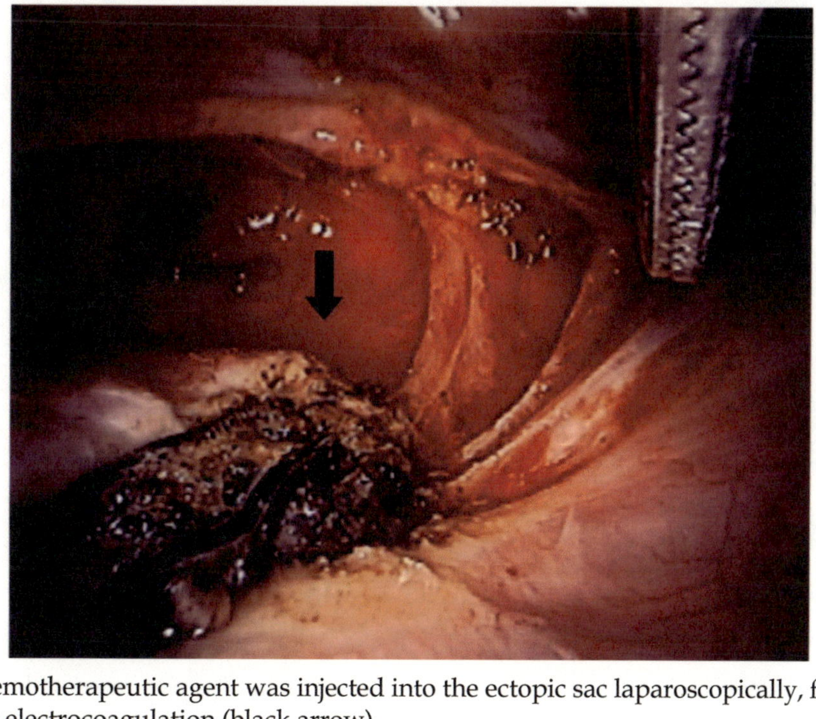

Fig. 1. Chemotherapeutic agent was injected into the ectopic sac laparoscopically, followed by bipolar electrocoagulation (black arrow).

a cesarean scar pregnancy. With the guidance of trans-vaginal sonography to precisely estimate the depth of the puncture site to the gestational sac, 100mg of etoposide was directly injected into the ectopic sac by laparoscopy (Figure 1). The puncture site was immediately sealed by bipolar electro-coagulation. The patient was followed up with serial trans-vaginal sonography and β-hCG level monitoring. The trans-vaginal sonography showed a progressive shrinkage of the mass, and the β-hCG levels declined continuously to 28.1 mIU/mL 9 days after the surgery, and 5.0 mIU/mL 17 days later. The patient experienced normal menstruation 45 days after the procedure.

Case II: A 33-year-old woman, gravida 1, para 0, had presented with a 7-week history of gestational amenorrhea and lower abdominal discomfort. Her general condition was fair. The serum b-hCG level was measured at 2,765 mIU/mL. The trans-vaginal sonography revealed an empty uterus and suggested an ectopic sac of 4.3 by 2.8 cm in diameter in the right ovarian region. The fluid in the Douglas pouch measured 2.0 x 1.8 cm in diameter. Based on these findings, an ovarian pregnancy was suspected. A laparoscopy was then performed. One hundred milliliters of bloody fluid was collected from the cul-de-sac. The two fallopian tubes were intact, and the uterus and left ovary were normal. A 4-cm diameter bluish and hemorrhagic mass on the right ovary indicated the possibility of an ovarian pregnancy. Punch with aspiration and direct injection of 100 mg of etoposide into the ectopic sac (Figure 2) was performed and the fluid aspirated from the hemorrhagic sac seen

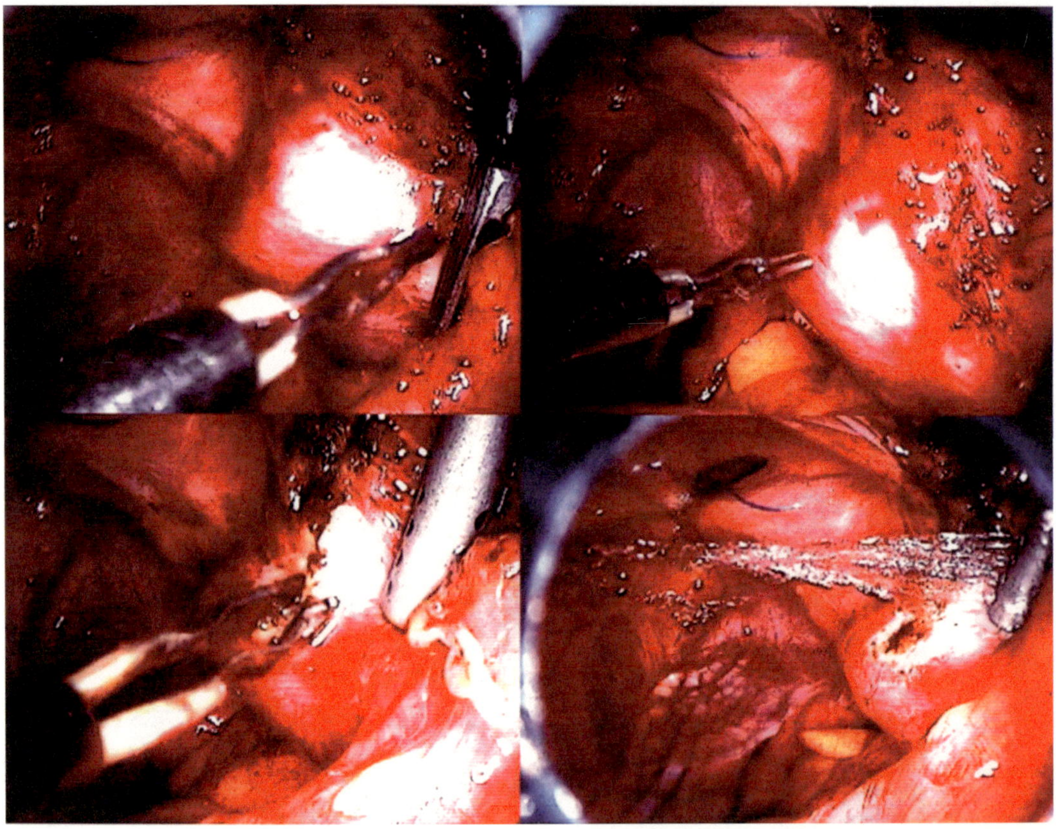

Fig. 2. After local injection of the chemotherapeutic agent, bipolar electro-coagulation was used to seal the puncture site.

at laparoscopy was sent for pathologic examination, which showed scant chorionic villi and granulosa cells (GC) in support of the diagnosis of ovarian pregnancy. The patient was followed up with serial trans-vaginal sonography and checking of b-hCG levels. The b-hCG levels declined continuously to 37.34 mIU/mL 8 days after surgery and 6.01 mIU/ mL 1 week later. The patient menstruated 25 days after the procedure.

The traditional treatments for ectopic pregnancies are considered more invasive procedures. Therefore, how to select one of the less invasive procedures to diagnose and treat this rare ectopic pregnancy is important. For example, in case I, a deeply implanted cesarean scar pregnancy was growing towards the abdominal cavity and bladder, thus we choose laparoscopy as a primary mean to approach the cesarean scar pregnancy (Vial, Petignat, & Hohlfeld, 2000; C. J. Wang, et al., 2006). Trans-vaginal sonography-guided local injection not only offers a precise localization of the injection site, but also offered a minimally invasive procedure for the case. Furthermore, local injection of etoposide bypasses the systemic side effects of the drug. Taken together, trans-vaginal sonography-guided laparoscopic local injection of etoposide for such cases are suggested.

4. The comparison of etoposide and methotrexate efficacies on tubal pregnancy treatment

Etoposide, an antineoplastic agent, can produce cytotoxic effects by damaging DNA, thereby inhibiting or altering DNA synthesis. The drug appears to be cell-cycle dependent and cycle-phase specific, inducing G2 phase arrest and killing cells in the G2 and late S phases. In 2002, Chen et al. successfully used a ultrasound-guided direct injection of etoposide to treat an interstitial pregnancy (C. L. Chen, et al., 2002). Based on the finding that etoposide was more effective and had fewer side effects in the management of low-risk gestational trophoblastic tumor, compared to methotrexate treatment (Matsui, et al., 2005), direct injection of etoposide for ectopic pregnancy is considered. Local administration of methotrexate was described in several cases (Hung, et al., 1996; Monteagudo, Minior, Stephenson, Monda, & Timor-Tritsch, 2005; Timor-Tritsch, et al., 1994). On the other aspect, the use of etoposide in ectopic pregnancy is relatively new. The standardized protocol is not yet available, although there were few cases used ultrasound-guided direct injection of etoposide to treat ectopic pregnancy (C. H. Chen, et al., 2009; C. L. Chen, et al., 2002; Juan, et al., 2008).

From 1993 through 2009, 28 patients of tubal pregnancy received local injection of methotrexate or etoposide were documented. In all cases, age, body weight, hemoglobin level and the operation time were recorded. The gestational age, cardiac activity of the conceptus, β-hCG levels before and after the treatment, and the occurrence and outcomes of subsequent pregnancies were evaluated. Among the enrolled patients, methotrexate has been administered locally to 11 patients and etoposide to 17 patients. In group (I), 50 mg of etoposide was injected into the ectopic sites by laparoscopy. In group (II), 50 mg of methotrexate was applied. All patients were followed up with serial β-hCG level monitoring. None of the patients had significant side effects of systemic treatment of the agents. More than 50% of the patients had a gestational size of greater than 30 mm.

The administration of methotrexate locally was chosen to avoid the adverse effect of systemic administration of methotrexate. Hung et al. observed that methotrexate alone or combined with procedures such as curettage or cervical tamponade is effective in ectopic pregnancies of up to 12 weeks (Hung, et al., 1996). In this survey, the median (range) of the time it took to decline to the non-pregnant β-hCG level (undetectable or below 5 mIU/mL) of methotrexate injection group was longer than the etoposide injection group, though not significant difference is observed (Table 1).

	Etoposide treatment (n=11) Median (range)	Methotrexate treatment (n=17) Median (range)	P Value
Age (years)	34 (26~37)	31 (22~38)	-
Body weight (kg)	52.3 (47.4~62.1)	49.7 (45~58)	-
Basal Hgb (g/dL)	11.1 (9.7~12.8)	10.6 (9.3~13.1)	-
β-hCG (mIU/mL)	2081 (430.1~55225)	7926 (250~27356)	0.50
Time of β-hCG level declined to below 5 mIU/mL (days)	19 (7~90)	37 (12~98)	0.28
Time of involution of gestational sac (days)	27 (18~116)	44 (19~134)	0.26

Table 1. Baseline characteristics of the enrolled women

There is still no consensus about the most appropriate treatment for ectopic pregnancy. Therefore, large prospective randomized trials are still needed to establish common selection criteria, dosage, and length of follow up of the therapies. Furthermore, to increase the success rate, experiences in invasive ultrasound-guided procedures is indeed crucial for the success of this treatment option, but careful selection of patients and their compliance is also important. In this study, local injection of 50 mg etoposide to treat ectopic pregnancy was evaluated and compared with local injection of methotrexate. In women who desire future pregnancy, these two types of conservative treatment may be an acceptable and promising alternative in the management of ectopic pregnancy. Taken together, a local injection of etoposide might be a good choice for ectopic pregnancy.

5. Summary

The advances in ultrasound equipment and easy access to quantitative β-hCG have made the diagnosis of early ectopic pregnancies possible. The efforts to improve the management of ectopic pregnancy have also stimulated many investigators to design new approaches to treat early ectopic pregnancy. This enables successful application of conservative therapies such as local treatment of chemotherapeutic agents such as etoposide or methotrexate. Not like methotrexate, etoposide is not yet considered as a standard treatment for ectopic pregnancy while there are still no criteria established. As compared to local methotrexate treatment, local etoposide treatment has the advantages of better efficacy to treat patients with higher β-hCG level. With the aid of laparoscopic injection, local treatment of etoposide is considered as a precise localization and the minimally invasive option to the management of ectopic pregnancy.

6. Acknowledgement

Part of the contents and research materials in this chapter were extracted from our previous works in Fertility and Sterility. We are giving full acknowledgment of the original publication of the article. Changes may have been made to this work since it was extended and re-edited to a book-length form.

7. References

Arslan, M., Pata, O., Dilek, T. U., Aktas, A., Aban, M., & Dilek, S. (2005). Treatment of viable cesarean scar ectopic pregnancy with suction curettage. *Int J Gynaecol Obstet, 89*(2), 163-166.

Bagga, R., Suri, V., Verma, P., Chopra, S., & Kalra, J. (2006). Failed medical management in ovarian pregnancy despite favorable prognostic factors--a case report. *MedGenMed, 8*(2), 35.

Chelmow, D., Gates, E., & Penzias, A. S. (1994). Laparoscopic diagnosis and methotrexate treatment of an ovarian pregnancy: a case report. *Fertil Steril, 62*(4), 879-881.

Chen, C. H., Wang, P. H., & Liu, W. M. (2009). Successful treatment of cesarean scar pregnancy using laparoscopically assisted local injection of etoposide with transvaginal ultrasound guidance. *Fertil Steril, 92*(5), 1747 e1749-1711.

Chen, C. L., Wang, P. H., Chiu, L. M., Yang, M. L., & Hung, J. H. (2002). Successful conservative treatment for advanced interstitial pregnancy. A case report. *J Reprod Med, 47*(5), 424-426.

Field, S. M., & Faraj, R. (2005). Ovarian pregnancy in the wall of corpus luteum. *J Obstet Gynaecol, 25*(6), 615-616.

Floridon, C., & Thomsen, S. G. (1994). Methotrexate treatment of ectopic pregnancy. *Acta Obstet Gynecol Scand, 73*(10), 746-752.

Habbu, J., & Read, M. D. (2006). Ovarian pregnancy successfully treated with methotrexate. *J Obstet Gynaecol, 26*(6), 587-588.

Hung, T. H., Jeng, C. J., Yang, Y. C., Wang, K. G., & Lan, C. C. (1996). Treatment of cervical pregnancy with methotrexate. *Int J Gynaecol Obstet, 53*(3), 243-247.

Hwu, Y. M., Hsu, C. Y., & Yang, H. Y. (2005). Conservative treatment of caesarean scar pregnancy with transvaginal needle aspiration of the embryo. *BJOG, 112*(6), 841-842.

Juan, Y. C., Wang, P. H., Chen, C. H., Ma, P. C., & Liu, W. M. (2008). Successful treatment of ovarian pregnancy with laparoscopy-assisted local injection of etoposide. *Fertil Steril, 90*(4), 1200 e1201-1202.

Lurie, S. (1992). The history of the diagnosis and treatment of ectopic pregnancy: a medical adventure. *Eur J Obstet Gynecol Reprod Biol, 43*(1), 1-7.

Mantalenakis, S., Tsalikis, T., Grimbizis, G., Aktsalis, A., Mamopoulos, M., & Farmakides, G. (1995). Successful pregnancy after treatment of cervical pregnancy with methotrexate and curettage. A case report. *J Reprod Med, 40*(5), 409-414.

Marcovici, I., Rosenzweig, B. A., Brill, A. I., Khan, M., & Scommegna, A. (1994). Cervical pregnancy: case reports and a current literature review. *Obstet Gynecol Surv, 49*(1), 49-55.

Matsui, H., Suzuka, K., Yamazawa, K., Tanaka, N., Mitsuhashi, A., Seki, K., et al. (2005). Relapse rate of patients with low-risk gestational trophoblastic tumor initially treated with single-agent chemotherapy. *Gynecol Oncol, 96*(3), 616-620.

Medical treatment of ectopic pregnancy. (2006). *Fertil Steril, 86*(5 Suppl 1), S96-102.

Monteagudo, A., Minior, V. K., Stephenson, C., Monda, S., & Timor-Tritsch, I. E. (2005). Non-surgical management of live ectopic pregnancy with ultrasound-guided local injection: a case series. *Ultrasound Obstet Gynecol, 25*(3), 282-288.

Ory, S. J. (1992). New options for diagnosis and treatment of ectopic pregnancy. *JAMA, 267*(4), 534-537.

Ravhon, A., Ben-Chetrit, A., Rabinowitz, R., Neuman, M., & Beller, U. (1997). Successful methotrexate treatment of a viable pregnancy within a thin uterine scar. *Br J Obstet Gynaecol, 104*(5), 628-629.

Seki, H., Kuromaki, K., Takeda, S., & Kinoshita, K. (1997). Ovarian pregnancy diagnosed in the third trimester: a case report. *J Obstet Gynaecol Res, 23*(6), 543-546.

Takashima, M., Yamasaki, M., Fujita, I., Ohashi, M., Matsuo, H., Mochizuki, M., et al. (1995). Enhanced magnetic resonance imaging in monitoring of conservative treatment of cervical pregnancy. *J Obstet Gynaecol, 21*(6), 545-550.

Te Linde, R. W., Rock, J. A., & Thompson, J. D. (1997). *Te Linde's operative gynecology* (8th ed.). Philadelphia: Lippincott-Raven.

Timor-Tritsch, I. E., Monteagudo, A., Mandeville, E. O., Peisner, D. B., Anaya, G. P., & Pirrone, E. C. (1994). Successful management of viable cervical pregnancy by local injection of methotrexate guided by transvaginal ultrasonography. *Am J Obstet Gynecol, 170*(3), 737-739.

Ushakov, F. B., Elchalal, U., Aceman, P. J., & Schenker, J. G. (1997). Cervical pregnancy: past and future. *Obstet Gynecol Surv, 52*(1), 45-59.

Vial, Y., Petignat, P., & Hohlfeld, P. (2000). Pregnancy in a cesarean scar. *Ultrasound Obstet Gynecol, 16*(6), 592-593.

Wang, C. B., & Tseng, C. J. (2006). Primary evacuation therapy for Cesarean scar pregnancy: three new cases and review. *Ultrasound Obstet Gynecol, 27*(2), 222-226.

Wang, C. J., Chao, A. S., Yuen, L. T., Wang, C. W., Soong, Y. K., & Lee, C. L. (2006). Endoscopic management of cesarean scar pregnancy. *Fertil Steril, 85*(2), 494 e491-494.

Wang, Y. L., Su, T. H., & Chen, H. S. (2006). Operative laparoscopy for unruptured ectopic pregnancy in a caesarean scar. *BJOG, 113*(9), 1035-1038.

Yen, M. S., & Wang, P. H. (2004). Primary ovarian ectopic pregnancy. *J Am Assoc Gynecol Laparosc, 11*(3), 287-288.

14

Fertility-Preserving Surgery for Cervical Ectopic Pregnancy, from Past to Present

Seiryu Kamoi, Nao Iwasaki and Toshiyuki Takeshita
Department of Obstetetrics and Gynecology, Nippon Medical School, Tokyo, Japan

1. Introduction

Cervical pregnancy is a rare form of ectopic pregnancy in which implantation occurs in the cervical mucosa below the level of the internal os of the uterus. In the past, especially when diagnostic tools like ultrasonography or MRI were unavailable, many patients frequently encountered life-threatening, uncontrollable hemorrhage either spontaneously or when the implant was evacuated by curettage with a presumptive diagnosis of incomplete or inevitable abortion[1]. Hysterectomy was the only measure that could save those patients [2, 3], although some surgeons challenged surgical methods to preserve fertility [4-8].

Many successful cases of fertility preservation have been reported since anti-chorionic villi drugs like methotrexate (MTX) became available and interventional radiology techniques were improved to reduce hemorrhage during curettage or evacuation. However, hysterectomy is still considered the final measure.

This chapter first describes the history of cervical ectopic pregnancy, followed by the history of its treatment in the past. Then, we present our novel fertility-preserving surgical technique in addition to a review of the uterine-conservation techniques which have been reported in the past.

2. Historical review of cervical ectopic pregnancy

According to Thomsen and Johansen, the first case of cervical pregnancy was reported in 1817 by Sir Everard Home, who found an early ovum in the cervical canal during post-mortem examination. Thereafter, more and more cases were reported soon after Karl Freiherr von Rokitansky described two cases in 1860 in the German literature. The maternal mortality rate early in the 1900s was exceptionally high mainly due to hemorrhage and sepsis (66% according to Hofsatter; 43% according to Zangemeister and Schilling; 13% according to Concetti), and was estimated to be an average of 30%[9].

However, this rate is not considered to have actually been this high, because of the limited ability of exact diagnosis in those days. That is, patients underwent evacuation of the uterus based on incorrect diagnosis, consequently suffering from massive hemorrhage, which was treated by hysterectomy. In 1946, Schneider defined "distal ectopic pregnancy" as a pregnancy in which the fetus resides in the cervical canal. He classified it into three categories by implantation site: (1) 'pure' cervical ectopic pregnancy; (2) isthmico-cervical pregnancy; and (3) endometrio-isthmico-cervical pregnancy[10]. With the probable inclusion of distal ectopic pregnancy other than true cervical pregnancy or other unconfirmed cases, Baptisti estimated the mortality rate to be only 6% of cases published between 1945 and 1953 and stated that this remarkable decline in the mortality rate was due to the development of blood transfusion in modern obstetrics[11].

Shinagawa, in his 10 years of experience, reported in 1969 about 19 cervical pregnancy cases, all of which resulted in abdominal hysterectomy after attempted vaginal treatment to save the uterus. He expressed his surprise for the discrepancy in the frequency of cases between the United States and Japan[12]. In the United States, a little over 80 cases had been reported up until 1967[13]. Sheldon et al. experienced two cases at the Mayo Clinic over a 15-year period, an incidence of approximately 1 in 16,000 pregnancies[7], while Paalman and McElin found only five cases in a series of 47,974 pregnancies at two American hospitals over a 10-year period—an incidence of 0.01%[14]. On the other hand, in Japan, in addition to Shinagawa's 19 cases of approximately 19,000 pregnancies reported at his university hospital and affiliated hospitals between 1958 and 1967, at least 119 cases had been reported throughout Japan between 1953 and 1967[12], suggesting the estimated incidence of the cervical ectopic pregnancy in Japan to be 0.1% (1:1000 pregnancies). Considering that no nulliparous woman was in his series and in 13 of the 19 cases of antecedent pregnancy were interrupted artificially, Shinagawa supposed that the difference in incidence was due to the higher number of legal abortions at that time in Japan. Therefore, the true incidence of cervical ectopic pregnancy is unknown, and comparison between countries is difficult because of the differences in cultures and eras.

Summarizing the past treatments in the literature, Thomsen and Johansen stated that most of the cases were treated based on incorrect original diagnosis[15]. Attempts to evacuate the uterus digitally or instrumentally usually produced violent hemorrhage, and in many cases it was so severe as to necessitate hysterectomy. Several authors reportedly controlled the bleeding by packing, sometimes with fibrin foam, or by amputating the cervix. Although utero-tonic agents are generally used against bleeding after delivery, Danforth pointed out that such agents are ineffective against hemorrhage as the open vessels could not be closed by contraction of the thin-walled, distended cervix, which contains few contractile elements[16]. Schneider and Drezin[17] and Steinbiss[18] also noted that tamponade may provide initial success of hemostasis, but a severe secondary hemorrhage may nevertheless occur up to six weeks later necessitating hysterectomy. By the 1950s, clinicians attempted to conserve the uterus during the treatment of cervical ectopic pregnancy with the establishment of blood transfusion methods[11].

3. Cases of cervical ectopic pregnancy with successful uterine conservation

In 1963, Sheldon and his colleagues reported two cases of cervical pregnancy[7]. One patient was a 42-year-old woman (gravida 3, para 2) who was treated with vigorous curettage when massive genital bleeding began. The pregnancy was terminated with little bleeding during the operation and with an uneventful postoperative follow-up. She had no further pregnancies.

The second patient was a 33-year-old woman (gravida 5, para 4) who underwent excision of the implantation site by sharp dissection and several sutures in the cervix; after curettage had caused heavy bleeding (>1000 ml), bleeding was controlled with tight packing by iodoform gauze. She was dismissed from the hospital on the fourth day and successfully gave birth to a girl.

In addition to these two cases, few cases have addressed efforts to determine a successful conservative therapy—one case by Whittle in 1976[8], four cases by Materacaru in 1968[19], and one case by Farghaly et al. in 1980[6].

The summary of the procedures for these cases are as follows. 1) The approach is vaginal. 2) The urinary bladder is moved upwards through a transverse incision of the anterior vaginal wall to make visible the whole anterior cervix. 3) Bleeding is controlled by clamping each side of the cervix to occlude the lateral cervical blood vessel. 4) The anterior cervical wall is incised longitudinally upwards from the external os to the internal os. 5) If the conceptive products have been implanted in the anterior wall, the local cervical wall is excised with the ectopic fetus, and both sides are sutured; if the implantation site is posterior, complete curettage is performed under direct visualization, usually requiring several sutures for the torn sites of the thin wall. 6) The procedure is achieved by removing the hemostasis clamp and packing the vaginal and cervical canal with gauze. During the procedure, blood transfusion of >1000 ml is usually necessary to maintain the patient's circulation.

Although such procedures involve a vaginal approach, abdominal surgery was also attempted during the same period. In 1969, Nelson applied ligation of the bilateral internal iliac arteries in two cases to perform successful curettage[20], following the idea of Dodeck[21].

The first case was a 17-year-old woman (gravida 1, para 0) who consulted a doctor because of low abdominal pain and abnormal vaginal bleeding. Although a 12-week pregnancy-sized pelvic mass was confirmed, the pregnancy test was negative. Therefore, exploratory laparotomy was indicated and it showed normal sized uterine corpus that had elevated out of the pelvis by a 10-cm soft cystic enlargement of the cervix. Cervical pregnancy was diagnosed. A large amount of necrotic placental tissue and an old clot was removed by vaginal curettage with 250 ml of blood loss after bilateral internal iliac artery ligation under laparotomy. Three years later, she became pregnant which ended in incomplete infected abortion. The following year, she received total abdominal hysterectomy and bilateral salpingo-oophorectomy because of a recurrent tubo-ovarian abscess.

The second case was a 33-year-old woman (gravida 3, para 2) who consulted a doctor with profuse vaginal bleeding at week 11 of gestation. With a diagnosis of threatened abortion, curettage was attempted. The first introduction of forceps into the cervical canal caused sudden loss of over 300 ml of blood, and further evacuation brought on uncontrollable hemorrhage. Laparotomy confirmed cervical pregnancy and bilateral internal iliac artery ligation was applied, followed by evacuation of the placental tissue by curettage. Estimated blood loss was 1200 ml, necessitating whole-blood transfusion.

Shinagawa stated that satisfactory hemostasis could not be achieved by internal iliac artery ligation, based on his reports of 19 cases which all received a hysterectomy after attempts to save the uterus; he did not indicate the number of cases that underwent this procedure.

As an alternative method to bilateral internal iliac artery ligation, Akashi et al. applied bilateral uterine artery ligation by the vaginal approach to stop bleeding in a case of massive hemorrhage. Akashi et al. further reviewed 29 successful cases of uterine conservation in Japan until 1976. These cases included curettage only in eight patients, curetting plus removal of the gestational sac in one, conservative treatment only in one (the method was not specified), curettage plus internal artery ligation in one, curettage plus cervical cerclage in one, cervicotomy only in one (the approach was not specified), abdominal cervicotomy in

six, removal of a vaginal portion in one, and vaginal cervicotomy in eight, to one of which was applied bilateral uterine artery ligation with a successful result.
These surgical treatments were less common following new methods of safe termination of cervical pregnancy by administration of MTX or application of interventional radiology [5, 22-24]. In 1994, Kudo et al. introduced vaginal surgery to conservatively treat cervical ectopic pregnancy in Japan[25]. This method is similar to those performed in the era without MTX. The only difference is that to reduce blood supply to the cervix, the main branches of both uterine arteries are identified and ligated by absorbable threads instead of being clamped by instruments. For the blood supply of subsequent pregnancies, these absorbable threads could be untied later. On the other hand, both main branches could be cut, as blood to the uterine corpus is supplied through ovarian arteries, or bypassed circulation could be established. This method may be less invasive and even superior if the surgeon is experienced and has good skills with the vaginal approach. Indications may not be favorable, however, when there is poor surgical visibility with heavy and massive bleeding. Therefore, surgical methods are needed that can be performed under any condition, with or without bleeding.

4. Recent surgical treatment: partial trachelectomy

We have recently experienced a case in which the size or blood supply of the gestational sac was increased despite MTX treatment[26]. In this case, curettage with angiographic occlusion of bilateral uterine arteries caused temporal hemorrhagic shock, and fertility was preserved by a novel surgical procedure referred to as "partial trachelectomy"[26]. In the past, the term partial trachelectomy was used for the procedure in which the whole vaginal portion of the uterine cervix was vaginally removed as an extension of deep conization [27, 28]. However, we would like to stress that our method of "partial trachelectomy" is completely different from those reported in the past.
We previously reported a 26-year-old woman (0-0-2-0) who was introduced to our hospital at 8 weeks of pregnancy, with suspected cervical ectopic pregnancy. On ultrasound, the gestational sac was located in the swollen cervix and a heart-beating fetus was visible (Fig. 1). Her serum β-human chorionic gonadotropin (β-hCG) level was 187,497 mIU/mL. We therefore started administration of MTX 20 mg daily for 5 days every 2 weeks, while checking her general condition including liver function. Fetal heart beat stopped after one course of administration, and her serum β-hCG level started to decline (Fig. 2).
Following chemotherapy, the gestational sac showed deformation but its size never decreased on B-mode scanning or MR imaging (Fig. 3a). The blood supply around the gestational sac appeared to increase on color flow mapping showing numerous dilated or pulsating vessels. Although her serum β-hCG level had declined to 4 mIU/mL after six courses of MTX administration, intermittent hemorrhaging occurred, sometimes being massive, necessitating blood transfusion. Spontaneous discharge of the conceptus content was expected but did not occur, resulting in only bleeding. Therefore, surgical evacuation was indicated with both internal iliac arteries temporally occluded angiographically using a balloon catheter. Even with these measures, instrumental evacuation caused uncontrollable hemorrhage and shock. Then, the curettage was interrupted and she received a blood transfusion shortly thereafter, for preparation of a new approach to preserve fertility by partial trachelectomy; informed consent was obtained before the procedure.

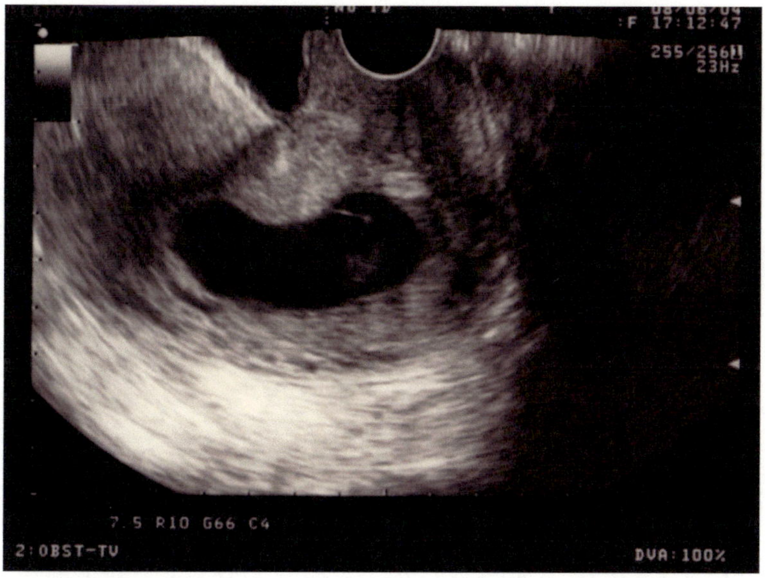

Fig. 1. B-mode ultrasound findings at admission. The gestational sac in the swollen cervix and a heart-beating fetus are visible.

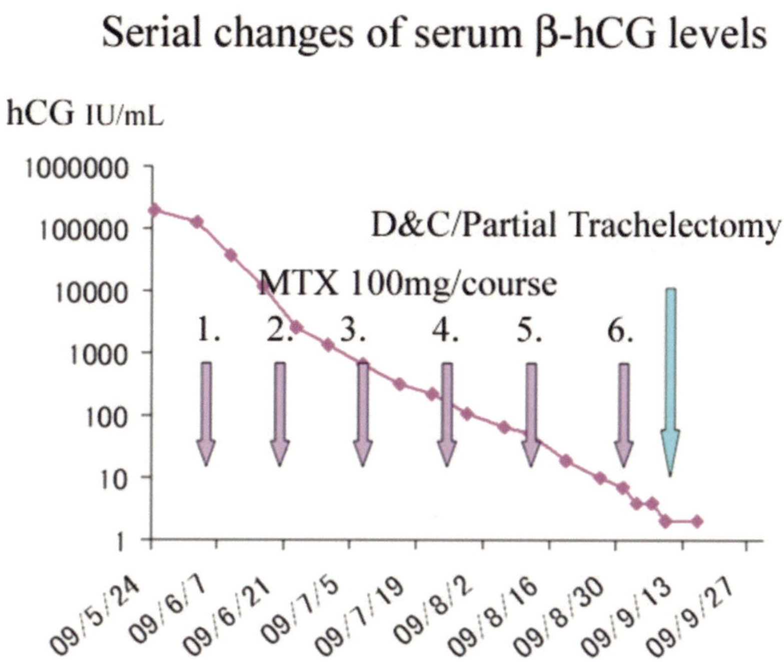

Fig. 2. Serial changes in serum β-hCG levels after admission
Serum β-hCG levels of the patient reduced from 187,497 to 4 U/mL by six courses of systemic administration of MTX (20 mmg/day × 5 days). After five courses of MTX treatment, frequent sporadic genital bleeding up to 500 ml occurred, indicating partial trachelectomy following dilatation and curettage (D&C).

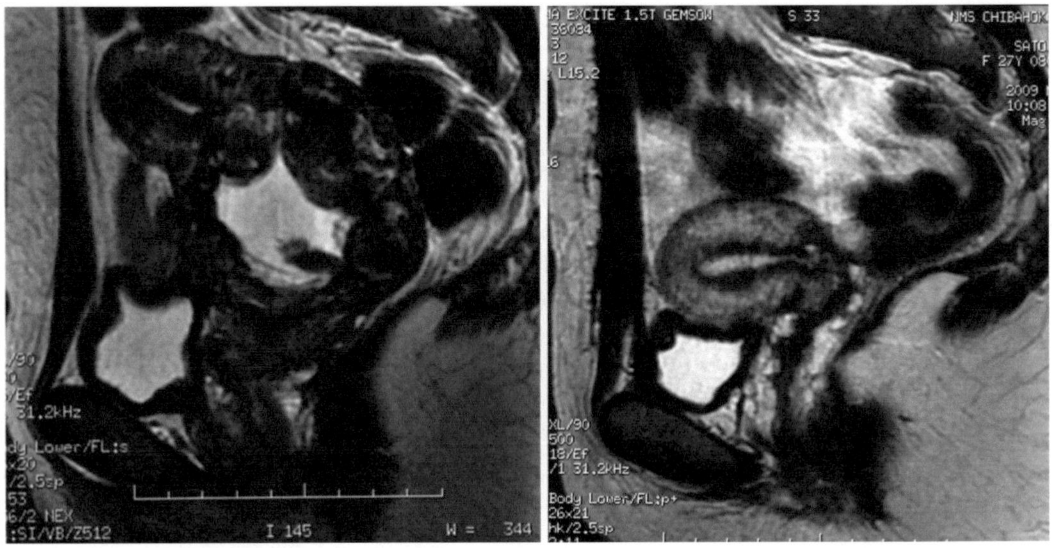

Fig. 3. MRI immediately prior to surgery and one year and two months post-surgery
a. MR image just before curettage showing a swollen cervix and an unclear border between the gestational sac and cervical wall. b. MR image one year and two months after fertility-preserving surgery showing a normal uterine corpus and small cervix.

The procedure was conducted under general anesthesia with an operation time of 6 h and 1300 ml of blood loss, most of which was considered to be from the vagina, not the surgical area. The postoperative surgical state was fairly good and she was discharged from the hospital on the tenth postoperative day. Her serum β-hCG level was undetectable immediately after surgery, and normal menstruation returned one month later. Six months later, the uterine shape appeared almost normal, and one year later, T2-weighted MRI findings (sagital view) were completely normal, presenting three zonal patterns of the corpus and clearer shape of the retained cervix (Fig. 3b).

For partial trachelectomy, the abdomen is opened with a median vertical subumbilical incision, confirming a normal-sized uterine corpus and a swollen cervix (Fig. 4a). The left round ligament is divided and the broad ligament is opened to enter the retroperitoneal space. The same procedure is performed on the right side. The uterovesical fold of the peritoneum is cut and the urinary bladder is displaced downwards to directly view the swollen cervix. The left uterine artery is identified following anterior division of the left hypogastric artery with special attention of the ureter. A careful dissection is made around the bifurcation into both ascending and descending branches of the uterine artery. The descending branch is ligated and cut just distal to the bifurcation to stop the blood supply into the cervix. The opposite side is ligated and cut in the same manner (Fig. 5). Circumcision of the vagina is then completed at the fornix using a translucent vaginal cylinder to distinguish between the vaginal vault and the uterus (Fig. 4b). In this state, the uterine corpus is attached to both adnexae and the blood supply maintained by both bilateral ovarian arteries and the bilateral ascending branches of the uterine arteries (Fig. 5). This procedure allows mobility of the cervix upwards to visualize the external os (Fig. 4c). If the implantation site is considered to be posterior, the anterior wall of the cervical canal is cut longitudinally upwards from the external cervical opening to view the ectopic gestational sac. The part of the posterior wall including the implantation site is excised in a spindle shape following the border from the normal structure (Figs. 4d and 6). If the implantation site is anterior, the posterior wall is excised in the same manner. Both the posterior and anterior walls are closed by vicryl (Ethicon, Inc., Somerville, NJ) -interrupted sutures (Fig. 4e), and the reconstructed cervix and amputated vaginal vault are connected again by vicryl-interrupted sutures. Finally, the procedure is completed by pelvic peritonealization including reconnection of both round ligaments (Fig. 4f).

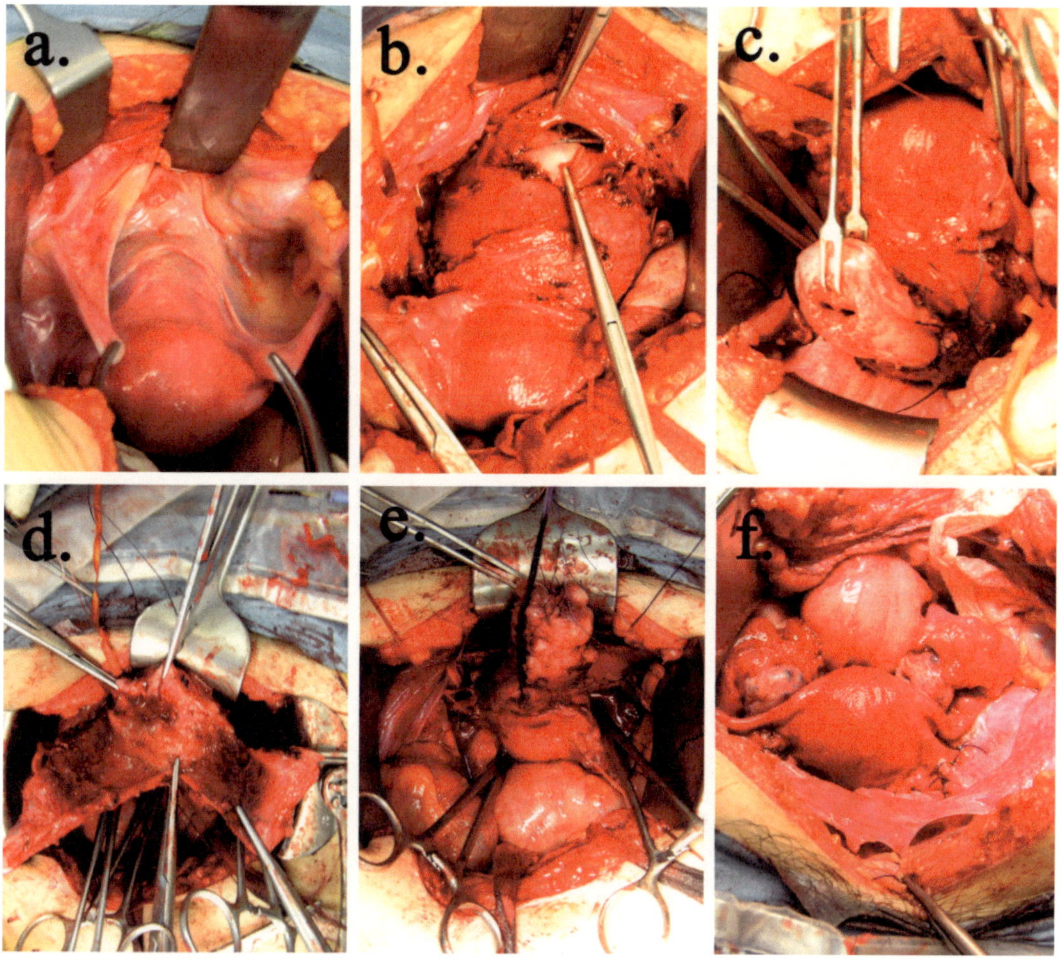

Fig. 4. Intraoperative photographs
a. Anterior view of the swollen cervix and corpus of the uterus when the abdomen was just opened. b. Anterior vaginal wall partially opened at the fornix after the blood supply was stopped by ligation of both descending branches of the uterine artery, guided by a translucent cylinder that had been inserted into the vagina. c. Whole ectocervix after circumcision of the vagina. d. Opened left and right bilateral flaps of the intact cervical wall after fusiform excision of the cervical wall with the ectopic pregnancy. e. Re-construction of the cervical canal by suturing both flaps at the anterior and posterior. f. Pelvic cavity after the cervix was anastomosed with the vagina.

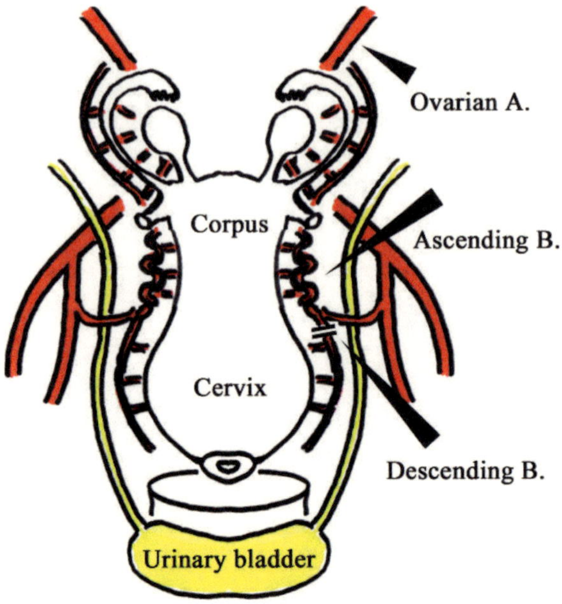

Fig. 5. Vascular anatomy of partial trachelectomy for cervical ectopic pregnancy
Each descending branch of the bilateral uterine artery is tied and cut just distal to the bifurcation indicated by the long arrowhead. The vagina is amputated at the fornix. The blood supply is provided by both uterine and ovarian arteries. B.: branch; A.: artery

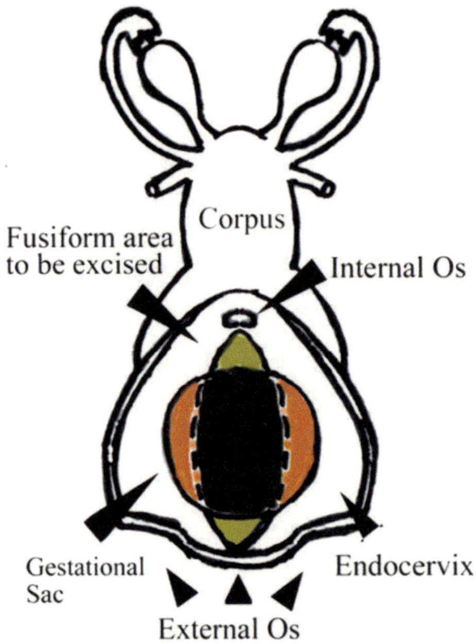

Fig. 6. Schematic of direct visualization of the conceptive product
The conceptus mass is directly visible by the opening of the longitudinal incision of the anterior cervical wall. The internal cervical os is also visible. The expected line of the fusiform incision at the posterior wall is indicated by the dashed line.

Figure 7a shows the product of conception removed by curettage and Fig. 7b shows the excised vaginal wall in a spindle shape. Histological examination of the excised specimen showed necrotic villi with hemorrhage at the surface and intermediate trophoblast invasion deeply in the cervix.

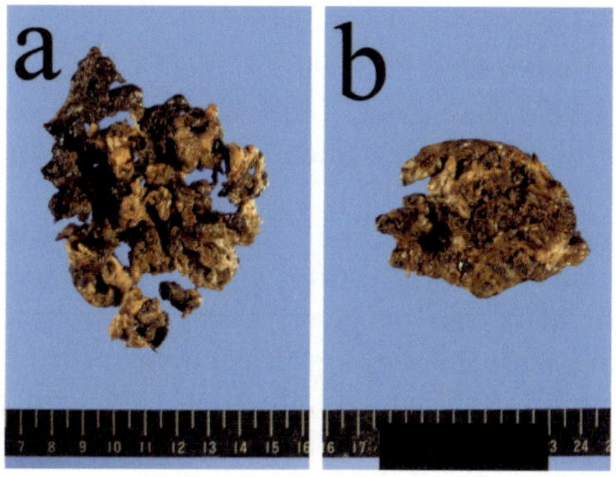

Fig. 7. Macroscopic findings of resected specimen
a. The gestational sac (the product of conception) broken into pieces by curettage. b. The vaginal wall with the implantation site excised in a spindle shape. The right side of the specimen is directed toward the internal os.

Our partial trachelectomy method was developed based on radical trachelectomy which is an established method for removal of the whole cervix with part of the vaginal wall in cervical cancer patients who hope to preserve their fertility[29, 30]. For patients with cervical pregnancy, but not cervical cancer, wide resection of the uterine cervix is unnecessary and only a small part, at the implantation site, should be excised from the cervix. This approach may thus be less invasive from the viewpoint of fertility.

Many precise diagnostic tools such as MRI, ultrasound and color flow mapping; villocidal agents such as MTX and actinomycin D with local or systemic delivery; and interventional radiology techniques such as transarterial embolization and balloon occlusion are currently available. These advances in medicine allow clinicians to treat patients conservatively and specifically by combining these methods. However, conservative treatment of patients with cervical ectopic pregnancy is still limited. Analysis of prognostic factors affecting the outcome of conservative MTX treatment showed that MTX therapy is generally associated with higher failure rates for cases of cervical pregnancy with 1) serum β-hCG levels greater than 10,000 IU/L, 2) gestational age > 9 weeks amenorrhea, 3) positive fetal cardiac activity or, 4) crown-rump length > 10 mm[31]. In our experience, we have successfully treated two patients with cervical ectopic pregnancy: one case with systemic MTX alone or another case with MTX and curettage (unpublished). However, in the present case, we experienced for the first time a case in which MTX was insufficient as a safe and conservative treatment. Leeman et al. divided treatment choices for cervical ectopic pregnancy conceptually into five categories: 1) tamponade (cervical/vaginal packing or Foley balloon), 2) reduction of blood supply (cervical cerclage, angiographic embolization, or large vessel ligation), 3) excision of trophoblastic tissue (dilation and curettage, hysteroscopic resection, or hysterectomy), 4) intra-amniotic feticide (potassium chloride or MTX), and 5) systemic chemotherapy (MTX intramuscularly or other chemotherapy regimens) and proposed one possible treatment algorithm. [32] In the case of hemorrhaging, hysterectomy is selected if bleeding cannot be stabilized by the measures such as Foley balloon tamponade, large vessel ligation, or angiographic embolization. In the clinically stable cases, measures are categorized into three groups by ultrasound examination. 1) Systemic MTX is recommended at less than 9 weeks of gestation with no cardiac activity. 2) Intra-amniotic potassium chloride with systemic MTX is chosen at 9 to 12 weeks or less than 9 weeks with cardiac activity. 3) Primary hysterectomy is indicated at more than 12 weeks. That is, at an advanced gestational age or after treatment failure, pregnancy should be terminated by hysterectomy.

In our case, serum β-hCG levels were over 10,000 IU/L and ultrasound examination showed positive fetal cardiac activity. Therefore, systemic MTX administration was chosen to treat the patient.

With regards to MTX administration, Barnhart pointed out that mainly two protocols were used for medical management for unruptured ectopic pregnancy: "single dose" regimen and "multidose" regimen. MTX can be given using a "multidose" regimen of 1mg/kg intramuscularly, alternating with 0.1 mg/kg of leucovorin intramuscularly for up to four daily doses of each drug[33]. Alternatively, methotrexate can be administered using a "single dose" method, based on body surface area, at 50 mg/m^2 without the need for leucovorin rescue. It is concluded that "single dose" regimen is milder than in side effect but has higher failure rate than "multidose" regimen. This "multidose" regimen has been used for a long time as MTX-leucovorin rescue regimen for the patients with low-risk gestational trophoblastic disease and it has slightly lower remission rate than 5-days MTX regimen[34]. Five-days MTX regimen, in which MTX is administered in a dose of 0.4mg/kg intramuscularly for five days with cycles repeated every 14 days, is another protocols that is frequently used for low-risk gestational trophoblastic disease[35]. With above consideration, we applied 5 days MTX regimen for our patient. The serum β-hCG level fell slowly to 4 mIU/mL before surgery, just as following the normal regression curve of β-hCG after molar evacuation[36]. However, it became undetected at the next day after surgery. According to Kamrava, the serum clearance of hCG by radioimmunoassay may take place at least up to 24 days after surgery if the lesion can be removed completely and the initial tilter of hCG is a significant factor in determining the length of time that it can be detected in the serum postoperatively[37]. In this means, the surgical excision of the trophoblastic tissue was considered to be complete with this procedure.

Although the surgery in our case was considered to be fairly long, i.e., 6 h (it was initiated as an emergency operation, late at night (21:00), due to continuous bleeding from the vagina), partial trachelectomy could be completed in less time upon improved techniques. In consideration of the new treatment option of partial trachelectomy, the treatment algorism should be revised to include more chances to preserve fertility, especially in difficult cases. Indications for partial trachelectomy include: 1) when measures for massive hemorrhage such as Foley balloon tamponade, large vessel ligation, and/or angiographic embolization are ineffective; 2) when MTX is ineffective indicating primary hysterectomy for cases at gestational age > 12 weeks; or 3) when systemic MTX plus intra-amniotic potassium is ineffective as a complete cure and additional surgical measures like curettage or suction evacuation are necessary. However, this surgical option might be accompanied with various risks, including relapse, premature delivery, and surgical wound rupture, although the risk should be less than that for radical trachelectomy indicated for the increasing number of cases of cervical cancer patients. Further studies are needed to determine the benefits and risks of partial trachelectomy before establishing it as a treatment for patients with cervical ectopic pregnancy.

5. Conclusions

In conclusion, "partial trachelectomy" is a new procedure that shares many similarities to previous procedures. It differs in the following two respects: 1) exact ligation or cut of the descending branch of the bilateral uterine artery and 2) excision of the spindle shaped-cervical wall of the implantation site under direct vision by temporally detaching the vaginal wall and cervix. This procedure preserves fertility under any condition although with more risk of complication for future pregnancies compared to previous methods in which fertility preservation is not always successful. However, it is less invasive compared to radical trachelectomy which is a common method of fertility preservation for cancer patients with non-cervical pregnancy.

6. Acknowledgments

The authors thank Drs. Michiaki Watanabe, Kenji Igarashi, Takashi Yamada, and Tadashi Asakura for help in treating this patient; Dr. Hiroshi Kawamata for angiographic management; and the late Dr. Yoshiharu Ohaki for his pathologic diagnosis.

7. References

[1] Flanagan, J.F. and C.R. Walsh, *Cervical pregnancy; report of a case.* Obstet Gynecol, 1954. 4(5): p. 511-3.

[2] Haans, L.C., P.H. van Kessel, and H.C. Kock, *Treatment of ectopic pregnancy with methotrexate.* Eur J Obstet Gynecol Reprod Biol, 1987. 24(1): p. 63-7.

[3] Kim, T.J., et al., *Clinical outcomes of patients treated for cervical pregnancy with or without methotrexate.* J Korean Med Sci, 2004. 19(6): p. 848-52.

[4] Akashi, E., N. Kawase, and M. Hashimoto, *The diagnosis and therapy for cervical pregnancy.* Sanfujinka no jissai, 1976. 33: p. 659-667.

[5] Cepni, I., et al., *Conservative treatment of cervical ectopic pregnancy with transvaginal ultrasound-guided aspiration and single-dose methotrexate.* Fertil Steril, 2004. 81(4): p. 1130-2.

[6] Farghaly, S.A. and J.G. Mathie, *Cervical pregnancy managed by local excision.* Postgrad Med J, 1980. 56(661): p. 789.

[7] Sheldon, R.S., L.A. Aaro, and J.S. Welch, *Conservative Management of Cervical Pregnancy.* Am J Obstet Gynecol, 1963. 87: p. 504-6.

[8] Whittle, M.J., *Cervical pregnancy managed by local excision.* Br Med J, 1976. 2(6039): p. 795-6.

[9] Studdiford, W., *Cervical Pregnancy.* Amer.J.Obstet.gynecol, 1945. 49: p. 169.

[10] Schneider, P., *Distal ectopic pregnancy; implantation of the ovum in the cervical mucosa.* Am J Surg, 1946. 72: p. 526-39.

[11] Baptisti, A., Jr., *Cervical pregnancy.* Obstet Gynecol, 1953. 1(3): p. 353-8.

[12] Shinagawa, S. and M. Nagayama, *Cervical pregnancy as a possible sequela of induced abortion. Report of 19 cases.* Am J Obstet Gynecol, 1969. 105(2): p. 282-4.

[13] Price, J.J. and A. Webster, *Cervical pregnancy.* Am J Obstet Gynecol, 1967. 99(1): p. 134-7.

[14] Paalman, R.J. and E.T. Mc, *Cervical pregnancy; review of the literature and presentation of cases.* Am J Obstet Gynecol, 1959. 77(6): p. 1261-70.

[15] Thomsen, M. and F. Johansen, *Two cases of cervical pregnancy.* Acta obstet gynec scandinav, 1961. 40: p. 99.

[16] Danforth, D.N., *The fibrous nature of the human cervix, and its relation to the isthmic segment in gravid and nongravid uteri.* Am J Obstet Gynecol, 1947. 53: p. 541-60.

[17] Schneider, P. and D.H. Dreizin, *Cervical pregnancy.* Am.J. Surg., 1957. 93: p. 27-40.

[18] Steinbiss, W., *Tod infolge einer Placenta cervicalis accreta unter falschem Verdacht auf Kriminalem Abort.* Deutsch. Ztschr. f. ges. gericht. Med., 1938. 12: p. 234.

[19] Matracaru, G., *A new method for the operative management of the cervical pregnancy.* Centralblatt for Gynecology, 1968. 37: p. 1264.

[20] Nelson, R.M., *Bilateral internal iliac artery ligation in cervical pregnancy: conservation of reproductive function.* Am J Obstet Gynecol, 1979. 134(2): p. 145-50.

[21] Dodeck, S.M., *Cevical Pregnancy: diagonaosis and Management.* South. Med.J, 1965. 58: p. 167-70.

[22] Honey, L., A. Leader, and P. Claman, *Uterine artery embolization--a successful treatment to control bleeding cervical pregnancy with a simultaneous intrauterine gestation.* Hum Reprod, 1999. 14(2): p. 553-5.

[23] Trambert, J.J., et al., *Uterine artery embolization in the management of vaginal bleeding from cervical pregnancy: a case series.* J Reprod Med, 2005. 50(11): p. 844-50.

[24] Yang, J.H., et al., *Combined treatment with temporary intraoperative balloon occlusion of common iliac arteries and hysteroscopic endocervical resection with postoperative cervical balloon for intractable cervical pregnancy in an infertile woman.* Fertil Steril, 2007. 88(5): p. 1438 e11-3.

[25] Kudo, R., et al., *A conservative surgical treatment of cervical pregnancy through vagina.* Sanfujinka Chiryou (in Japanese) (gyenecological management), 1994. 69: p. 8-21.

[26] Kamoi, S., et al., *Partial Trachelectomy :A New and Final Option for Fertility-Preserving Management of Cervical Ectopic Pregnancy.* J Gynecol Surg, 2009. 25: p. 139-146.

[27] Jeng, C.J., J. Shen, and S.H. Huang, *Partial trachelectomy: a new treatment choice for persistent or recurrent high grade cervical intraepithelial neoplasia.* Gynecol Oncol, 2006. 100(2): p. 231-2.

[28] Krebs, H.B., M.A. Wilstrup, and J.B. Wheelock, *Partial trachelectomy in the elderly patient with abnormal cytology.* Obstet Gynecol, 1985. 65(4): p. 579-84.

[29] Abu-Rustum, N.R., et al., *Fertility-sparing radical abdominal trachelectomy for cervical carcinoma: technique and review of the literature.* Gynecol Oncol, 2006. 103(3): p. 807-13.

[30] Smith, J.R., et al., *Abdominal radical trachelectomy: a new surgical technique for the conservative management of cervical carcinoma.* Br J Obstet Gynaecol, 1997. 104(10): p. 1196-200.

[31] Hung, T.H., et al., *Prognostic factors for an unsatisfactory primary methotrexate treatment of cervical pregnancy: a quantitative review.* Hum Reprod, 1998. 13(9): p. 2636-42.

[32] Leeman, L.M. and C.L. Wendland, *Cervical ectopic pregnancy. Diagnosis with endovaginal ultrasound examination and successful treatment with methotrexate.* Arch Fam Med, 2000. 9(1): p. 72-7.

[33] Barnhart, K.T. and A.C. Hummel, *Pitfalls of partial meta-analysis: single- versus multidose for the treatment of ectopic pregnancy.* Am J Obstet Gynecol, 2007. 196(1): p. e22; author reply e22-3.

[34] Bagshawe, K.D., et al., *The role of low-dose methotrexate and folinic acid in gestational trophoblastic tumours (GTT).* Br J Obstet Gynaecol, 1989. 96(7): p. 795-802.

[35] Hammond, C.B., et al., *Primary chemotherapy for nonmetastatic gestational trophoblastic neoplasms.* Am J Obstet Gynecol, 1967. 98(1): p. 71-8.

[36] Morrow, C.P., et al., *Clinical and laboratory correlates of molar pregnancy and trophoblastic disease.* Am J Obstet Gynecol, 1977. 128(4): p. 424-30.

[37] Kamrava, M.M., et al., *Disappearance of human chorionic gonadotropin following removal of ectopic pregnancy.* Obstet Gynecol, 1983. 62(4): p. 486-8.

15

Modern Management of Cornual Ectopic Pregnancy

Maged Shendy[1] and Rami Atalla[2]
[1]*MRCOG, Royal Berkshire Hospital, Reading*
[2]*FRCOG, Queen Elizabeth II Hospital, Welwyn Garden City*
UK

1. Introduction

Corneal ectopic or interstitial ectopic is a pregnancy that implants in the intrauterine portion of fallopian tube. Due to its location, there is an inherit difficulty in the diagnosis and treatment leading to high mortality compared with other ectopic pregnancies.
Transvaginal Ultrasound scan is the most useful diagnostic tool for establishing the diagnosis though serial β-HCG and even laparoscopy are sometimes needed to confirm the diagnosis.
Due to the high risk of rupture with serious or fatal bleeding, there is no role for the expectant management. Surgery is the most common management option. Though traditionally laparotomy is the main surgical intervention, recently increasing number of laparoscopic or even hysteroscopic approach have been used. Injection of Methotrexate locally or systemically has also been used successfully.

2. Anatomy

Each Fallopian tube is usually 10 cm long with variations in length from 7 to 14 cm. The abdominal ostium is situated at the base of a funnel-shaped expansion of the tube, the infundibulum. Medially, it opens into the thin-walled ampulla forming more than half the length of the tube and 1 or 2 cm in outer diameter; it is succeeded by the isthmus, a round and cord-like structure constituting the medial one-third of the tube and 0.5-1 cm in outer diameter. The isthmus continues through the uterine wall to the uterine cavity forming the interstitial or conual portion of the tube. This segment of the tube is about 1 cm in length and 1 mm in diameter.(Diamond, 1988)

3. Epidemiology

Interstitial (cornual) pregnancy is a rare type of ectopic pregnancy, accounting for 2–4% of all tubal pregnancies (Lau S& Tulandi T, 1999) .The surrounding myometrial tissue allows progression of the pregnancy into the second trimester but rupture at such an advanced gestation may result in catastrophic haemorrhage with a mortality rate of up to 2 %. This high mortality rate is partially due to the difficult challenging diagnosis as well as the speed of haemorrhage. (Tulandi T&Al-Jaroudi D, 2004; Vicino M et al, 2000; Dilbaz S et al, 2005; Rock J et al, 2003)

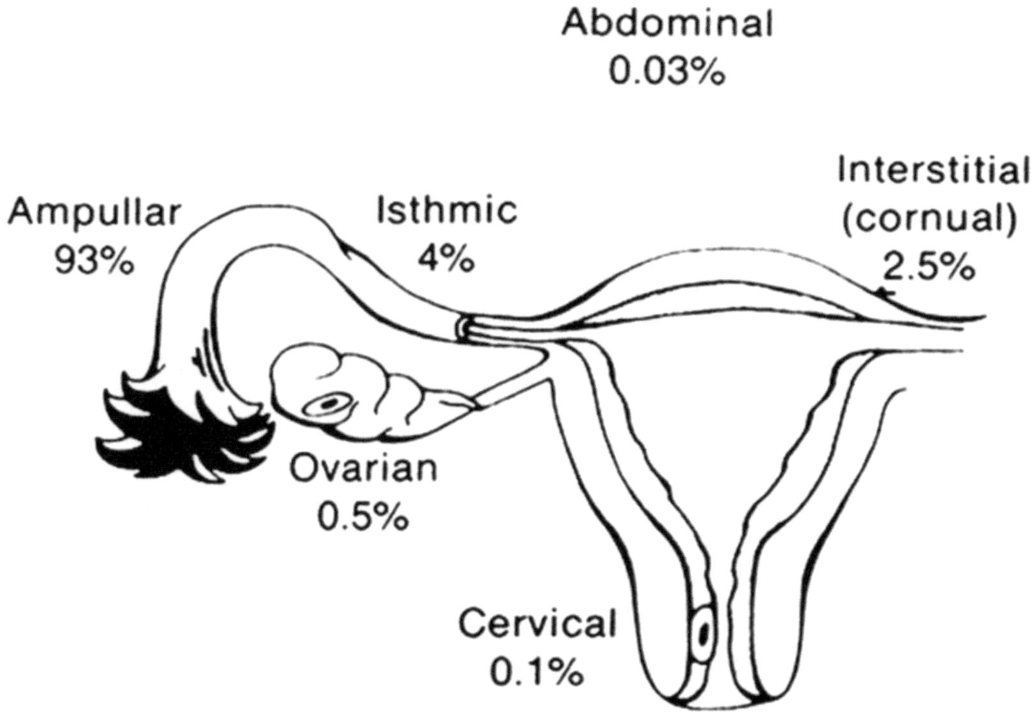

Fig. 1. Sites and frequencies of ectopic pregnancy.

4. Risk factors

Cornual ectopics share the common risk factors of other ectopic pregnancies which are:

4.1 Pelvic inflammatory disease (PID)

The incidence of tubal damage after the first episode of PID is 13%. This incidence increases to 35% after the second episode of PID and to 75% after the third episode. A history of salpingitis increases the risk of ectopic pregnancy by 4 fold. (Westrom L et al, 1981)

4.2 History of previous ectopic pregnancy

After one ectopic pregnancy, patients have a 7-13 fold increase in the likelihood of another ectopic pregnancy. Method of management of previous ectopic pregnancy influences the chance of recurrence. The incidence is increased according to the size of the ectopic pregnancy specially if treated salpingostomy. The incidence of recurrence of ectopic is 18% and 8% after treatment with sapingotomy and salpingectomy respectively though the chance of future intrauterine pregnancy is 89% after salpingostomy compared with 66% after salpingectomy. (Silva Pet al, 1993)

4.3 History of tubal surgery and conception after tubal ligation

Salpingectomy, salpingostomy, neosalpingostomy, fimbrioplasty, tubal reanastomosis, and lysis of peritubal or periovarian adhesions are associated with an increased risk of ectopic pregnancies.

One third of patients who conceive after a tubal ligation are reported to experience an ectopic pregnancy. Ectopic pregnancies following tubal ligation usually occur 2 or more years after sterilization, rather than immediately after. In the first year, only about 6% of sterilization failures result in ectopic pregnancy. (DeStefano F, 1982)

4.4 Assisted reproductive technology

The risk of ectopic pregnancy increases if the patient has conceived following an assisted reproductive technique, such as in vitro fertilization (IVF) or gamete intrafallopian transfer (GIFT). The ectopic pregnancy rate quoted as 1.6% and the heterotopic pregnancy rate as 13%.

4.5 Use of an intrauterine contraceptive device (IUD)

Conception with an IUD in place is coupled with 3-4% risk of ectopic pregnancy which again more than double the background risk. This is more prominent as IUD decreases the intrauterine conception rate. (Ory HW, 1981)

4.6 Increasing age

Women over 40 years of age have a 3 - 4 fold increase in the risk for developing an ectopic pregnancy compared to women aged 15-24 years. This has been attributed to a possible progressive loss of myoelectrical activity along the fallopian tube with ageing or to the deterioration in the quality of the fertilised egg.

4.7 Smoking

Smoking has been shown to increase the risk of ectopic pregnancy by 3 fold. To date, no study has supported a specific mechanism by which cigarette smoking affects the incidence of ectopic pregnancy however, delayed ovulation, altered tubal motility, or altered immunity have been suggested. (Coste J et al, 1991)

4.8 Previous pelvic surgeries

Previous pelvic surgeries have shown to increase the risk of ectopic pregnancy. Right ectopic pregnancy seems to be more frequent than left due to history of appendicitis or even subclinical subacute inflammation of the appendix.

4.9 Other

Salpingitis isthmica nodosum like any other inflammation of the tubes has been thought to be associated with increase incidence of ectopic pregnancy.

5. Presentation

The wide spread of specialised early pregnancy units and the abundance of ultrasound facilities led to early diagnosis of cornual ectopics. There is an increasing incidence of asymptomatic ectopics compared with more traditional presentation of lower abdominal pains and vaginal bleeding.

Ruptured ectopics can however present with typical signs of haemorrhagic shock, which include pallor, tachycardia, hypotension and oliguria. The assessment of the uterine size is rarely helpful and cervical excitation is not a specific sign in cornual ectopic.

6. Diagnosis

6.1 Ultrasound

Trans vaginal ultrasound scan is the corner stone for the early diagnosis of cornual ecopic. The ultrasonographic diagnosis of cornual ectopic is challenging and needs expert hands. The eccentric position of the gestational sac with an empty uterine cavity and the presence of a thin (less than 5 mm) or even absent myometrium surrounding the sac are highly suggestive of cornual ectopic pregnancy. (Timor-Tritsch IE et al, 1992; Johnson PT& Shah C). The diagnosis may be helped with the use of Doppler studies showing increase vasculature around the gestational sac. (Abraham D& Silkowski C, 2010). This is sometimes described as a ring of vessels (Ring of fire). It also helps to exclude pseudosac due to endometrial reaction. The gestational sac is usually seen away from the thickened endometrium associated with the pregnancy.

The ultrasound picture of cornual ectopic can be very similar to that of an early pregnancy in a bicornuate uterus or a fibroid uterus. Therefore the diagnosis of cornual ectopic should be made with caution, keeping in mind the possible differential diagnosis. (Abraham D& Silkowski C, 2010).

In experienced hands, trans-vaginal ultrasound can establish diagnosis of cornual ectopics in nearly 71% of cases. (Tulandi T& Al-Jaroudi D, 2004).

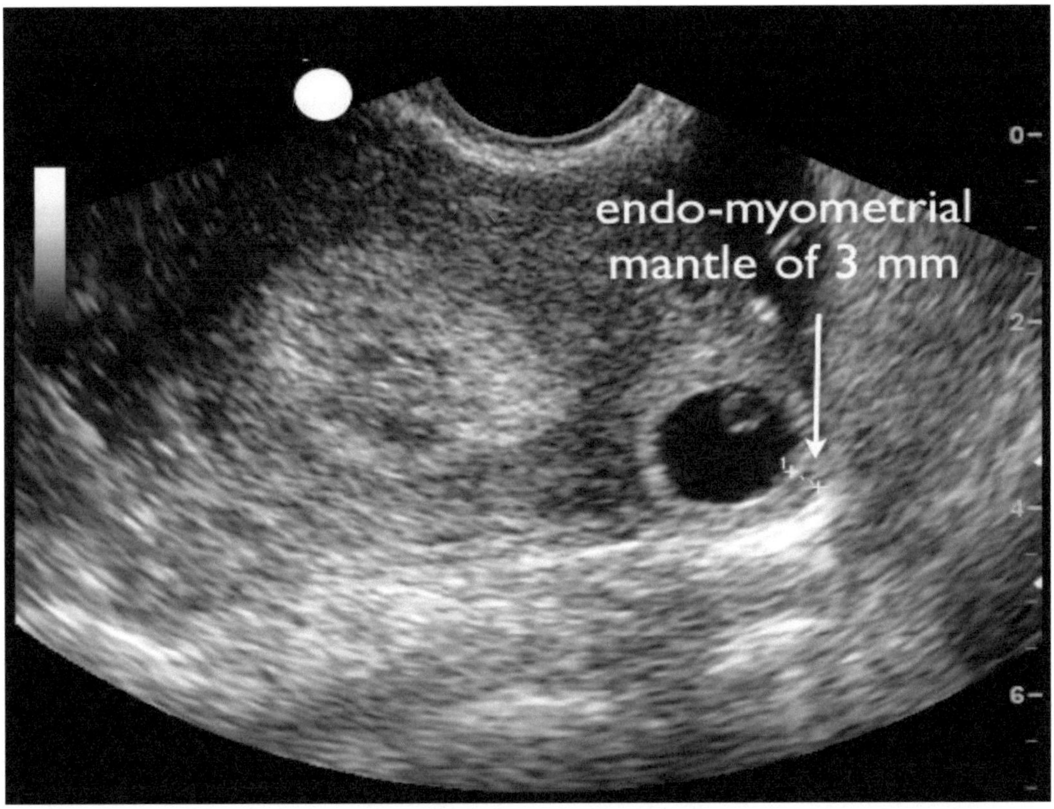

Fig. 2. Cornual ectopic located eccentrically within uterine cavity. Note the thin layer of myometrial tissue on the lateral aspect of gestational sac.

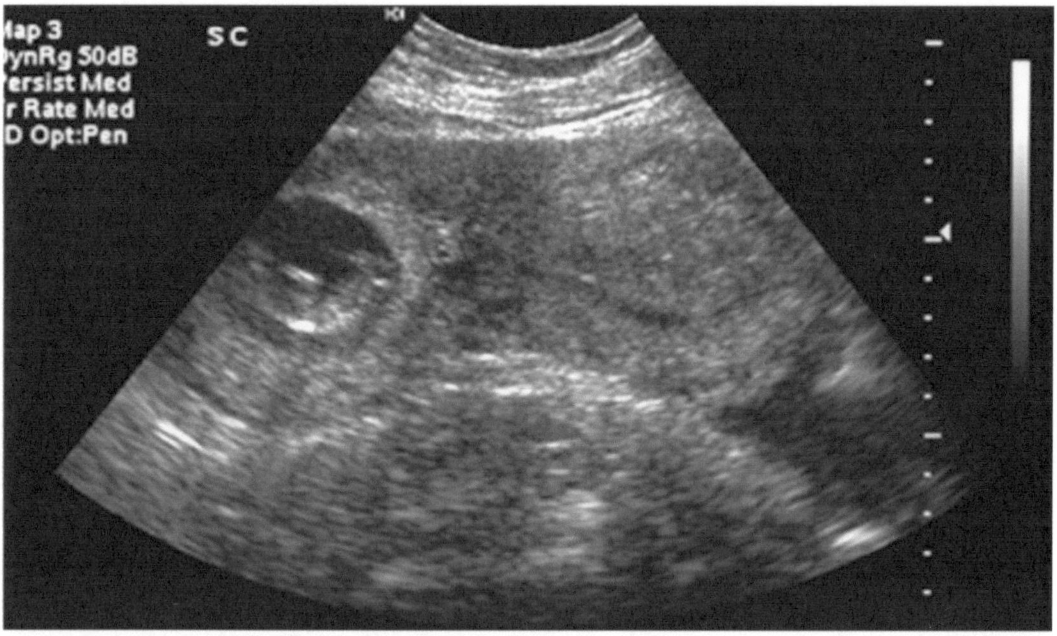

Fig. 3. Bicornuate uterus mimicking cornual ectopic pregnancy. Transverse transabdominal view shows bicornuate uterus with a pregnancy in right horn

The use of 3-D and 4-D improves sensitivity of establishing the diagnosis especially when contrast is used. (Lee GS et al, 2005; Chou MM et al, 2005). However, lack of its availability in many units limits their use as the recommended methods.

6.2 Serial β hCG

Ectopic pregnancy is known to be associated with a suboptimal increase or plateau of serum β hCG. (Banerjee S et al, 1999; Hajenius P et al, 1995) With a detection rate of 97% and a specificity of 77%, serial serum β hCG is useful to establish the diagnosis of ectopic pregnancy in association of the sonographic findings. (Cacciatore B et al, 1990)

In cornual ectopics, there are reports of doubling of serum β hCG, therefore the value of performing serial serum β hCG is doubtful and the results should be interpreted with caution. (Abraham D & Silkowski C, 2010)

6.3 Role of laparoscopy

Laparoscopy is an essential diagnostic tool as well as a possible treatment method route for suspected cornual ectopics. However, in cornual ectopics, difficulty arises with small ectopic masses that can be missed.

Experienced laparoscopic operator is crucial in such cases in order to have the ability to deal with possible high risk of heavy bleeding when treatment of cornual ectopics is accomplished laparoscopically.

7. Management of cornual ectopic

Early diagnosis allows a varied choice of treatment options with a high possibility of preserving fertility.

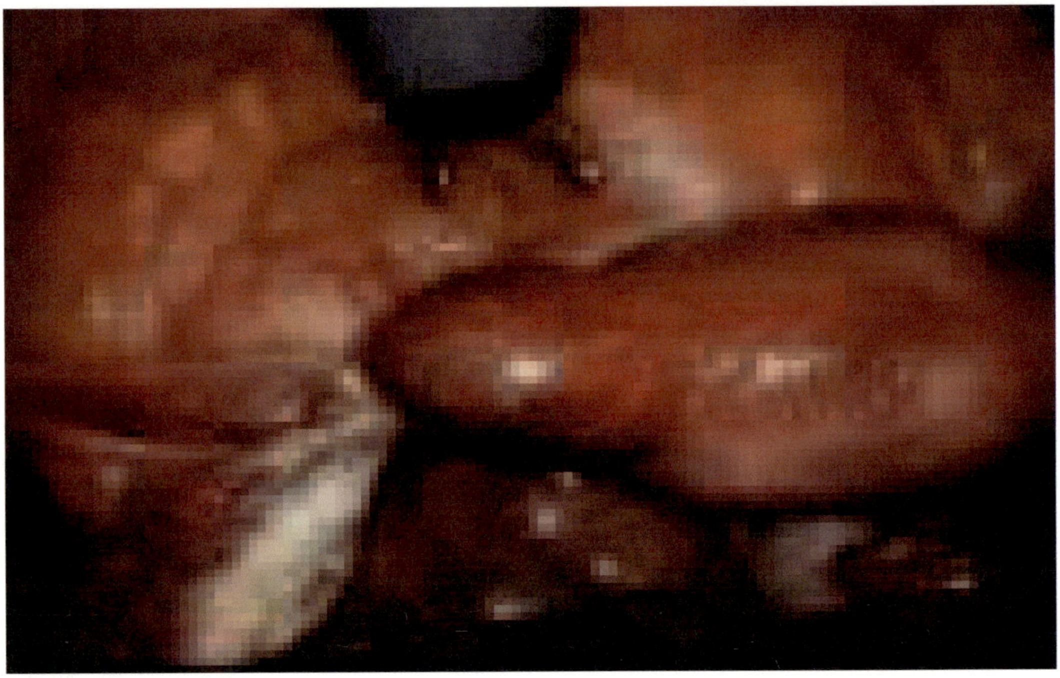

Fig. 4. Left cornual ectopic

7.1 Medical treatment

7.1.1 Systemic methotrexate

An increasing number of cornual ectopic have been treated with Methotrexate. This is mainly due to the accuracy of the ultrasound scan in confirming the diagnosis as well as the wide spread experience in the use of Methotrexate in the management of ectopic pregnancies.

Patients suitable for medical management should have minimal or no symptoms, be haemodynamically stable (Royal College of Obstetricians and Gynaecologists, 2004) , and with β hCG < 3000 IU. (Yao M& Tulandi T, 1997; Sowter M& Frappell J, 2002; Kelly H et al, 2006; Teal SB, 2006). It is more successful if no fetal heart beats(Yao M& Tulandi T, 1997; Sowter M& Frappell J, 2002) are detected in the ectopic pregnancy and the ectopic size is < 4 cm. Patients should be willing to attend regular follow up and have no contraindication for Methotrexate. (Royal College of Obstetricians and Gynaecologists, 2004)

There is no clear data regarding the effect of ectopic size on the treatment outcome but the larger the ectopic the more likely the treatment fails. (Lipscomb G et al, 1999)The patient should be given clear and written information about the Methotrexate treatment protocol, its success rate and the possible adverse effects. (Royal College of Obstetricians and Gynaecologists, 2004) A clear follow-up protocol should be explained to the women with explanation of possible symptoms or ruptured ectopic. (Royal College of Obstetricians and Gynaecologists, 2004) The possible need for further treatment either electively or as an in case of emergency should be documented and the women should be given a contact number for advice or emergency. (Royal College of Obstetricians and Gynaecologists, 2004)

Identified patients for medical treatment should have blood tests for Full Blood Count, Liver Function Tests and Renal function tests before starting the Methotrexate treatment. (Royal College of Obstetricians and Gynaecologists, 2004; Kelly H et al, 2006; Teal SB, 2006).

The Body surface area is calculated and a single dose 50 mg/m^2 is given Intra-muscularly. This dose has been shown to be effective with < 15% needs additional treatment with least side effects compared to other regimens. (Royal College of Obstetricians and Gynaecologists, 2004; Yao M& Tulandi T, 1997; Sowter M& Frappell J, 2002; Kelly H et al, 2006; Teal SB, 2006) The possible side effects of Methotrexate includes, GIT upset, Conjunctivitis and photosensitivity, pneumonitis, reversible alopecia, liver or renal impairment, myelosuppression and possible teratogenicity, so the patient should not conceive within 3 months of completion of treatment. (Royal College of Obstetricians and Gynaecologists, 2004; Barnhart KT et al, 2003).

Following the injection of Methotrexate, follow-up β hCG should be done on day 4 and day 7 after the treatment aiming check to for the decreasing levels. An initial rise may be observed but an expected drop of > 15% is expected between day 4 and day 7 in successfully treated ectopics. (Yao M& Tulandi T, 1997; Sowter M& Frappell J, 2002)A weekly follow-up is needed till non pregnant levels of β hCG. (Royal College of Obstetricians and Gynaecologists, 2004)

Liver function tests may need to be repeated at the same time as the β hCG due to the possible side effects of Methotrexate on Liver Function. Throughout the follow-up duration, the patients should maintain an easy access to the hospital and informed to come back if they experience pain or bleeding. (Sowter M et al, 2001; Mol B et al, 1999)

The systemic route of administration offers advantages over local injection of the ectopic gestation as it is less invasive and not operator dependent. (Royal College of Obstetricians and Gynaecologists, 2004)

7.1.2 Local methotrexate

Methoterxate can be injected directly into the ectopic sac through the myometrium under transvaginal ultrasound guidance or alternatively during the laparoscopic procedure. (Timor-Tritsch IE, 1997; Benifla JL et al, 1996; Onderoglu LS et al, 2006)

Either of these treatment options aimed to reduce the systemic exposure and side effects of Methotrexate with a chance of spontaneous resolution of ectopics in some studies can be as high as 100%. (Monteagudo A et al, 2005)

Local potassium chloride injection has been used as alternative to Local Methotrexate with promising results. It is used mainly if the patient is keen on conceiving soon after the ectopic. (Doubilet PM et al, 2004)

7.2 Surgical management

7.2.1 Surgical techniques

Surgical management depends mainly on the presenting condition of the patient and the skills of the operating surgeon. Cornual ectopic has been reported to be treated by variation of procedures mainly cornuotomy, cornual resection and a more radically a hysterectomy. The latter has only a role in a life saving condition when other methods has been tried and exhausted. However, in experienced hand, it is nearly always possible to avoid a hysterectomy even in haemodynamically unstable patients with ruptured ectopic pregnancy.

In cornuotomy or cornual resection, the usage of diathermy or harmonic scalpel in the dissection can help in the reduction of blood loss. Intracorporeal knots of the PDS or Vicryl stitches can be used to close the cornual resection site. The round ligament could be used to

cover the cornual resection site aiming to reduce post operative adhesions and to facilitate the closure of resection site especially when large size ectopics are removed. (Api M& Api O, 2010; MacRae R et al, 2009; Tinelli A et al, 2010; Moon HS et al, 2000).
No clear data is available to compare risks of subsequent ectopic and the chances of persistent trophoblastic disease after cornual resection versus cornuotomy. Preservation of fertility following these surgical techniques has been confirmed. However, there is an expected reduction in chances of conception due to loss of the function of that tube. Future pregnancy is usually ending by a caesarean section due to the risk of uterine rupture. (Lindheim SR et al, 2006)
Uterine artery ligation may help to conserve the uterus in ruptued corneal ectopic as it can aid the homeostasis if conservative surgery attempted via open approach (Khawaja N et al, 2005).

7.2.2 Open approach versus laparscopic approach

Laparotomy is preferred in hemodynamically unstable patients with signs and symptoms of hypovolaemic shock. Senior operator is necessary in such situation where the bleeding might be sever and life threatening because of the enormous blood supply to the uterine cornue especially when the gestation is advanced at time of ectopic rupture. (Grimbizis GF et al, 2004)
Laparoscopic approach is preferred over the laparotomy for unruptured cases provided a skilled laparoscopic surgeon is available. (Hill GA et al, 1989; Grobman WA& MP Milad , 1998) Laparoscopic approach is associated with less intra-operative bleeding, less post operative pain and analgesia requirement, shorter hospital stay and fewer post operative adhesions. (Royal College of Obstetricians and Gynaecologists, 2004)
No clear data available to compare chances of having a subsequent intrauterine pregnancy between the open versus the laparoscopic approaches for cornual ectopics however the latter is though to be possibly associated with less risk of recurrent ectopics.

7.2.3 Vaginal approach

In the last decade, trans-cervical approach for the treatment of cornual ectopic has been advocated. The cornual ectopic is disturbed under hyteroscopic, laparoscopic or even ultrasound guidance. (Thakur Y et al, 2004)
It avoids extensive surgery and can be useful for women who are reluctant to undergo medical treatment with Methorexate or in whom this treatment failed.(Pal B et al, 2003)
The approach involves identification and disturbance of ectopic sac through a vaginal approach using a curette. The products of conception then removed using polyp forceps or a suction curette. (Minelli L et al, 2003; MeyerWR& Mitchell DE, 1989; Sanz LE& Verosko J, 2002) The use of laparoscopic or ultrasonic guidance is recommended due to the high risk of perforation. (Marian Morgan et al, 2009) Also this approach is not aimed at evacuation of all the product of conception as this could be associated with perforation. It is only aiming at disturbing the pregnancy and removing some of the product safely. (Marian Morgan et al, 2009) Therefore, follow-up is essential to ensure complete resolution of the pregnancy. In severe bleeding, laparoscopic local injection of vasopressin may reduce intraoperative bleeding. (Pal B et al, 2003)
This approach is simple and associated with less morbidity than abdominal approach. It is associated with less bleeding as the myometrium remained undisturbed, rapid recovery and a shorter post-operative stay resulting in financial and psychological benefits.

It is also possible that it would have less effect on fertility than abdominal approach and further intrauterine pregnancies could be managed as low risk with no increase chance of uterine rupture and hence normal vaginal delivery could be the choice of the mode of delivery.

7.2.4 Serum β hCG clearance

Serial serum β hCG should be measured after any conservative surgical treatment of corneal ectopic to ensure complete resolution. The duration of the monitoring is of little significant but a declining titre is essential and needs monitoring at intervals till resolution. (Kamrava MM et al, 1983)

7.3 Expectant management

Cornual ectopics are associated with high risk of rupture that could occur as late as 10 - 16 weeks. . (Abraham D& Silkowski C, 2010).Rupture of a corneal ectopic at that late gestation can cause profuse intraperitoneal bleeding which can be life threading. The Confidential Enquiry into Maternal and Child Health (CEMACH) report for 2000–02 confirmed that 4 out of 11 deaths due to ectopic pregnancies (36%) were corneal ectopics. (Confidential Enquiry into Maternal and Child Health, 2004)
Therefore, expectant management has no place in confirmed cornual ectopic.(Kok-Min S et al, 2004)

8. Effect of cornual ectopic treatment on future fertility

With regard future fertility, cornual ectopic is associated with higher risk of recurrent ectopic compared with other types of ectopic pregnancy. If the uterus is conserved, there is an increased incidence of uterine rupture at the surgical site in future pregnancies in the 2nd and 3rd trimesters especially in the cases where the sac excision leads to defective myo-metrium &/or the uterine cavity has been opened. However, the data about the absolute increase in such risk is still conflicting. (Lau S& Tulandi T, 1999; Weissman A& Fishman A, 1992)
There is a view about reinforcing the uterine wall with the use of round ligament especially if the cavity is opened. Again, no evidence yet has shown a proven benefit of such techniques.(Chatterjee J et al, 2009)
With regard the mood of delivery in subsequent pregnancy, caesarean section is recommended by many clinicians however, no evidence yet available to evaluate the safety of caesarean section versus vaginal delivery after cornual ectopic treatment. (Downey GP& Tuck S, 1994)

9. References

Abraham D, & Silkowski C .(2010). Emergency Medicine Sonography 1st ed, 264-274
Api M, & Api O.(2010). Laparoscopic cornuotomy in the management of an advanced interstitial ectopic pregnancy: a case report. Gynecol Endocrinol.;26(3):208–212.
Banerjee S, Aslam N, Zosmer N, Woelfer B, & Jurkovic D. (1999) The expectant management of women with early pregnancy of unknown location. Ultrasound Obstet Gynecol, 14:231–6.

Barnhart KT, Gosman G, Ashby R, & Sammel M. (2003).The medical management of ectopic pregnancy: a meta-analysis comparing "single dose" and "multidose" regimens. Obstet Gynecol , 101:778.

Benifla JL, Fernandez H, Sebban E, Darai E, Frydman R, & Madelenat P. (1996) Alternative to surgery of treatment of unruptured interstitial pregnancy: 15 cases of medical treatment. Eur J Obstet Gynecol Reprod Biol, 70:151-6

Cacciatore B, Stenman U, & Ylöstolalo P. (1990) .Diagnosis of ectopic pregnancy by vaginal ultrasonography in combination with a discriminatory serum hCG level of 1000 iu/l (IRP). Br J Obstet Gynaecol ,97:904–8.

Chatterjee J, Abdullah A, Irvine L, & Griffin D. (2009).A rare sequel following cornual ectopic pregnancy: a case report . BMJ Case Reports ,doi:10.1136/bcr.02.2009.1614

Confidential Enquiry into Maternal and Child Health. Why Mothers Die 2000–2002. The Sixth Report of the Confidential Enquiries into Maternal Deaths in the United Kingdom. London: RCOG Press; 2004.

Coste J, Job-Spira N, Fernandez H. (1991). Increased risk of ectopic pregnancy with maternal cigarette smoking. Am J Public Health,81:199–201.

Chou MM, Tseng JJ, Yi YC, Chen WC, & Ho ES. (2005). Diagnosis of an interstitial pregnancy with 4-dimensional volume contrast imaging. Am J Obstet Gynecol ,193:1551–3. doi:10.1016/j.ajog.2005.02.088

DeStefano F, Peterson HB, Layde PM, et al. (1982). Risk of ectopic pregnancy following tubal sterilization. Obstet Gynecol ,60:326–330.

Diamond, M. P. (1988). Surgical aspects of infertility. In Gynecology and Obstetrics (j. W. Sciarra, Ed.), pp. 1-23. Harper & Row, Philadelphia.

Dilbaz S, Katas B, Demir B, & Dilbaz B. (2005). Treating cornual ectopic pregnancy with a single methotrexate injection. J Reprod Med,50(2): 141-143

Doubilet PM, Benson CB, Frates MC, & Ginsburg E. (2004). Sonographically guided minimally invasive treatment of unusual ectopic pregnancies. J Ultrasound Med ,23:359–70.

Downey GP, & Tuck S. (1994) Spontaneous uterine rupture during subsequent pregnancy following non-excision of an interstitial ectopic gestation. Br J Obstet Gynaecol ,101:162–3.

Grimbizis GF, Tsalikis T, Mikos T, Zepiridis L, Athanasiadis A, Tarlatzis BC, & Bontis JN. (2004) Case report: laparoscopic treatment of a ruptured interstitial pregnancy. Reprod Biomed Online ,9:447–51.

Grobman WA, & MP Milad. (1998). Conservative laparoscopic management of a large cornual ectopic pregnancy. Hum Reprod ,13:2002–4.

Hajenius P, Mol B, Ankum W, Van der Veen F, Bossuyt P, & Lammes F. (1995). Suspected ectopic pregnancy: expectant management in patients with negative sonographic findings and low serum β-hCG concentrations. Early Pregnancy ,1:258–62.

Hill GA, Segars JH, & Herbert CA. (1989). Laparoscopic management of interstitial pregnancy. J Gynecol Surg ,5:209–12.

Johnson PT, Shah C. Ectopic pregnancy-role of ultrasound , Available from [www.sonoworld.com/Article/ShowArticleDetails.aspx?aid=28].

Kamrava MM, Taymor ML, Berger MJ, Thompson IE,& Seibel MM.(1983) Disappearance of human chorionic gonadotropin following removal of ectopic pregnancy. Obstet Gynecol. ,62(4):486-8.

Kelly H, Harvey D, & Moll S. (2006). A cautionary tale: fatal outcome of methotrexate therapy given for management of ,ectopic pregnancy. Obstet Gynecol ,107:439.

Khawaja N, Walsh T, & Gill B. (2005).Uterine artery ligation for the management of ruptured cornual ectopic pregnancy. Eur J Obstet Gynecol Reprod Biol 118:269.

Kok-Min S, Bin-Chwen Hsieh YL-A, Tsai L-W, Huang L-W, &Hwang J-L. (2004). Expectant management of a cornual pregnancy followed up by serialtransvaginal color power Doppler angiography and serum beta humanchorionic gonadotropin levels. Acta Obstet Gynecol Scan ,83:1221.

Lau S, & Tulandi T. (1999). Conservative medical and surgical management of interstitial ectopic pregnancy. Fertil Steril 72:207–15.

Lee GS, HurSY, Kown I, Shin JC, Kim SP, & Kim SJ. (2005). Diagnosis of early intramural ectopic pregnancy. J Clin Ultrasound ,33:190–2. doi:10.1002/jcu.20107

Lindheim SR, Olive DL, & Pritts EA. (2006). Cornual gestation: a systematic literature review and two case reports of a novel treatment regimen. J Minim Invasive Gynecol ,13:74–8.

Lipscomb G, McCord M, Stovall T, Huff G, Portera S, & Ling F. (1999). Predictors of success of methotrexate treatment inwomen with tubal ectopic pregnancies. N Engl J Med ,341:1974–8.

MacRae R, Olowu O, Rizzuto MI, Odejinmi F. (2009).Diagnosis and laparoscopic management of 11 consecutive cases of cornual ectopic pregnancy. Arch Gynecol Obstet. ,280(1):59–64.

Marian Morgan, M. Aziz, M. Mikhail, R. Atalla, & M. Henein. (2009) .Ultrasound guided treatment of cornual ectopic pregnancy. European Journal of Obstetrics & Gynecology and Reproductive Biology 143 ;126–129

MeyerWR, & Mitchell DE. (1989). Hysteroscopic removal of an interstitial ectopic gestation. A case report. J Reprod Med ,34:928–9.

Minelli L, Landi S, Trivella G, Fiaccavento A, & Barbieri F. (2003).Cornual pregnancy successfully treated by suction curettage and operative hysteroscopy. BJOG ,110:1132–4.

Mol B, Hajenius P, Engelsbel S, Ankum W, Hemrika D, Van der Veen F, et al. (1999).Treatment of tubal pregnancy in the Netherlands: an economic comparison of systemic methotrexate administration and laparoscopic salpingostomy. Am J Obstet Gynecol ,181:945–51.

Monteagudo A, MiniorVK, Stephenson C, Monda S, & Timor-Tritsch IE. (2005).Nonsurgical management of live ectopic pregnancy with ultrasound-guided local injection: a case series. Ultrasound Obstet Gynecol ,25:282–8.

Moon HS, Choi YJ, Park YH, & Kim SG. (2000).New simple endoscopic operations for interstitial pregnancies. Am J Obstet Gynecol ,182:114–21.

Onderoglu LS, Salman MC, Ozyuncu O, & Bozdag G. (2006).Successful management of a cornual pregnancy with a single high-dose laparoscopic methotrexate injection. Gynecol Surg ,3:31–3. doi:10.1007/s10397-005-0159-8

Ory HW. The Women's Health Study. (1981)Ectopic pregnancy and intrauterine contraceptivedevices: new perspectives. Obstet Gynecol ,57:137–144.

Pal B, Akinfenwa O, & Kevin H. (2003). Hysteroscopic management of cornual ectopic pregnancy. BJOG ,110:879–80.

Rock J, & Thompson J. (2003).Telinde's Operative Gynecology. 9th ed. Philadelphia, PA: Lippincott-Raven.

Royal College of Obstetricians and Gynaecologists.(2004). The Management of Tubal Pregnancy. Green Top Guideline No. 21.

Sanz LE, & Verosko J. (2002) Hysteroscopic management of cornual ectopic pregnancy. Obstet Gynecol ,99:941–4.

Silva P, Schaper A, & Rooney B. (1993). Reproductive outcome after 143 laparoscopic procedures for ectopic pregnancy. Fertil Steril ,81:710–5.Langer R, Bukovsky I,

Sowter M, Farquhar C, & Gudex G. (2001). An economic evaluation of single dose systemic methotrexate and laparoscopic surgery for the treatment of unruptured ectopic pregnancy. Br J Obstet Gynaecol, 108:204–12.

Sowter M, & Frappell J. (2002).The role of laparoscopy in the management of ectopic pregnancy. Rev Gynaecol Practice ,2:73–82.

Teal SB. (2006). A cautionary tale: fatal outcome of methotrexate therapy given for management of ectopic pregnancy. Obstet Gynecol ,107:1420

Thakur Y, Coker A, Morris J, & Oliver R. (2004).Laparoscopic and ultrasound-guided transcervical evacuation of cornual ectopic pregnancy: an alternative approach. J Obstet Gynaecol ,24(October (7)):809–10.

Timor-Tritsch IE, Monteagudo A, & Lerner JP. (1997). A 'potentially safer' route for puncture and injection of cornual ectopic pregnancies. Ultrasound Obstet Gynecol , 7:353–5. doi:10.1046/j.1469- 0705.1996.07050353.

Timor-Tritsch IE, Monteagudo A, Matera C, & Veit CR. (1992). Sonographic evolution of cornual pregnancies treated without surgery. Obstet Gynecol , 79:1044–9.

Tinelli A, Malvasi A, Pellegrino M, Pontrelli G, Martulli B, & Tsin DA. (2010). Laparoscopical management of cornual pregnancies: a report of three cases. Eur J Obstet Gynecol Reprod Biol. , 151(2):199-202

Tulandi T, & Al-Jaroudi D. (2004). Interstitial pregnancy: results generated from The Society of Reproductive Surgeons Registry. Obstet Gynecol , 103: 47-50

Weissman A, & Fishman A. (1992). Uterine rupture following conservative surgery for interstitial pregnancy. Eur J Obstet Gynecol Reprod Biol ,44: 237–9.

Westrom L, Bengtsson LPH, & Mardh P-A. (1981). Incidence, trends, and risks of ectopic pregnancy in a population of women. BMJ , 282:15–18.

Vicino M, Loverro G, Resta L, Bettocchi S, Vimercati A, & Selvaggi L. (2000). Laparoscopic cornual excision in a viable large interstitial pregnancy without blood flow detected by color Doppler ultrasonography. Fertil Steril , 74(2): 407-409

Yao M, & Tulandi T. (1997). Current status of surgical and nonsurgical management of ectopic pregnancy. Fertil Steril,67: 421–33.